Pediatric Voice Disorders

DIAGNOSIS AND TREATMENT

Pediatric Voice Disorders

DIAGNOSIS AND TREATMENT

Christopher J. Hartnick, MS, MD
Mark E. Boseley, MS, MD

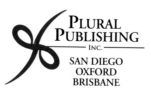

PLURAL
PUBLISHING
INC.
SAN DIEGO
OXFORD
BRISBANE

MW

PLURAL PUBLISHING
INC.

5521 Ruffin Road
San Diego, CA 92123

e-mail: info@pluralpublishing.com
Web site: http://www.pluralpublishing.com

49 Bath Street
Abingdon, Oxfordshire OX14 1EA
United Kingdom

Library of Congress Cataloging-in-Publication Data:
Pediatric voice disorders / edited by Christopher Hartnick and Mark Boseley.
     p. ; cm.
  Includes bibliographical references.
  ISBN-13: 978-1-59756-178-5 (pbk.)
  ISBN-10: 1-59756-178-9 (pbk.)
  1. Voice disorders in children. I. Hartnick, Christopher. II. Boseley, Mark.
  [DNLM: 1. Voice Disorders—diagnosis. 2. Child. 3. Voice—physiology. 4. Voice Disorders—therapy. WV 500 P371 2007]
  RF511.C45P43 2007
  618.92'855—dc22
                                          2007039910

6/3/10

Contents

Preface

This book is the product of hard work from a diverse group of authors across a range of specialties. What binds this group of pediatric otolarygnologists, pulmonologists, gastroenterologists, psychologists, psychiatrists, and speech-language pathologists is an interest in caring for children with a wide variety of voice disorders. We hope this book is novel, exciting, and educational in its cross-fertilization of thoughts and ideas that results from the coming together of a seemingly diverse group of specialists to focus on specific pediatric disease-based and pediatric voice pathology-based topics. For example, when faced with a child with paradoxical vocal fold motion, how would a pulmonologist or otolaryngologist each approach such a child and what tests might each employ to arrive at a diagnosis? After a diagnosis has been made: who should the pulmonologist or otolaryngologist refer to —a speech pathologist, a psychologist, or a psychiatrist? These are not simple questions and there are no pat answers. In this book, members of different specialties attend to these questions and comment on how they can best work together toward obtaining diagnoses and rendering unified and comprehensive treatment. The book allows for multimedia discussions from text, images, or videos so that each author can best render his or her material and aid the reader in the exploration of a given topic. We hope you enjoy!

About the Editors

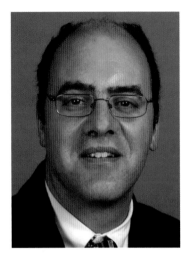

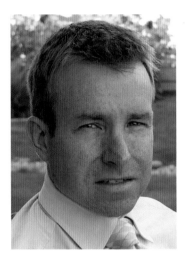

Christopher Hartnick, M.D., M.S. is an associate professor of Otology and Laryngology at the Massachusetts Eye and Ear Infirmary and Harvard Medical School in Boston, MA. Dr. Hartnick directs the Pediatric Otolaryngology fellowship at the Massachusetts Eye and Ear Infirmary and co-directs the Pediatric Airway, Voice, and Swallowing Center in collaboration with his Pulmonary and Gastroenterology colleagues at the Massachusetts General Hospital for Children. Dr. Hartnick has published numerous book chapters on pediatric voice and airway conditions and has approximately 50 publications in the pediatric otolaryngology literature. Dr. Hartnick received his M.D. degree at the Albert Einstein Medical School in New York in 1994 and completed his otolaryngology residency at Montefiore Medical Center in 1999. Dr. Hartnick completed a pediatric otolaryngology fellowship at Cincinnati Children's Hospital in 2001 and obtained a Master's Degree in Epidemiology at the Harvard School of Public Health in 2001.

Lieutenant Colonel Mark E. Boseley, M.D., M.S. is an associate professor of surgery at the Uniformed Services University of the Health Sciences in Washington D.C. and the Assistant Chief of Otolaryngology/research director at Madigan Army Medical Center in Tacoma, WA. Dr. Boseley also has a clinical appointment at Children's Hospital and Regional Medical Center in Seattle, WA. Dr. Boseley has published numerous book chapters on pediatric voice and airway conditions and has approximately 20 publications in the pediatric otolaryngology literature. Dr. Boseley received his M.D. degree at Tulane University in 1995 and completed his otolaryngology residency at the University of Cincinnati in 2001. Dr. Boseley completed a pediatric otolaryngology fellowship at the Massachusetts Eye and Ear Infirmary and Children's Hospital Boston and obtained a Master's Degree in Epidemiology at the Harvard School of Public Health in 2006.

Contributors

Jennifer Allegro, MSc, SLP (C), Reg. CASLPO
Speech-Language Pathologist
Centre for Paediatric Voice and Laryngeal
    Function
Hospital for Sick Children
555 University Avenue
    Toronto, ON   M5G 1X8
Chapter 12

Jennifer G. Andrus, MD
Clinical Fellow, Division of Laryngology
Massachusetts Eye and Ear Infirmary
Chapter 4

Barbara M. Wilson Arboleda, MS, CCC-SLP
Beth Israel Deaconess Medical Center
Boston, Massachusetts
Voicewize
Dedham, Massachusetts
Chapter 7

Mark E. Boseley, MD, MS
Pediatric Otolaryngology
Madigan Army Medical Center
Building 9040
Fitzsimmons Drive
Tacoma, WA 98431
Children's Hospital and Regional Medical
    Center
4800 Sand Point Way NE
Seattle, WA 98105
Assistant Professor
Department of Surgery
Uniformed Services University of the
    Health Sciences
Washington D.C.
Chapters 1, 6, and 9

Paolo Campisi, MSc, MD, FRCSC, FAAP
Director, Centre for Pediatric Voice and
    Laryngeal Function
Hospital for Sick Children
Assistant Professor
Dept. of Otolaryngology-Head and Neck
    Surgery
University of Toronto
Toronto, Canada
Chapter 5

Venu Divi, MD
Assistant Professor
Department of Otolaryngology
Drexel University
Philadelphia, Pennsylvania
Chapter 19

Abigail L. Donovan, MD
Child and Adolescent Psychiatry Fellow,
    Massachusetts General Hospital and
    McLean Hospital
Clinical Fellow in Psychiatry, Harvard
    Medical School
Chapter 20

Robert Edwin
Robert Edwin Studio
Associate Editor, *Journal of Singing*
National Association of Teachers of
    Singing (NATS)
American Academy of Teachers of Singing
    (AATS)
Chapter 13

Ramon A. Franco Jr, MD
Director, Division of Laryngology
Massachusetts Eye and Ear Infirmary
Chapter 4

Shirley Gherson, MA, CCC-SLP
Speech-Language Pathologist
Voice Specialist
Voicewize
Massachusetts Eye and Ear Infirmiry
Chapter 7

Stephen C. Hardy, MD
Pediatric Gastroenterology and Nutrition
Massachusetts General Hospital for Children
Assistant Professor of Pediatrics
Harvard Medical School
Boston, MA
Chapter 10

Christopher J. Hartnick, MD, MS
Associate Professor
Department of Otolaryngology
Massachusetts Eye and Ear Infirmary
Chapters 1, 6, 9, and 16

Kenan Haver, MD
Co-Director, Pediatric Airway, Voice &
    Swallowing Center
Massachusetts Eye & Ear Infirmary
Pediatric Pulmonary Unit
Massachusetts General Hospital
Assistant Professor of Pediatrics
Harvard Medical School
Chapter 11

Mary J. Hawkshaw, RN, BSN, CORLN
Research Associate Professor
Drexel University College of Medicine
Department of Otolaryngology-Head and
    Neck Surgery
Philadelphia, Pennsylvania
Chapter 19

Al Hillel, MD
Professor, Otolaryngology-Head and Neck
    Surgery
University of Washington Medical Center
Seattle, Washington
Chapter 8

Joseph E. Kerschner, MD
Professor and Chief, Division of Pediatric
    Otolaryngology
Department of Otolaryngology and
    Communication Sciences
Medical College of Wisconsin
Children's Hospital of Wisconsin
Chapter 3

Bruce J. Masek, PhD, ABPP
Clinical Director of Outpatient Child and
    Adolescent Psychiatry Massachusetts
    General Hospital
Associate Professor of Psychology
    (Psychiatry), Harvard Medical School
Chapter 20

J. Scott McMurray, MD
Associate Professor
Pediatric Otolaryngology Head and Neck
    Surgery
Department of Surgery
University of Wisconsin School of
    Medicine and Public Health
Madison, Wisconsin
Chapter 14

Albert L. Merati, MD
Associate Professor and Chief,
    Laryngology
Department of Otolaryngology-Head and
    Neck Surgery
University of Washington School of
    Medicine
Chapter 3

Matthew B. Patterson, MD
Chapter 15

Seth M. Pransky, MD
Director
Pediatric Otolaryngology
Children's Specialists San Diego
Rady Children's Hospital, San Diego
San Diego, California
Chapter 15

Nelson Roy, Ph.D, CCC-SLP
Department of Communication Sciences
    and Disorders
The University of Utah
Salt Lake City, Utah
Chapter 18

Robert T. Sataloff, MD, DM, FACS
Professor and Chairman
Department of Otolaryngology-Head and
    Neck Surgery
Associate Dean for Clinical Academic
    Specialties
Drexel University College of Medicine
Philadelphia, Pennsylvania
Introduction, Chapters 4 and 19

Cara Sauder, MA, CCC-SLP
University Hospital
The University of Utah
Salt Lake City, Utah
Chapter 18

J. Andrew Sipp, MD
Pediatric Otolaryngologist
Pediatric ENT of Atlanta
Chapter 16

Marshall E. Smith, MD
Division of Otolaryngology/Head and
    Neck Surgery
University of Utah School of Medicine
The University of Utah
Salt Lake City, Utah
Chapter 18

Susan L. Thibeault, PhD, CCC/SLP
Assistant Professor
Director, Voice and Swallow Clinics
Division of Otolaryngology-Head and Neck
    Surgery, Department of Surgery
University of Wisconsin—Madison
Madison, Wisconsin
Chapter 2

Karen B. Zur, MD
Assistant Professor, Department of
    Otorhinolaryngology: Head and Neck
    Surgery
University of Pennsylvania School of
    Medicine
Director, Voice Program
Associate Director, The Center for
    Pediatric Airway Disorders
The Children's Hospital of Philadelphia
Philadelphia, Pennsylvania
Chapter 17

Introduction

The Pediatric Larynx and Voice: Anatomy, Development, and Emerging Developments

Robert T. Sataloff

Voice medicine and surgery have advanced remarkably since the late 1970s. Most of the innovations were inspired by adult professional voice users. Interest in the "Olympic athletes" of the voice world has led to advances in physical examination, objective voice assessment, medical treatment, voice therapy, voice surgery, and research (clinical and basic). Voice also has evolved into an established subspecialty of otolaryngology. Although the standard of care has improved dramatically for all voice patients, the application of new knowledge and technology to the care of pediatric patients with voice disorders has lagged behind the integration of new approaches into the care of adult voice patients. Most otolaryngologists who subspecialize in laryngology treat children as well as adults, but a high percentage of children with dysphonia are managed by pediatric otolaryngologists. In general, the sophisticated, multidisciplinary teams and protocols that are now routine for adult voice patients have not been available widely in pediatric otolaryngology divisions. This deficiency has been recognized for at least 2 decades. It should be noted that the problem exists not only for pediatric voice disorders, but also for all areas of pediatric arts medicine. Although arts medicine centers have been established since the early 1980s and adult arts medicine is a well established field,[1] the first arts medicine center based at a pediatric hospital is being developed only now. To understand the evolution of pediatric laryngology/voice as it emerges as a subspecialty, it helps to consider it in the context of the development of voice care in general.

HISTORY

In the past 3 decades, increasing interest and new technology have generated unprecedented activity within a number of disciplines that address the voice. Since 1972, laryngologists, voice scientists, physicists, computer scientists, speech-language pathologists, singing teachers, acting teachers, voice coaches, singers, actors, and other professionals have met at the Voice Foundation's week-long annual Symposium on Care of the Professional Voice, started by Dr. Wilbur James Gould. At this unique meeting, experts have gathered to report their research and share their ideas. The resultant interdisciplinary understanding and cooperation have produced great advances and hold even greater promise for future understanding. These activities have rendered care of the professional voice the most advanced discipline within the new specialty of arts medicine. They have also inspired numerous successful interdisciplinary publications, including the *Journal of Voice*. Although the majority of presentations at the Voice Foundation and publications in the *Journal of Voice* have addressed adult subjects, many are applicable to adults and children; and numerous pediatric voice topics have been included.

In many ways, the status of voice care is still analogous to that of otology 30 years ago. Until recently, voice evaluation was reminiscent of ear examinations with a head mirror instead of a microscope or whispered voice tests instead of audiograms. In many places, it still is. Fortunately, expert research has led to greater understating of the voice and development of instrumentation for sophisticated assessment and quantitative analysis to facilitate clinical management and research. Although efforts have focused largely on adult professional singers and actors, the knowledge developed through clinical and basic research has advanced our understanding of voice in general and modified substantially the state of the art in clinical care of all persons with voice disorders including pediatric performers, and other children with voice abnormalities. Still, the field is new. The first extensive article in English literature intended to teach clinicians how to approach professional singers was not published until 1981,[2] and the first major American general textbook of otolaryngology containing a chapter on care of the professional voice was not published until 1986.[3] This first modern comprehensive textbook in English on medical care of the professional voice was not published until 1991.[4] However, it should be remembered that, although these contributions in English helped signal the arrival and acceptance of voice as a subspecialty, there were noteworthy predecessors who discussed voice; and some even addressed the professional voice user.[5-11]

The importance of interdisciplinary voice care to the evolution of modern voice care cannot be overemphasized. Although there were a few scattered collaborations in the 19th and 20th centuries, the first formal, academically based interdisciplinary voice clinic in the United States was established by Drs. Hans von Leden and Paul Moore at Northwestern University Medical School, Chicago, Illinois in 1954. This concept was expanded in Philadelphia in 1981 when the author hired a singing teacher and speech-language pathologist as employees of his medical practice. Today, our interdisciplinary voice team now includes singing teachers, speech-language pathologists, a psychologist, a voice scientist, an acting-voice trainer, and otolaryngologic nurse-clinicians. It also includes very close collaboration with arts-medicine colleagues located nearby, including a pulmonologist, psychiatrist, neurologist, gastroenterologist, endocrinologist, ophthalmologist, complementary medicine practitioners, and others. We anticipate further expansion of this interdisciplinary approach because it has proven so valuable in advancing patient care, and stimulating creative research. The author has also advocated the development of analogous multidisciplinary pediatric voice care teams utilizing similar diagnostic instrumentation since the early 1980s. Although there have been promising plans over the years, such programs have been slow to develop. Hence, much of the sophisticated pediatric voice care has been delivered by voice centers that treat more adults than children.

In the past few years, many new centers and academic training programs have acquired voice laboratories and begun practicing and teaching modern, advanced voice care; but more time still will be required before state-of-the-art care is available in most geographical areas.

At present, new understanding of the special aspects of the history and physical examination of voice patients has been supplemented by technological advances in voice analysis, which are available readily to interested clinicians. Flexible fiberoptic laryngoscopy has been indispensable, and the advent of chip-tip technology has enhanced image quality. This is especially important for pediatric laryngology, as it is frequently impossible to obtain stroboscopic images on children (especially infants and very young children) through transoral examination using a laryngeal rigid telescope. Hence, improved flexible endoscopic resolution is an exceedingly important advancement for pediatric laryngology. It should be noted that chip-tip resolution and magnification are still not comparable to laryngeal telescopic images, and further advances in chip-tip technology are needed. The development and refinement of laryngeal stroboscopy are singularly important advancements. Strobovideolaryngoscopic evaluation of vocal fold function in slow motion allows diagnoses that are simply missed without it. High-speed video and videokymography are valuable newer techniques that improve our ability to assess the mucosal wave. These high-speed imaging techniques also may be particularly important to pediatric otolaryngology as the phonatory segments available for stroboscopic analysis are often considerably shorter in infants than in adults. So, the ability to analyze individual waves in greater detail may prove espe-cially helpful. Spectrography, electroglot-tography, electromyography, airflow analysis, and other techniques have enhanced our ability to analyze and treat voice disorders reliably in both adults and children. Laryngeal electromyography can be performed in patients of any age, even infants. In most cases, experienced electromyographers can perform the necessary studies in an office setting. However, there are occasions when laryngeal electromyography under sedation or light anesthesia is more effective.

When physicians encounter a patient with a voice problem, they approach the problem using a combination of art (style, empathy, intuition) and science (objective analysis based on facts). Both components are important; and no physician, speech-language pathologist, singing teacher, or acting voice teacher can be considered excellent if she or he abandons the art of practice in favor of dispassionate scientific analysis alone. However, care is at least as bad when we are forced to depend on intu-ition almost exclusively, because of insuffi-cient knowledge. Fortunately, science has provided us with an understanding that the voice consists of at least three principal components (power source, oscillator, res-onator); that each component is designed to control specific aspects of voice produc-tion, and that there are ways to identify and quantify the performance of each compo-nent. This information provides voice care professionals with a framework and language with which we can think about voice prob-lems. This has permitted us to add not only scientific fact, but also scientific thought to voice care. Unfortunately, the objective and scientific components of voice evaluation protocols have been applied much more consistently to adults than to children, espe-cially in departments or divisions of pedi-atric otolaryngology that are not affiliated with an adult voice center.

Farsighted pediatric otolaryngologists have recognized the problem, and many have addressed it, at least in part. Since the 1980s, the author has discussed the subject with several leading pediatric otolaryngologists who have expressed interest and attempted to address the problem, with varying degrees of intensity. For example, in the mid-1980s, Robin Cotton committed to a serious effort to develop a pediatric voice center. He hired Robert Coleman, PhD, an outstanding voice scientist. Shortly before Bob Coleman was to move to Cincinnati, he developed serious health problems that prevented his relocation, and forced his retirement. A similar major effort was never resumed in Cincinnati, but Robin Cotton has remained consistently interested in and attentive to voice problems, particularly the potential for preserving or improving voices in children who have required laryngotracheal reconstruction. His department has continued to explore opportunities to develop a pediatric voice division. Gerald Healy, MD and his associates at Boston Children's Hospital also have attended to pediatric laryngology, as have Lauren Holinger, MD in Chicago, Illinois, Lucinda Holstead in Charleston, South Carolina, Christopher Hartnick in Boston, Massachusetts, James Riley in Wilmington, Delaware, and others. However, even the best of these centers is not comparable to the leading adult voice centers with regard to consistent, multidisciplinary, practical, and effective use of strobovideolaryngoscopy and other vocal fold imaging and dynamic voice assessment techniques, laboratory evaluation for voice disorders, laryngeal electromyography, development and routine application of age-appropriate multidisciplinary voice therapy and training, and intensive clinical and basic voice research. There is no question in this writer's mind that a full commitment to pediatric voice care analogous to the commitment made by adult voice centers will result in improvement in diagnosis and treatment of children with voice disorders. There is also no doubt that it will expose shortcomings for the pediatric population of technologies and techniques currently used in adults, and that these revelations will inspire new approaches that will improve not only pediatric laryngologic care, but that also enhance the way we treat adults.

CONCLUSION

Great progress has been made toward understanding the function, dysfunction, and treatment of the human voice. Because so many of the advances have involved collaboration among physicians, voice scientists, speech-language pathologists, singing and acting teachers, singers, and actors, they have applied practically much more quality than usual. The dramatic progress that has occurred in the last 3 decades has resulted in great diagnostic and therapeutic benefits for all patients with voice complaints and the emergence of a new medical specialty in voice. Scientific advances and collaboration have not given us merely new tools, but rather a whole new approach to the voice. No longer must we depend on intuition and mysticism in the medical office or voice studio. We now have the knowledge and vocabulary necessary for accurate analysis of voice problems and systematic, logical solutions. Thus, we finally have enough information to include effectively in our voice armamentarium the most important missing component: rational thought. It has raised the standard of voice care and training forever, and advanced care should be applied to children as consistently as it is to adults. This book represents an important step toward the development of pediatric laryngology/voice care as a field. It summarizes current knowledge and offers practical approaches toward application of a state-of-the-art voice care to children in a practical fashion. One hopes it will help pediatric otolaryngologists bring optimal care routinely to children with voice disorders, as well as help them advance the state-of-the-art of pediatric laryngology.

REFERENCES

1. Sataloff RT, Brandfonbrener A, Lederman R. (eds.) *Performing Arts Medicine*, 2nd ed. San Diego, Calif: Singular Publishing Group; 1998.

2. Sataloff RT. The professional singer: the science and art of clinical care. *Am J Otolaryngol.* 1981; 2(3):251–266.

3. Sataloff RT. The professional voice. In: Cummings CV, Frederickson JM, Harker LA, et al, eds. *Otolaryngology-Head and Neck Surgery.* St. Louis, Mo: CV Mosby; 1986; 3:2029–2053.

4. Sataloff RT. *Professional Voice: The Science and Art of Clinical Care.* New York, NY: Raven Press; 1991.

5. Rush J. *The Philosophy of Human Voice,* 4th ed. Philadelphia, Pa: Lippincott, Grambo & Co; 1855.

6. Punt NA. The singers and actors throat: the vocal mechanism of the professional voice user and its care. In: *Health and Disease.* London/Melbourne: William Heinemann Medical Books; 1952.

7. Brodnitz FS. *Vocal Rehabilitation.* Rochester, Minn: American Academy of Otolaryngology; 1959.

8. Damste PH, Lerman JW. *An Introduction to Voice Pathology.* Springfield, Mass: Thomas; 1975.

9. Hirano M. *Clinical Examination of the Voice.* Wien/New York: Springer-Verlag; 1981.

10. Luchsinger R. *Handbuch der Stimm- und Sprachheilkunde. Vol. 1. Die Stimme und ihre storugen.* Wein/New York: Springer-Verlag; 1970.

11. Schonhard E. *Die Stroboskopie in der praktischen Laryngologic.* Stuttgart, Germany: Geroge Thieme-Verlag; 1960.

*To our families without whose patience and support
this book would never have been completed.*

1

Developmental, Gross, and Histologic Anatomy of the Larynx

Mark E. Boseley
Christopher J. Hartnick

INTRODUCTION

Understanding the embryologic development of the larynx is important when trying to comprehend the pathophysiology and treatment options we face as pediatric voice specialists. This chapter first focuses on the maturation of the anatomic structures. We then discuss the gross and histologic development of the true vocal folds ex utero. Our specific aims are to provide an anatomic review, as well as to add additional facts that might prove helpful in a clinical context.

EMBRYOLOGIC ANATOMY OF THE LARYNX

The larynx and pharynx are derived from the branchial arches in utero. Each branchial arch consists of mesenchyme, and is covered externally by ectoderm and internally by endoderm. Neural crest cells migrate into the branchial arches and eventually surround the central core of mesenchyme. It is important to note here that each branchial arch has an associated nerve, muscle, and skeletal structure.[1] These relationships are shown in Table 1–1.

The laryngeal framework, consisting of the epiglottis, hyoid bone, and the laryngeal and cricoid cartilages, begins to develop during the fourth week of gestation. These structures form from the mesenchyme of the second through fifth branchial arches. The cartilage of the epiglottis actually forms from the mesenchyme in the hypobranchial eminence (third and fourth brancial arches). The hyoid bone is also derived from two branchial arches (the second and third). The second arch contributes to the lesser cornu and superior part of the body. The

Table 1–1. Structures Derived from the Branchial Arches

Arch	Nerve	Muscles	Skeletal Structures
First	Trigeminal (V)	Muscles of mastication, mylohyoid and anterior belly of the diagastric, tensor tympani, and tensor veli palatini	Malleus and incus
Second	Facial (VII)	Muscles of facial expression, stapedius, stylohyoid, and posterior belly of diagastric	Stapes, styloid process, lesser cornu and upper part of body of hyoid
Third	Glossopharyngeal (IX)	Stylopharyngeus	Greater cornu and lower part of hyoid
Fourth, fifth and sixth	Superior laryngeal and recurrent laryngeal branches of vagus (X)	Cricthyroid, levator veli palatini, constrictors of the pharynx, intrinsic muscles of the larynx, and striated muscles of the esophagus	Thyroid cartilage, cricoid cartilage, arytenoid cartilage, corniculate cartilage, and cuneiform cartilage

third arch becomes the greater cornu and inferior portion of the body of the hyoid. Finally, the fourth and six arch mesenchyme fuse to form both the laryngeal and cricoid cartilages.[1]

The internal structures of the larynx also begin to develop during the fourth week of gestation. The endoderm lining the laryngotracheal groove begins to invaginate, forming a laryngotracheal diverticulum. Longitudinal folds then fuse to become the tracheoesophageal septum. Proliferating mesenchyme at the cranial end of the laryngotracheal apparatus diiferentiates into what will become the arytenoid, corniculate, and cuneiform cartilages. This process changes the narrow slitlike glottic aperture into a T-shaped opening. Also of note is that the laryngeal epithelium is rapidly proliferating during this time and actually obliterates the lumen of the larynx before later recanalizing by the 10th week of gestation. This recanalization is instrumental in the maturation of the false and true vocal folds, as well as the laryngeal ventricles. Failure of this to occur leads to congenital cartilaginous subglottic stenosis. When present, the cricoid cartilage is usually abnormally shaped with prominent lateral shelves obstructing the subglottic lumen. A further consequence of failure of recanalization is the presence of a supraglottic or glottic web. Glottic webs are the more common of the two and often extend into the subglottis. They are subdivided into types I to IV, with a type I representing a thin anterior web involving up to 50% of the glottis, progressing to a type IV which is a thick web involving 75 to 90% of the glottis and often extending into the subglottis.[2]

GROSS ANATOMY OF THE LARYNX

Muscles of the Larynx

The laryngeal muscles are derived from the fourth and sixth branchial arches and are innervated by the nerves that supply each (see Table 1-1).[1] The muscles of the larynx can be divided into extrinsic and intrinsic. The extrinsic muscles move the larynx as a whole. These include the depressors of larynx which are the omohyoid, sternohyoid, and sternothyroid. The elevators of the larynx are the stylohyoid, diagastric, and mylohyoid. There are also muscles that modify the pharyngeal inlet. The stylopharyngeus and palatopharyngeus elevate the pharynx, whereas the middle and inferior pharyngeal constrictors participate in changing the shape of the air passage.[3]

The intrinsic muscles of the larynx are the cricothyroid, posterior and lateral cricoarytenoids, interarytenoid, thyroarytenoid, and vocalis (Figs 1-1 and 1-2). The posterior cricoarytenoid muscle slides the arytenoids laterally and is the only abductor of the true vocal folds. The cricothyroid muscle tilts the cricoid lamina in a backward direction and thus lengthens, tenses, and adducts the true vocal folds. The lateral cricoarytenoid muscle pulls the vocalis process of the vocal fold forward and laterally and therefore adducts the folds. The interarytenoid muscle approximates the arytenoid cartilages and subsequently is also an adductor of the vocal folds. The thyroarytenoid muscle

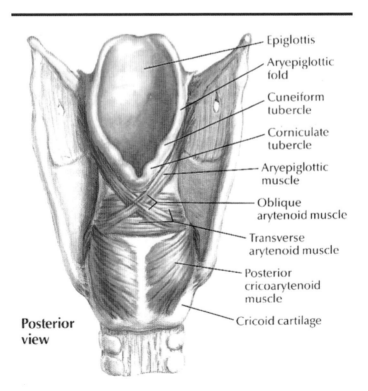

Epiglottis

Aryepiglottic fold

Cuneiform tubercle

Corniculate tubercle

Aryepiglottic muscle

Oblique arytenoid muscle

Transverse arytenoid muscle

Posterior cricoarytenoid muscle

Cricoid cartilage

Posterior view

Fig 1–1. Intrinsic muscles of the larynx—posterior view.

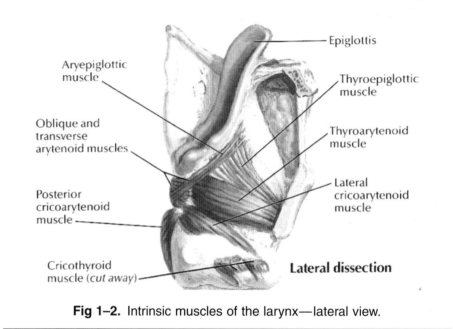

Aryepiglottic muscle

Oblique and transverse arytenoid muscles

Posterior cricoarytenoid muscle

Cricothyroid muscle (*cut away*)

Epiglottis

Thyroepiglottic muscle

Thyroarytenoid muscle

Lateral cricoarytenoid muscle

Lateral dissection

Fig 1–2. Intrinsic muscles of the larynx—lateral view.

draws the arytenoids forward and medially and adducts the true and false folds. The last of the intrinsic laryngeal muscles is the vocalis. This muscle is difficult to discern anatomically from the thyroarytenoid, but is instrumental in adducting and tensing the true vocal folds.[3]

Blood Supply of the Larynx

The larynx's blood supply is supplied from the superior and inferior laryngeal arteries. The superior laryngeal artery arises from the superior thyroid artery and runs horizontally across the thyrohyoid membrane. The artery then penetrates the membrane and lies in the submucosa of the lateral wall and floor of the piriform sinus; supplying the mucosa and musculature of the larynx. The inferior laryngeal artery is a branch of

the inferior thyroid artery (itself a branch of the thyrocervical trunk) and enters the larynx below the inferior constrictor muscle. This artery anastomoses with the superior laryngeal artery to also supply the laryngeal mucosa and muscles.[3]

Nerves of the Larynx

The innervation to the larynx is via the superior and inferior laryngeal nerves (Fig 1-3). Both of these nerves are branches of the vagus nerve. The superior laryngeal nerve passes down the vagal trunk and lies medial to the internal and external carotid arteries. This nerve has an external and internal branch. The external branch travels down the lateral surface of the inferior constrictor and ends at the cricothyroid muscle. The internal branch takes a similar course to

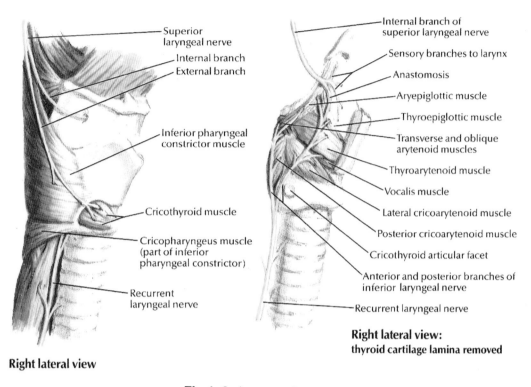

Superior laryngeal nerve
Internal branch
External branch
Inferior pharyngeal constrictor muscle
Cricothyroid muscle
Cricopharyngeus muscle (part of inferior pharyngeal constrictor)
Recurrent laryngeal nerve

Right lateral view

Internal branch of superior laryngeal nerve
Sensory branches to larynx
Anastomosis
Aryepiglottic muscle
Thyroepiglottic muscle
Transverse and oblique arytenoid muscles
Thyroarytenoid muscle
Vocalis muscle
Lateral cricoarytenoid muscle
Posterior cricoarytenoid muscle
Cricothyroid articular facet
Anterior and posterior branches of inferior laryngeal nerve
Recurrent laryngeal nerve

Right lateral view:
thyroid cartilage lamina removed

Fig 1–3. Laryngeal nerves.

the superior laryngeal artery, penetrating the thyrohyoid membrane. Sensory fibers from the internal branch supply the posterior aspect of the tongue, valleculae, epiglottis, piriform recesses, vestibular folds, ventricles, and the posterior laryngeal and anterior pharyngeal walls at the level of the cricoid cartilage.[3]

The inferior laryngeal nerve is an extension of the recurrent laryngeal nerve. It enters the larynx with the inferior thyroid artery just posterior to the cricothyroid articulation. There are usually at least two branches from this nerve which may occur before or after it enters the larynx. The anterior branch, or adductor of the larynx, supplies the lateral cricoarytenoid, thyroarytenoid, and vocalis muscles. The posterior branch, or abductor of the larynx, supplies the posterior cricoarytenoid and the interarytenoid musculature.[3]

Framework of the Larynx

External changes in position and structure of the larynx itself can be seen as a child matures. The larynx descends in the neck in relationship to the cervical vertebrae from infancy (where the inferior aspect of the cricoid approximates the fourth cervical vertebra) to the mature position (C6-C7) by mid-adolescence (see Fig 1–2).[4] Kahane[5] discovered that the laryngeal and cricoid cartilages also undergo significant changes as a child grows. He compared specimens before and after puberty and noted changes that included increase in length, height, width, and weight of both cartilages. As one might expect, these changes were greater in male than in female specimens.

Internal laryngeal changes are equally important as the child grows. There have been two studies published utilizing MRI scans to examine changes in laryngeal anatomy over time.[6,7] One of these was a report from the anesthesia literature which looked at 99 children between the ages of 2 months to 13 years. They determined that the anterior-posterior and transverse measurements at the levels of the true vocal folds, subglottis, and cricoid all increased linearly with age. The narrowest region was the transverse dimension at the true vocal fold level.[6] A second study compared serial MRI scans in two pediatric patients over the first 4 years of life. Their most significant finding was that laryngeal and tongue descent appeared to be the most influential in vocal fold lengthening over time.[7]

The actual growth of the true vocal folds has also been studied. Male vocal folds undergo over twice the growth of female true vocal folds.[5] Hirano[8] measured the length of the developing vocal fold and its anatomic components, namely, the membranous and cartilaginous portions. The measurements comparing newborn with adult male and female vocal folds are presented in Table 1–2. Important to note is the vocal fold at birth has nearly equal contribution of the membranous and cartilaginous portions. The membranous portion of the vocal fold is dominant by 3 years of age (Fig 1–4).[8]

HISTOLOGIC ANATOMY OF THE LARYNX

The "modern" description of the micro-anatomy of the human vocal folds has been properly attributed to Dr. Hirano with his seminal work in 1975 entitled "Phono-surgery: Basic and Clinical Investigations."[9] It was here that Hirano defined the trilaminar structure of the human vocal fold. He labeled these the superficial, intermediate and deep layers of the lamina propria. The layers were defined by examining the elastin and collagen concentrations within each layer in adult autopsy specimens (Fig 1–5).[9-11]

Lamina Propria Development

The lamina propria is instrumental in modulating voice. This is often explained with the cover-body theory of phonation. Defin-

Table 1–2. True Vocal Fold Lengths

Age	Overall Vocal Fold Length	Membranous Vocal Fold Length	Cartilaginous Vocal Fold Length
Newborn	2.5–3.0 mm	1.3–2.0 mm	1.0–1.4 mm
Adult Males	17–21 mm	14.5–18 mm	2.5–3.5 mm
Adult Females	11–15 mm	8.5–12 mm	2.0–3.0 mm

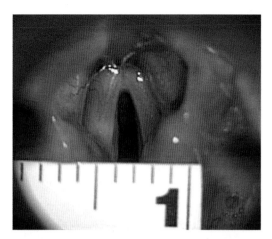

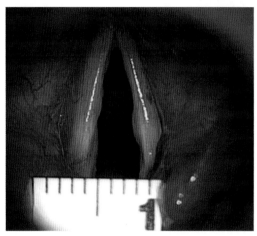

Fig 1–4. Suspension laryngoscopy of an infant (*top*) and adolescent (*bottom*) larynx. Note that ratio of the length of the arytenoid cartilage to membranous vocal fold changes significantly with age as the membranous vocal fold lengthens.

itions of what layers of the vocal fold make up the cover and body vary. Perhaps the most common definition is that the cover consists of the epithelium and superficial portion of the intermediate layers of the lamina propria. This relatively pliant layer moves over the stiffer vocal ligament (composed of the middle and deep layers of the lamina propria), rests upon the vocalis muscle, and allows the vocal fold to vibrate with consistency and control.[8]

As the lamina propria has such an important role in voice production, it is important that we attempt to understand both how and when it develops into its final three-layered form. We know that the lamina is not fully developed in the newborn. Studies have shown that it appears to be a uniform, one-layered structure at birth.[12-15]

There are areas of more abundant cells in the anterior and posterior portions of the fold that are adjacent to the thyroid cartilage and vocalis process. These areas are labeled the anterior and posterior macula flavae, respectively. Cells within the macula flavae appear to be important in the growth and maturation of lamina propria.[12-14]

Macula Flavae and Lamina Propria Cells

Immature fibroblasts are the primary cells found within the infant macula flavae. They appear to be more abundant than the mature form seen in the adult. The mechanism of how these cells differentiate into mature cells has yet to be elucidated. One theory is that the trauma produced as a child begins to develop speech might stimulate dif-ferentiation of the cells within the lamina propria. These fibroblasts produce collagen, elastin, and reticular fibers, as well as glycoprotein (fibronectin) or ground substance; substances that are vital for maintenance of strength and elasticity of the vocal fold.[12-13]

The cells within the lamina propria layers are also believed to be important in the differentiation of the three-layered vocal fold. Fibroblasts are again the most prominent cell type.[12,13] Macrophages and myofibroblasts

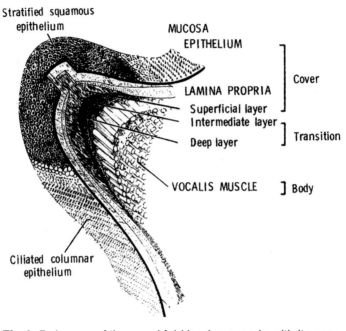

Fig 1–5. Layers of the vocal fold lamina propria with its overlying epithelium. Also labeled are the layers that are typically thought to make up the cover and body of the vocal fold.

(differentiated fibroblasts believed to be important in the reorganization of tissues) are also found within the lamina. The discovery that the cytoplasm of these cells contain proteoglycans indicates that they, along with fibroblasts, are involved with the development and maintenance of the vocal fold.[16]

Catten[17] expanded on this work by looking at the concentration of fibroblasts, myofibroblasts, and macrophages in each layer of the lamina propria. He found that fibroblasts were most abundant in the deepest layer of the lamina propria and myofibroblasts were found in more superficial regions. Macrophages were only seen in 36% of his specimens and, when present, were also found in the superficial layer.[17] The cell signaling mechanisms that are

instrumental in cell differentiation have yet to be determined.

The early work by Catten looking at differences in cellular concentration in the three layers of the lamina propria was important as before that time the layers were defined only by elastin and collagen concentrations. Hartnick[15] was the first to look cellular differences as the vocal fold develops from infancy until adolescence He found that the newborn vocal fold contained only a monolayer of cells, which agreed with what had been previously described by Sato and Hirano.[12,13] This became two layers of cells by 5 months and three layers by 7 years (Fig 1–6). The results of the study helped support the notion that the three-layered vocal fold might develop earlier than what had previously been

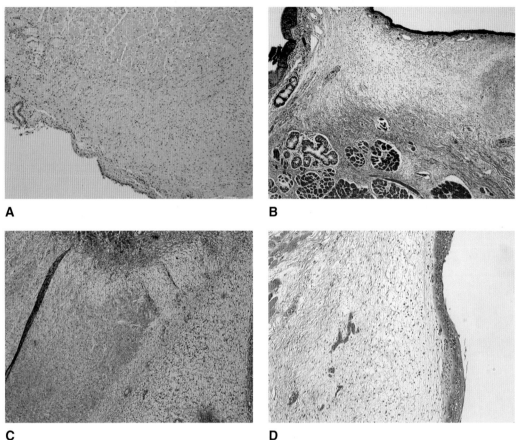

Fig 1–6. Four micrometer sections of 2-day-old (*A*), 2-year-old (*B*), 7-year-old (*C*), and 13-year-old (*D*) true vocal folds. **A.** Hematoxylin-eosin stain at 10x magnification showing single hypocellular layer of the lamina propria. **B.** Alcian blue stain at 40× magnification showing two distinct cellular populations within the lamina propria. **C.** Trichrome stain at 100x magnification showing the beginning of middle layer of the lamina propria. There are superficial and deep areas of hypocellularity with a middle layer that is more cellular. **D.** Hematoxylin-eosin stain at 40x magnification showing the fully developed three-layered lamina propria.

described by using elastin and collagen content.[15]

Boseley and Hartnick[18] later duplicated Catten's study, looking specifically at the concentrations of macrophages and myofibroblasts in the lamina propria. These cells were first seen by the age of 11 months.

This work provided additional evidence that both are predominately found in the superficial layers of the lamina.

Measurements of the depth of the entire lamina propria and the superficial lamina propria were also reported. The superficial layer appeared to become thinner with age, encompassing approximately 20% of the entire lamina propria in the 7-year-old specimen. In addition, the total depth of the lamina propria reached 1,300 μm in the specimen of a 10-year-old child (Fig 1–7). These two measurements approximate what is seen in the adult. Therefore, one could conclude that the vocal fold may be fully developed at some point within this age range. The small sample size in the study, however, prevents making definitive conclusions.[18]

Lamina Propria Proteins

Elastin

Elastin plays a significant role in the biomechanics of the lamina propria. These fibers are primarily found in the intermediate layer of the lamina propria in the fully developed vocal fold and are intimately associated with a glycosaminoglycan (hyaluronic acid) and a proteoglycan (fibromodulin). Here elastin can stretch up to two times its resting length.[19]

Elastin is found in low concentrations in the newborn, but its fibers aren't fully developed (thin, coiled fibers). The concentration increases with age, with the highest concentrations found in geriatric male and female specimens. This fact doesn't necessarily mean that vocal fold elasticity is increased with age. One theory is that cross-linking may cause decreased elasticity despite the higher concentrations. It should also be noted here that there does not appear to be gender-related differences in elastin concentrations.[19]

Collagen

Collagen is another important protein found in the lamina propria. Unlike elastin, collagen is typically found immediately under the surface epithelium and also in the deep layer of the lamina propria. The deep layer and the underlying vocalis muscle make up part of the vocal ligament (in addition to the deep portion of the intermediate layer). This accounts for the relatively stable body, over which the cover of the vocal fold can move.[20]

Collagen concentration within the basement membrane of the epithelium is actually greater in infant specimens than what is found in adult and geriatric specimens. However, the collagen within the deep layer of the lamina propria increases significantly until adulthood and then appears to level off. Furthermore, there seems to be a significantly higher concentration of collagen in males compared to females. The reason for this is not completely understood. This is particularly puzzling if one suspects that collagen production is in response to tension exerted on the fold which should be the same in both sexes. Other gender specific environmental (voice use) and

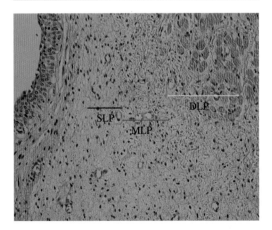

Fig 1–7. Histologic photomicrograph of a 10-year-old child's TVF. Lines are drawn to demonstrate how the individual layers of the lamina were measured using an optical analysis computer software program. The total depth of the three layers was 1300 μm.

physiologic (hormones, etc) factors may also play a role, although this has not been definitively proven.[20]

CONCLUSION

Although much knowledge has been gained regarding the development of the human vocal fold, there are still many questions to be answered. Thus far, definitive conclusions have been difficult to reach due, in part, to the small sample size restraints in most published studies. To this end, new technologies are being developed that may allow us to examine the histologic make-up of the vocal fold in vivo. In addition to continuing to examine the anatomic development of the vocal fold, we also need to examine the mechanisms of cellular differentiation and the biomechanical properties of the various layers of the vocal fold. The hope is that this information will be helpful in treating various pathologies that are seen in the pediatric population.

REFERENCES

1. Moore KL. *The Developing Human*. Philadelphia, Pa: Saunders; 1988:170–210.
2. Cotton RT, Myer CM. *Practical Pediatric Otolaryngology*. Philadelphia, Pa: Lippincott-Raven; 1999:497–513.
3. Hollinshead WH. *Anatomy for Surgeons The Head and Neck*. Philadelphia,Pa: Lippincott, Williams & Wilkins; 1982:418–432.
4. Cummings CW, Fredrickson JM, Harker LA, Krause CJ, Richardson MA, Schuller DE. *Otolaryngology-Head and Neck Surgery*. St. Louis, Mo: Mosby; 1998.
5. Kahane JC. Histologic structure and properties of the human vocal folds. *Ear Nose Throat J*. 1988;67:322–330.
6. Litman RS, Weissend EE, Shibata D, Westesson P. Developmental changes of laryngeal dimensions in unparalyzed, sedated children. *Anesthesiology*. 2003;98:41–45.
7. Vorperian HK, Kent RD, Gentry LR, Yandell BS. Magnetic resonance imaging procedures to study the concurrent anatomic development of vocal tract structures: preliminary results. *Int J Pediatr Otorhinolaryngol*. 1999;49:197–206.
8. Hirano M. Growth, development, and aging of human vocal folds. In: Abbs J. *Vocal Fold Physiology*. San Diego,Calif: College-Hill Press; 1983:23–43.
9. Hirano M. Phonosurgery. Basic and clinical Investigations. *Otologia (Fukuoka)*. 1975; 21(suppl 1):239–260.
10. Hirano M. Structure and vibratory behavior of the vocal folds. In: Sawashima M, Franklin S, eds. *Dynamic Aspects of Speech Production*. Tokyo, Japan: University of Tokyo Press; 1977:13–30.
11. Hirano M. Structure of the vocal fold in normal and disease states: anatomical and physical studies. *ASHA Reports*. 1981;11:11–30.
12. Sato K, Hirano M. Histologic investigation of the maculae flava of the human vocal fold. *Ann Otol Rhinol Laryngol*. 1995;104: 556–562
13. Sato K, Hirano M, Nakashima T. Fine structure of the human newborn and infant vocal fold mucosae. *Ann Otol Rhinol Laryngol*. 2001;110:417–424.
14. Ishii K, Akita M, Yamashita K, Hirose H. Age-related development of the arrangement of connective tissue fibers in the lamina propria of the human vocal fold. *Ann Otol Rhinol Laryngol*. 2000;109:1055–1064.
15. Hartnick CJ, Rehbar R, Prasad V. Development and maturation of the pediatric human vocal fold lamina propria. *Laryngoscope*. 2005;115:4–15.
16. Pawlak A, Hammond TH, Hammond E, Gray SD. Immunocytochemical study of proteoglycans in vocal folds. *Ann Otol Rhinol Laryngol*. 1996;105:6–11.
17. Catten M, Gray SD, Hammond TH, Zhou R, Hammond E. Analysis of cellular location

and concentration in vocal fold lamina propria. *Otolaryngol Head Neck Surg.* 1998; 118:663-667.

18. Boseley ME, Hartnick CJ. Development of the human vocal fold: depth of cell layers and quantifying cell types within the lamina propria. *Ann Otol Rhinol Laryngol.* 2006; 115:784-788.

19. Hammond TH, Gray SD, Butler J, Zhou R, Hammond E. Age- and gender-related elastin distribution changes in human vocal folds. *Otolaryngol Head Neck Surg.* 1998;119:314-322.

20. Hammond TH, Gray SD, Butler JE. Age- and gender-related collagen distribution in human vocal folds. *Ann Otol Rhinol Laryngol.* 2000;109:913-920.

Emerging Science Regarding the Human Vocal Fold

Susan L. Thibeault

INTRODUCTION

Research and science in the field of laryngology is at an exciting point in its evolution. There has been an increased acknowledgment, demonstrated by recent research creativity, that this is a multifaceted area of study that requires consideration of a multidisciplinary approach. This is becoming increasingly more common in medical research in so much that this cross-discipline, team-based research approach has been previously proposed in an NIH Roadmap for Medical Research laid out in 2003 by Dr Elias A. Zerhouni, Director of the NIH.[1] We are at a crossroads in laryngology research such that the emerging science regarding the human vocal fold has began to demonstrate a greater focus on understanding basic science through a variety of disciplines and translating the findings to the clinical realm.

It is difficult to write a chapter such as this, with its inclusive pediatric focus, as there is a paucity of literature specific to pediatric vocal fold science. Research specific to the pediatric vocal fold and its development has lagged behind that regarding the adult vocal fold. Not withstanding, however, the multidisciplinary concept has started to appear in pediatric research. This chapter presents approaches in the emerging science regarding the vocal fold. State-of-the-art science with translational application is presented. The reader should note, however, that many of the research areas investigated for the adult larynx could, should, and need to be replicated for the pediatric larynx.

RESEARCH IN LARYNGEAL DEVELOPMENT

The earliest viewing into the development of the larynx is just that, with the use of sonographic examination of the fetus. Assessment of the prenatal patterns of growth and function of upper airway structures including the pharyngeal and laryngeal regions, provide the structural foundation for later phonatory, ingestive, and respiratory functions.[2] Miller et al, using sonographic technology, have found that it is important to identify when structural differences first emerge in the upper airway, their developmental sequence, and what casual factors (if any) provide indices for early identification and clinical intervention. For example, it has been reported the complex oral-motor and upper airway skills merged earlier in females, suggesting a sex-specific trajectory of motor development.[3] The lag measured in males corresponded to follow-up postnatal data with males exhibiting a greater percentage of postnatal feeding-related difficulties.

Magnetic resonance imaging has been utilized to denote the physical changes that the vocal tract structures undergo during development. A research group at the University of Wisconsin-Madison led by Dr. Vorperian, has developed this technology with the goal to qualitatively characterize the macroanatomic developmental changes in the bony and soft tissue structures of the vocal tract during the first two decades of life.[4,5] Such data would have translational implications for developmental voice acoustics and for increasing our understanding of the anatomic bases of motor adjustments in speech development.

There has been a keen interest in the role of vitamin A in the development of the larynx and specifically the vocal folds. Vitamin A is a liposoluble vitamin, stored in lipid droplets in cytoplasm and is generally accepted to be a morphogen that controls the differentiation and morphogenesis of cells. Newborn vocal folds have immature macula flavae that contain oval-shaped fibroblasts with limited vitamin A-containing cells.[6] Vitamin A-containing lipid droplets become more prevalent at 3 and 8 months old in the macula flava portion of the vocal fold.[7] In a unique study aimed to determine if vitamin A deficiency affects prenatal laryngeal development by Tateya et al, pregnant rats (five vitamin A-deficient rats and five control rats) were studied.[8] Eighteen percent of the vitamin A-deficient embryos collected at embryonic day 18.5 were alive and demonstrated laryngotracheal cartilage malformation, incomplete separation of the glottis, and laryngoesophageal cleft. Tateya et al[7] also determined that prenatal vitamin A deficiency causes laryngeal malformations whereas postnatal vitamin A deficiency causes a thickening of the epithelium. To further study whether or not vitamin A plays a role in development Tateya et al, determined that retinoic acid receptors (RARs) (retinoic acid is the active form of vitamin A) are expressed in human vocal folds. [9] The expression of RARs in vocal folds suggests that vitamin A is not only stored in the vocal folds but also acts as a regulatory factor.

Initial research in understanding the basic structure and function of the pediatric larynx, especially the vocal folds, focused on describing the histologic layering and changes through maturation.[10-13] There is general consensus that the newborn larynx is without a layered structure and is predominantly cellular. As the vocal folds age, a layered structure becomes evident concomitantly with the development of a vocal ligament by the end of the teenage years. All of this work is seminal; however, the investigation's outcomes generate more questions that require study. The reasons for changes in the vocal fold through maturation are not known, nor are the mechanism or mechanisms that cause these changes. Hartnick et al[12] have proposed that molecular biology techniques will be able to assist in the elucidation of how and why the vocal fold structure develops. Areas in need of investigation include cell signaling, the effects of mechanical forces on development, relationship of hormones to maturation, and gender differences. Lastly, an improved understanding of the basis of development and maturation will be able to assist with surgical and therapeutic diagnosis and treatment. The relationship between the layered structure and disease development, such as benign lesions, is an entirely unstudied area in pediatrics. Unfortunately, we cannot assume that what we know regarding adults in terms of the etiology, diagnosis, and treatment of benign lesions is the same for children. A different layered structure of the vocal folds may preclude differing patterns of etiology and allow for varying approaches to treatment.

GENOMICS AND PROTEOMICS

Genomics and proteomics are two areas of study that have promising applications in laryngology. Genomics is the study of an organism's entire genome and complementary DNA microarray (MA) a powerful tool, is used in these investigations. The advent of MA in the mid-1990s made it possible for high throughput monitoring of the expression of many genes in parallel, allowing for the opportunity to define gene patterns at the level of the whole genome. This has also been called transcription or expression profiling and represents an innovative method for searching broadly for genotypes that are responsible for disease. The use of MA has been utilized to establish expression profiles among diseases with similar phenotypes, such as multiple sclerosis,[14,15] diffuse large B-cell lymphoma,[16,17] melanoma,[18] breast cancer,[19] and squamous cell carcinoma.[20] In laryngology, MA has been recently utilized by Thibeault et al[21] and Duflo et al [22] to establish distinct gene expression profiles for vocal fold lesions. Established transcript profiles can provide insight into the molecular and cellular processes involved in these diseases. Furthermore MA may be used for improved diagnosis and treatment of benign lesions.

Until recently, gene expression studies were limited by the size of tissue obtainable. Recently, however, linear amplification of mRNA has yielded approaches that enable the production of large amounts of RNA from minimal starting quantities for use in gene expression studies. mRNA extraction is now possible from even single cells using laser capture microdissection. Laser capture microdissection provides a method to extract exact areas of tissue (for multiple types of assays) without contamination from unwanted tissue. Amplification expands the amount of mRNA and consequently the numbers of experiments that can be conducted from precious vocal fold samples. Amplified RNA (aRNA) can be readily used for microarray analysis. The capacity to amplify mRNA has significant consequences on vocal fold biology because until now the size of most vocal fold samples were too small for complete gene expression or microarray analysis. As a consequence no vocal fold sample now need be regarded as too small. The ability to amplify RNA from even a single sample will allow us to interrogate clinical material in a fashion not previously feasible. This may allow identification of precisely what is different between a normal ECM and diseased ECM. Furthermore, this will allow for identification of clinical genes that direct synthesis of key components and allow for ascertaining genetic changes that take a cell from normalcy to disease. Understanding and identifying these genes will make it possible to devise strategies to treat and potentially ameliorate dysphonias.

Proteomic methodologies offer promise in elucidating the system-wide cellular and molecular processes that characterize normal and diseased tissue of the vocal folds at a given time. Proteomics is often considered the next step in the study of biological systems, after genomics. Proteomics has been introduced to voice research by several research labs. Li et al[23] used these methodologies to determine changes in protein expression in denervated laryngeal muscles with hopes of identifying proteins for future therapeutic gene transfer. Welham et al[24] has assessed protein expression changes in the thyroid arytenoid muscle of a rat following the injection of botulinum toxin serotype A (BoNT/A). BoNT/A was investigated as it is a commonly used therapeutic agent in the treatment of spasmodic dysphonia, and appears to induce molecular changes in skeletal muscle (via neurotoxic and/or myotoxic processes) that are distinct from those observed following other modes of denervation. Four postinjection time points were studied: 72 h, 7 days, 14 days, and 56 days. Injection of BoNT/A resulted in biologically significant variations in individual protein expression throughout the rat TA muscle proteome. Furthermore, variation in the rat TA proteome was observed as a function of time postinjection.

Regarding future approaches, as genes and proteins play a central role in the life of an organism, both methodologies—genomics and proteomics will be instrumental in discovery of biomarkers that indicate a particular disease. These biomarkers may be used in isolation or together to develop biochips that are used for diagnosis. Tissue may be obtained from needle aspirates or biopsies that may provide sufficient tissue for analysis without causing injury. Gray et al were the first to introduce this concept in 2002.[25] This area of research and translational application requires more investigation before it becomes clinically ready.

VOCAL FOLD IMAGING

During the past 10 years there has been a rapid increase in the scientific literature and reported use of high-speed videoendoscopy (HSV). This rapid increase may be contributed to the cheaper, practical, improved technology that is now available. HSV allows view of true intracycle vibration through a full view of the vocal folds. HSV is considered by some a secondary technique that supplements videostroboscopy. There are some limitations at this time that restrict the technology from becoming widely accessible, including development of optimal camera specifications, effective segmentation methods, and intuitive facilitative playback techniques.[26] To date there have been no reports of use of HSV in the pediatric population.

Optical coherence tomography (OCT) is a relatively new imaging modality that measures infrared light backscattered from within tissue to provide cross-sectional images resembling vertical sections in histology. It is analogous to ultrasound imaging but it uses infrared light instead of acoustic waves. The technology allows for low depth penetration and ultrahigh tissue resolution. In the larynx, preliminary reports have found usefulness for in vivo imaging of the microstructure of the vocal folds (several millimeters in depth).[27,28] The most promising is visualization of epithelial and superficial layers of the vocal folds particularly of malignant and benign lesions. The use of OCT in adults and pediatrics is promising with a multitude of possibilities for applications are technology improves.

LARYNGOPHARYNGEAL REFLUX

The association between gastroesophageal reflux disease (GERD) and laryngeal disorders in children is not well established and there is still a lack of data concerning the true extent of the laryngeal complications of GERD in children, in addition to diagnosis and treatment of such. The role of pepsin, bile acids, pancreatic enzymes, motility disorders, and food allergies in GERD in children has only recently been recognized. There is an emphasis in the recently published research regarding the basic biology of pepsin, its diagnosis, and its role in upper airway inflammation. Johnston et al[29-32] have published a number of papers that investigate the presence of laryngeal stress proteins and their response to pepsin. She has concluded that receptor-mediated uptake of pepsin by laryngeal epithelial cells, as may occur in LPR, causes a change in the normal acid-mediated stress protein response. This altered stress protein response may lead to cellular injury and thus play a role in the development of disease. This work is the first to document the molecular pathways for pepsin-induced LPR. Other molecularly based studies by Ylitalo et al[33] have investigated the laryngeal fibroblast responses to varying the pH of acid and pepsin at different time points. Lastly, an immunoassay that can detect pepsin in throat sputum has been developed.[34] This appears to be a sensitive, non-invasive method for diagnosis of pepsin-related LPR. This translation application of pepsin biology will have a useful role in the clinic setting for pediatrics and adults.

REGENERATION, ENGINEERING, AND WOUND HEALING

Research focusing on nerve regeneration for the recurrent laryngeal nerve has been very active with different approaches utilizing tissue engineering techniques—application of application of growth hormones,[35] application of neurotrophins,[36-38] gene therapy,[39,40] and electrical stimulation.[41,42] Each approach has demonstrated some improvement and recognizes the need for further investigation. Moreover, the need to overlap approaches—application of growth hormones and nerve grafting together may provide synergistic results.

Emerging technology has emerged with labs across the country actively involved in tissue engineering research of the vocal fold lamina propria and tracheal cartilage. Tissue engineering of the vocal fold lamina propria extracellular matrix (ECM) is a comprehensive area of study that requires consideration of material composition, size, shape, surface properties, viscoelastic properties, mechanical loading, and surgical technique. Each of these areas deserves active research to be able to provide varying biomaterials and constructs to be used clinically. Three main principles for tissue engineering exist—development using scaffolds, cells, or a combination of scaffolds or cells. Various constructs and approaches have been reported for the vocal folds including a synthetic extracellular matrix,[43-45] hydrogels,[46,47] acellular xenografts,[48,49] autologous fibroblasts,[50] and stem cells.[51,52] To date, all reports have been in vitro or animal trials.

Vocal fold injury and repair or wound healing research in laryngology has focused on defining the wound healing processes and its ensuing manifestations—hemostasis, inflammation, mesenchymal cell migration and proliferation, angiogenesis, epithelialization, collagen and proteoglycan synthesis, and wound contraction and remodeling. More recently there has been a push for a molecular characterization of wound healing which involves molecular approaches to understanding complex pathways. The most active area is that of vocal fold scarring. Present treatments for this clinical condition are inconsistent and often produce suboptimal results. A number of studies have characterized the histologic and molecular manifestations of vocal fold scarring at different points postinjury and in a number of animal models.[53-58] Various studies have investigated the potential of treating vocal fold injury with growth factors, namely, hepatocyte growth factor,[59,60] hyaluronic acid,[43,46,61] or various collagen matrices,[47] in animal models, with varying benefits. Human trials have been limited to inconsistent improvement with collagen-based, fat, or HA-based injectables.[62,63] As the basic science in wound healing provides us with more insight into the disease process, our treatment options will produce more dependable results and favorable clinical outcomes.

A common methodology that measures functional return in tissue properties is rheology. Vocal fold lamina propria has been described as viscoelastic, demonstrating both viscous and elastic properties. It has been shown that the viscoelastic properties of vocal fold tissues critically determine the vibratory characteristics of the vocal folds, affecting such variables as phonation threshold pressure.[64] This suggests that under-

standing the relationship between tissue biology and viscoelastic properties might provide valuable information regarding treatment options. Rheologic methodology is one way to investigate the viscoelastic shear properties of vocal fold tissues and injectable bioimplants in vitro.[65-67] For a viscoelastic material, elastic shear modulus (μ or G') is a quantification of the energy storage component of the material in shear deformation (the material's stiffness in shear), whereas dynamic viscosity (η or η') is a quantification of the energy loss component of the material (the material's resistance to shear flow). Chan and Titze[65-67] related shear stiffness and viscosity to the ease of relative displacement and slippage between molecules of the material, which are determined by different kinds of intramolecular and intermolecular interactions. For example, conceptually, tissue scarring would seem to decrease the "slippage" between molecules because of an unorganized matrix deposition as well as a distorted relationship between the molecules. In other words, the scarred arrangement may alter molecular interactions, resulting in increased viscosity and decreased compliance (increased stiffness), which may correspond to the clinical findings of stiffness and loss of mucosal wave.[68,69] Rheology has been used as an outcome measure for a number of research papers. One of the limitations of rheology, however, is that it is an ex vivo technique, such that the tissue needs to be removed prior to being tested, thereby limiting its applicability.

Most recently there has been a focus on in vivo assessment of vocal fold viscoelasticity. Several publications have demonstrated potential using a linear skin rheometer.[70] This rheometer would allow assessment of viscoelasticity properties in vivo—in patients in the operating room or in the outpatient clinic. If achieved this would provide an objective measurement for which outcomes could be measured for research and in clinical practice.

BIOLOGICAL EFFICACY OF VOICE THERAPY

A novel new area of research involves determining and defining the biological mechanisms active in vibration that can be correlated to voice therapy. This work has included modeling and use of vibration or strain in vitro paradigms to assess change in cell behavior. The main question is how vocal fold cells respond to mechanical forces. Titze at al[71] recently described the development of a novel bioreactor approximately phonatory forces (200 Hz) and demonstrated altered gene expression of human vocal fold fibroblasts with varying levels of strain and vibration. Branski et al[72] also demonstrated that low levels of mechanical signals (<1 Hz) improved inflammatory profiles in rabbit vocal fold fibroblasts. As in other parts of the body, vocal fold fibroblasts do respond to mechanical forces. Optimizing those mechanical forces for desired production from the fibroblasts will be an exciting challenge. Our understanding of mechanical forces and their importance in development, maintenance, and pathology of the vocal folds is an area that has yet to be studied.

CONCLUSIONS

There are a tremendous number of avenues that are emerging for investigation in vocal fold biology. As scientists we are charged with translating the basic science phenomenon into clinical possibilities. We hope that you as readers will follow the research closely—you will not be disappointed.

REFERENCES

1. Zerhouni EA. *NIH Roadmap for Medical Research: A Briefing by the NIH Director and Senior Staff.* Retrieved May 7, 2007 from: http://grants.nih.gov/grants/guide/notice-files/NOT-RM-04-010.html .
2. Miller JL, Sonies BC, Macedonia C. Emergence of oropharyngeal, laryngeal and swallowing activity in the developing fetal upper aerodigestive tract: an ultrasound evaluation. *Early Hum Dev.* 2003;71(1):61–87.
3. Miller JL, Macedonia C, Sonies BC. Sex differences in prenatal oral-motor function and development. *Dev Med Child Neurol.* 2006; 48(6):465–470.
4. Vorperian HK, Kent RD, Lindstrom MJ, Kalina CM, Gentry LR, Yandell BS. Development of vocal tract length during early childhood: a magnetic resonance imaging study. *J Acoust Soc Am.* 2005;117(1):338–350.
5. Vorperian HK, Kent RD, Gentry LR, Yandell BS. Magnetic resonance imaging procedures to study the concurrent anatomic development of vocal tract structures: preliminary results. *Int J Pediatr Otorhinolaryngol.* 1999;49(3):197–206.
6. Sato K, Nakashima T. Vitamin A-storing stellate cells in the human newborn vocal fold. *Ann Otol Rhinol Laryngol.* 2005;114(7): 517–524.
7. Tateya T, Tateya I, Munoz-del-Rio A, Bless DM. Postnatal development of rat vocal folds. *Ann Otol Rhinol Laryngol.* 2006; 115(3):215–224.
8. Tateya I, Tateya T, Bless DM. Prenatal vitamin A deficiency causes laryngeal malformation; a rat study. *Ann Otol Rhinol Laryngol.* Manuscript submitted for publication.
9. Tateya I, Tateya T, Bless DM. Expression of retinoic acid receptors in human and rat vocal folds. *Ann Otol Rhinol Laryngol.* Manuscript submitted for publication.

10. Hammond TH, Gray SD, Butler J. Age and gender related collagen distribution in human vocal folds. *Ann Otol Rhinol Laryngol*. 2000;109:913-920.

11. Hammond TH, Gray SD, Butler J, Zhou R, Hammond E. Age- and gender-related elastin distribution changes in human vocal folds. *Otolaryngol Head Neck Surg*. 1998;119(4): 314-322.

12. Hartnick CJ, Rehbar R, Prasad V. Development and maturation of the pediatric human vocal fold lamina propria. *Laryngoscope*. 2005;115(1):4-15.

13. Ishii K, Yamashita K, Akita M, Hirose H. Age-related development of the arrangement of connective tissue fibers in the lamina propria of the human vocal fold. *Ann Otol Rhinol Laryngol*. 2000;109(11):1055-1064.

14. Lock C, Hermans G, Pedotti R, et al. Gene-microarray analysis of multiple sclerosis lesions yields new targets validated in autoimmune encephalomyelitis. *Nat Med*. 2002; 8(5):500-508.

15. Tompkins SM, Miller SD. An array of possibilities for multiple sclerosis. *Nat Med*. 2002;8(5):451-453.

16. Wright G, Tan B, Rosenwald A, Hurt EH, Wiestner A, Staudt LM. A gene expression-based method to diagnose clinically distinct subgroups of diffuse large B cell lymphoma. *Proc Natl Acad Sci U S A*. 2003;100(17): 9991-9996.

17. Shipp MA, Ross KN, Tamayo P, et al. Diffuse large B-cell lymphoma outcome prediction by gene-expression profiling and supervised machine learning. *Nat Med*. 2002;8(1): 68-74.

18. Bittner M, Meltzer P, Chen Y, et al. Molecular classification of cutaneous malignant melanoma by gene expression profiling. *Nature*. 2000;406(6795):536-540.

19. Ma XJ, Salunga R, Tuggle JT, et al. Gene expression profiles of human breast cancer progression. *Proc Natl Acad Sci U S A*. 2003;100(10):5974-5979.

20. Leethanakul C. Distinct pattern of expression of differentiation and growth-related genes in squamous cell carcinomas of the head and neck revealed by the use of laser capture microdissection and cDNA arrays. *Oncogene*. 2000;19:3220-3224.

21. Thibeault SL, Hirschi SD, Gray SD. DNA microarray gene expression analysis of a vocal fold polyp and granuloma. *J Speech Lang Hear Res*. 2003;46(2):491-502.

22. Duflo S, Thibeault S, Li W, Smith ME, Shade G, Hess M. Differential gene expression profiling of vocal fold polyps and Reinke's edema by cDNA microarray. *Ann Otol Rhinol Laryngol*. Manuscript submitted for publication.

23. Li ZB, Lehar M, Samlan R, Flint PW. Proteomic analysis of rat laryngeal muscle following denervation. *Proteomics*. 2005; 5(18):4764-4776.

24. Welham NV. *Proteomic profiling of laryngeal muscle*. [dissertation]. Madison, WI: University of Wisconsin;2006.

25. Gray SD, Thibeault SL, Tresco PA. Witnessing a revolution in voice research: genomics, tissue engineering, biochips and what's next! *Logop Phoniat Voco*. 2003;28(7): 7-13; Discussion 14-17.

26. Deliyski D. Clinical feasibility of high speed videoendoscopy. *Perspec Voice Voice Dis*. 2007;17(7):12-16.

27. Kraft M, Luerssen K, Lubatschowski H, Glanz H, Arens C. Technique of optical coherence tomography of the larynx during microlaryngoscopy. *Laryngoscope*. 2007; 117(5):950-952.

28. Klein AM, Pierce MC, Zeitels SM, et al. Imaging the human vocal folds in vivo with optical coherence tomography: a preliminary experience. *Ann Otol Rhinol Laryngol*. 2006;115(4):277-284.

29. Johnston N, Dettmar PW, Bishwokarma B, Lively MO, Koufman JA. Activity/stability of human pepsin: implications for reflux attributed laryngeal disease. *Laryngoscope*. In press

30. Johnston N, Dettmar PW, Lively MO, et al. Effect of pepsin on laryngeal stress protein (Sep70, Sep53, and Hsp70) response: role in laryngopharyngeal reflux disease. *Ann Otol Rhinol Laryngol*. 2006;115(1):47-58.

31. Gill GA, Johnston N, Buda A, et al. Laryngeal epithelial defenses against laryngopharyngeal reflux: investigations of E-cadherin, carbonic anhydrase isoenzyme III, and pepsin. *Ann Otol Rhinol Laryngol.* 2005;114(12): 913-921.

32. Johnston N, Knight J, Dettmar PW, Lively MO, Koufman J. Pepsin and carbonic anhydrase isoenzyme III as diagnostic markers for laryngopharyngeal reflux disease. *Laryngoscope.* 2004;114(12):2129-2134.

33. Ylitalo R, Baugh A, Thibeault SL, Li W. Effect of acid and pepsin on gene expression in laryngeal fibroblasts. *Ann Otol Rhinol Laryngol.* 2004;113(11):866-871.

34. Knight J, Lively MO, Johnston N, Dettmar PW, Koufman JA. Sensitive pepsin immunoassay for detection of laryngopharyngeal reflux. *Laryngoscope.* 2005;115(8):1473-1478.

35. Flint PW, Nakagawa H, Shiotani A, Coleman ME, O'Malley BW Jr. Effects of insulin-like growth factor-1 gene transfer on myosin heavy chains in denervated rat laryngeal muscle. *Laryngoscope.* 2004;114(2):368-371.

36. Kingham PJ, Hughes A, Mitchard L, et al. Effect of neurotrophin-3 on reinnervation of the larynx using the phrenic nerve transfer technique. *Eur J Neurosci.* 2007;25(2): 331-340.

37. Kingham PJ, Terenghi G. Bioengineered nerve regeneration and muscle reinnervation. *J Anat.* 2006;209(4):511-526.

38. Kingham PJ, Terenghi G, Birchall MA. Tissue engineering strategies for reinnervation of the larynx. *Clin Otolaryngol.* 2006;31(3):245.

39. Shiotani A, Saito K, Araki K, Moro K, Watabe K. Gene therapy for laryngeal paralysis. *Ann Otol Rhinol Laryngol.* 2007;116(2):115-122.

40. Araki K, Shiotani A, Watabe K, Saito K, Moro K, Ogawa K. Adenoviral GDNF gene transfer enhances neurofunctional recovery after recurrent laryngeal nerve injury. *Gene Ther.* 2006;13(4):296-303.

41. Zealear DL, Billante CL, Chongkolwatana C, Herzon GD. The effects of chronic electrical stimulation on laryngeal muscle reinnervation. *ORL J Otorhinolaryngol Relat Spec.* 2000;62(2):87-95.

42. Zealear DL, Billante CR, Chongkolwatana C, Rho YS, Hamdan AL, Herzon GD. The effects of chronic electrical stimulation on laryngeal muscle physiology and histochemistry. *ORL J Otorhinolaryngol Relat Spec.* 2000; 62(2):81-86.

43. Hansen JK, Thibeault SL, Walsh JF, Shu XZ, Prestwich GD. In vivo engineering of the vocal fold extracellular matrix with injectable hyaluronic acid hydrogels: early effects on tissue repair and biomechanics in a rabbit model. *Ann Otol Rhinol Laryngol.* 2005;114(9):662-670.

44. Duflo S, Thibeault SL, Li W, Shu XZ, Prestwich GD. Vocal fold tissue repair in vivo using a synthetic extracellular matrix. *Tissue Eng.* 2006;12(8):2171-2180.

45. Duflo S, Thibeault SL, Li W, Shu XZ, Prestwich G. Effect of a synthetic extracellular matrix on vocal fold lamina propria gene expression in early wound healing. *Tissue Eng.* 2006;12(11):3201-3207.

46. Jia X, Yeo Y, Clifton RJ, et al. Hyaluronic acid-based microgels and microgel networks for vocal fold regeneration. *Biomacromolecules.* 2006;7(12):3336-3344.

47. Hahn MS, Teply BA, Stevens MM, Zeitels SM, Langer R. Collagen composite hydrogels for vocal fold lamina propria restoration. *Biomaterials.* 2006;27(7):1104-1109.

48. Xu CC, Chan RW, Tirunagari N. A biodegradable, acellular xenogeneic scaffold for regeneration of the vocal fold lamina propria. *Tissue Eng.* 2007;13(3):551-566.

49. Ringel RL, Kahane JC, Hillsamer PJ, Lee AS, Badylak SF. The application of tissue engineering procedures to repair the larynx. *J Speech Lang Hear Res.* 2006;49(1): 194-208.

50. Chhetri DK, Head C, Revazova E, Hart S, Bhuta S, Berke GS. Lamina propria replacement therapy with cultured autologous fibroblasts for vocal fold scars. *Otolaryngol Head Neck Surg.* 2004;131(6):864-870.

51. Kanemaru S, Nakamura T, Omori K, et al. Regeneration of the vocal fold using autologous mesenchymal stem cells. *Ann Otol Rhinol Laryngol.* 2003;112(11):915-920.

52. Kanemaru S, Nakamura T, Yamashita M, et al. Destiny of autologous bone marrow-derived stromal cells implanted in the vocal fold. *Ann Otol Rhinol Laryngol.* 2005;114(12): 907-912.

53. Tateya T, Tateya I, Sohn JH, Bless DM. Histologic characterization of rat vocal fold scarring. *Ann Otol Rhinol Laryngol.* 2005; 114(3):183-191.

54. Rousseau B, Hirano S, Chan RW, et al. Characterization of chronic vocal fold scarring in a rabbit model. *J Voice.* 2004;18(1):116-124.

55. Thibeault SL, Rousseau B, Welham NV, Hirano S, Bless DM. Hyaluronan levels in acute vocal fold scar. *Laryngoscope.* 2004; 114(4):760-764.

56. Thibeault SL, Gray SD, Bless DM, Chan RW, Ford C. Histologic and rheologic characterization of vocal fold scarring. *J Voice.* 2002;16(1):96-104.

57. Rousseau B, Sohn J, Montequin DW, Tateya I, Bless DM. Functional outcomes of reduced hyaluronan in acute vocal fold scar. *Ann Otol Rhinol Laryngol.* 2004;113(10): 767-776.

58. Rousseau B, Hirano S, Scheidt TD, et al. Characterization of vocal fold scarring in a canine model. *Laryngoscope.* 2003;113: 620-627.

59. Hirano S, Bless DM, Nagai H, et al. Growth factor therapy for vocal fold scarring in a canine model. *Ann Otol Rhinol Laryngol.* 2004;113(10):777-785.

60. Hirano S, Bless DM, Rousseau B, et al. Prevention of vocal fold scarring by topical injection of hepatocyte growth factor in a rabbit model. *Laryngoscope.* 2004;114(3): 548-556.

61. Borzacchiello A, Mayol L, Garskog O, Dahlqvist A, Ambrosio L. Evaluation of injection augmentation treatment of hyaluronic acid based materials on rabbit vocal folds viscoelasticity. *J Mater Sci Mater Med.* 2005;16(6):553-557.

62. Hertegard S, Hallen L, Laurent C, et al. Cross-linked hyaluronan versus collagen for injection treatment of glottal insufficiency: 2-year follow-up. *Acta Otolaryngol.* 2004;124(10): 1208-1214.

63. Hertegard S, Hallen L, Laurent C, Lindstrom E, Olofsson K, Dahlqvist A. Cross-linked Hyaluronan used as augmentation substance for treatment of glottal insufficiency: Safety aspects and vocal fold function. *Laryngoscope.* 2002;112:2211-2219.

64. Chan RW, Titze IR, Titze MR. Further studies of phonation threshold pressure in a physical model of the vocal fold mucosa. *J Acoust Soc Am.* 1997;101(6):3722-3727.

65. Chan RW, Titze IR. Viscosities of implantable biomaterials in vocal fold augmentation surgery. *Laryngoscope.* 1998;108(5):725-731.

66. Chan RW, Titze IR. Hyaluronic acid (with fibronectin) as a bioimplant for the vocal fold mucosa. *Laryngoscope.* 1999;109(7 t 1): 1142-1149.

67. Chan RW, Titze IR. Viscoelastic shear properties of human vocal fold mucosa: measurement methodology and empirical results. *J Acoust Soc Am.* 1999;106(4 pt1): 2008-2021.

68. Benninger MS, Alessi D, Archer S, et al. Vocal fold scarring: current concepts and management. *Otolaryngol Head Neck Surg.* 1996; 115(5):474-482.

69. Hirano M, Bless DM. *Videostroboscopic Examination of the Larynx.* San Diego, Calif: Singular Publishing Group; 1993.

70. Dailey SH, Tateya I, Montequin D, Welham N, Goodyer E. Viscoelastic measurements of vocal folds using the linear skin rheometer. *J Voice.* In press.

71. Titze IR, Hitchcock RW, Broadhead K, et al. Design and validation of a bioreactor for engineering vocal fold tissues under combined tensile and vibrational stresses. *J Biomech.* 2004;37(10):1521-1529.

72. Branski RC, Perera P, Verdolini K, Rosen CA, Hebda PA, Agarwal S. Dynamic biomechanical strain inhibits IL-1 beta-induced inflammation in vocal fold fibroblasts. *J Voice.* In press.

Science of Voice Production from Infancy Through Adolescence

Joseph E. Kerschner
Albert L. Merati

INTRODUCTION

The science of voice production in children is conspicuous in its absence of depth, breadth, and overall general attention. However, as the field of pediatric laryngology continues to emerge as its own discipline there has been an increased emphasis on understanding speech, language, and voice production in children with respect to normal physiology and in the presence of pathology. Application of scientific principles to achieve insight about the development and function of voice is unique in that voice cannot be encompassed by a single organ and involves a complex coordination of numerous systems including the respiratory system, digestive system, and nervous system.[1] Given this complexity and the difficulties in studying pediatric patients, the underlying mechanics of voice production in children has, to a large degree, relied on discoveries in the field of adult laryngology until very recently. General anatomic principles, neuromuscular control, and the physics of voice production are highly conserved in humans across many age brackets. However, there are clearly many differences between adults and children with the potential to impact our understanding of pediatric laryngology and ultimately refine interventions in the pediatric patient. In the academic pursuit of knowledge about the pediatric voice it has become well accepted that adult models of laryngeal function are inadequate in predicting behavior and function in children.[2] Furthermore, the inherent nature of laryngeal development with growth and puberty further identifies pediatric laryngology as a discipline with unique parameters and considerations for study. In this chapter, active pathways toward understanding pediatric laryngeal function and dysfunction are discussed. This includes both broad and focused examples of active investigation in voice science, as well as specific characterizations of growth and maturation such as occurs in infancy and puberty.

AREAS OF ACTIVE INVESTIGATION IN PEDIATRIC VOICE SCIENCE

The development of surgical instrumentation and diagnostic evaluation tools specifically for children has provided a significant impetus for increased discovery in pediatric laryngology. Advances in molecular biology, physical modeling, and computer modeling have all been decisive in producing new directions in the science of laryngology and hold significant promise for future increased understanding. In addition, there have been important advances in clinical assessment tools for pediatric patients including both technologic advances and performance instruments. Anatomic changes between infancy and adulthood in the larynx proper have received a reasonable amount of attention in scientific investigation. However, changes in many other areas of the developing child have the potential to impact voice production and eventual susceptibility to pathology. Although a systematic examination of many of these areas is still lacking, initial investigations have provided ample starting ground for future work.

The development of speech and language is intimately associated with the study of voice in children. Understanding the interplay of speech acquisition and laryngeal physiology requires a broad knowledge of neuronal development encompassing both afferent and efferent signaling between the central nervous system and the larynx. The development of the central

nervous system and the many aspects of that development as related to speech and voice is beyond the scope of this text; however, several points of particular emphasis warrant discussion. Primate studies have demonstrated that imitative neurons or "mirror neurons" in the central nervous system may underlie the ability to transfer auditory perception to motor activity in the production of voice.[3]

A more thorough understanding and dissection of imitative neuronal physiology undoubtedly will yield significant advances in the understanding of speech and voice. However, even at this early stage, the concept of auditory input, imitation, and voice production provides explanations as to the potential of the developing child to acquire both normal physiologic and pathologic mechanics.[4] These findings also have specific implications with respect to particular pediatric populations and may provide for meaningful interventions.

Therapies aimed at productive imitations have been advocated for patients with stuttering disorders and vocal impairment associated with autism with some promise of success.[5,6] In addition, computational modeling with these concepts in mind has demonstrated that preferred motor parameters to allow for speech and prototypically perceived sounds develop concurrently. Furthermore, exposure to an ambient language modifies perception to coincide with the sounds from the language.[3]

An additional related area of intense study with respect to these concepts is in cochlear implant patients. The limited, but controlled auditory input in this patient population provides a potential study group to assess concepts around speech and voice development. Systematic studies of cochlear implant patients have demonstrated that auditory deprivation results in poor long-term control of frequency and amplitude during sustained phonation which can be restored with cochlear implantation.[7] Additionally, control over pitch and loudness with reduced jitter and shimmer is achieved rapidly after cochlear implantation.[8] Thoughtful investigations such as these hold the promise of not only improved understanding of auditory science, but also advances in comprehension of voice, speech, and language.

The ability to increasingly preserve functional abilities in infants with significant pathologic conditions early in life has resulted in several other areas of investigative importance with respect to laryngology and voice. These subjects are dealt with in detail in other sections of this text; however, two specific areas bear mention at this juncture.

Neuronal recovery following injury is of particular interest with respect to the developing voice and larynx. Infants and young children can demonstrate remarkable capabilities to recover from the sequelae of neurologic injury, and the same appears to be true with respect to the pediatric larynx. Vocal fold paralysis, with nearly universal severe morbidity in adults, demonstrates far less overall morbidity in children.[9] Specific causative or responsive phenomena potentially related to these findings in infants may include mechanism of injury, neuronal recruitment, differential ability in maintaining muscular tone, and increased plasticity in development of compensatory mechanics. These concepts and others need additional in-depth exploration, but may provide clues to therapeutic intervention for this relatively common pathologic entity in the larynx. In addition, preservation of voice in this high-risk infant population has prompted significant scientific investigation with respect to voice in patients requiring surgical intervention to maintain an adequate airway. Some of these findings

have included that tracheostomy placement in infants has the potential for long-term negative voice outcomes and that changes in glottic vibratory patterns after laryngotracheal reconstruction can negatively impact voice. These changes, however, may be amenable to therapy.[10]

DIFFERENCES BETWEEN THE PEDIATRIC AND ADULT LARYNX

A number of anatomic factors associated with the pediatric larynx create a general mechanical disadvantage compared to the adult larynx. Histologically, the infant vocal fold has been shown to have increased cellularity with a monolayer of cells and decreased cellular differentiation and organization compared with adult vocal folds.[11] Differentiation occurs gradually throughout childhood, and the microanatomy of the vocal fold progresses to incorporate a superficial, intermediate (or middle), and deep layer of the lamina propria (SLP, MLP, and DLP) by approximately 7 years of age. However, the lamina propria continues to mature and develop in size and depth toward adolescence. It is important to understand the development of the lamina propria in children (especially the superficial level), as many areas of pathology including nodules, polyps, and cysts involve the SLP. Theses developmental changes have important implications with respect to therapy and potential phonosurgery in this area.[12] Further biochemical differences in the maturing larynx have not been well studied. However, significant resources are being devoted to discover the underlying molecular regulation and homeostasis of the extracellular matrix in the superficial lamina propria.[13] Understanding developmental differences in these areas of the larynx will be important as future clinical interventions will be based on knowledge of how these biologic features are disturbed in the vocal folds of patients with dysphonia and how these changes relate to vocal symptoms.

Apart from histologic disadvantages, pediatric larynges also have disadvantages in voice production on a gross anatomic level. The child's larynx has a less rigid cartilaginous framework, a decreased ratio of membranous vocal fold length to total vocal fold length, and decreased efficiency in maintaining glottic competence with increased incidence and degree of posterior glottic chink.[14] These factors have gradual resolution over time, but clear developmental "milestones" or characteristics related to these features have yet to be thoroughly defined.

Other anatomic sites and systems outside of the larynx make important contributions to voice production. The lower respiratory system and surrounding anatomy is important in allowing the developing child to overcome some of its anatomic disadvantages. Overall subglottic pressures in children are elevated in comparison to that of adults. This increased pressure is attained by recruitment of a greater percentage of pulmonary capacity.[15] As children approach puberty and develop cartilage elasticity, laryngeal size, and vocal fold characteristics more resembling those of adult larynges, these subglottic pressures may also be reduced. However, these differences in the intensity of subglottic pressures and vocal fold energy undoubtedly contribute to unique opportunities for pathology in the pediatric larynx and are areas that require further investigation.

In addition to these anatomic and histologic changes of the developing larynx, attention has been given to spectral analysis in the developing child's voice. These studies have demonstrated the ability to predict chronologic age based on voice characteristics associated with changes in laryngeal energy levels as the developing larynx achieves more complete glottal closure, resulting in a reduction in frictional noise.[16] Additional investigations have used such techniques to assess gender differences in the developing voice and to assess changes in specific populations including patients with cleft-palate repair to specifically quantify hypernasality.[17]

One final scientific frontier in the assessment of voice in children that warrants discussion is the arena of quality-of-life (QOL) investigations. Recently, several pediatric specific tools have been developed to allow for QOL assessment in pathologic conditions, such as paradoxic vocal fold dysfunction and velopharyngeal insufficiency, as well as to collect data in normative populations.[18-21] These tools are particularly important in assessing the baseline impact of laryngeal pathology in children and to allow for the collection of objective data in making comparative assessments between various interventions required to treat these pathologic conditions.

TRANSITION TO ADULTHOOD: PUBERTY AND ITS EFFECT ON THE MALE AND FEMALE LARYNX

Puberty is certainly a conspicuous time for laryngeal development. Prior to puberty, the female and male larynx are not significantly different.[22] Although the changes that occur during puberty are more dramatic in males, the female vocal tract also undergoes development. In a cadaver study of laryngeal measurements, female postpubertal vocal folds were 24% longer than their prepubertal counterparts. The male vocal folds increased by 67% as determined by anatomic measurements of pre- and postpubertal specimens.[23] Amidst the characteristic changes of primary and secondary sexual changes, the testosterone produced first by the adrenal glands and subsequently by the testicles is also responsible for laryngeal maturation. These androgen-driven changes are irreversible in both males and females. This fact may be welcome for teenage boys; however, the unsuspecting adult female receiving testosterone for libido or other medical indications may find herself with unwanted pitch lowering. Anatomically, androgen receptors are found in the cytoplasm of laryngeal glands and progesterone receptors are found in the nuclei of the same cells. In contrast, estrogen receptors are found in epithelial cells of the larynx.[24]

There are several major structural alterations of the larynx that are driven by pubertal androgen increases.[25] The development of an acute laryngeal angle anteriorly (the "Adam's apple") results from an increase in the anteroposterior length of the thyroid ala. Within the larynx, the vocal folds become more rounded as they lengthen (in concert with the lengthening of the framework). As noted above, the microstructure of the vocal folds becomes more refined with the appearance of distinct layers. Finally, the arytenoids enlarge along with expansion of the intrinsic muscles and ligaments of the larynx.[22,26] The deepening of the male voice is highly dependent on vocal tract lengthening that occurs following puberty.[22]

The female voice also changes with puberty. Although the framework of the larynx has completed development by the end of the teenage years,[22] the pitch progressively declines by about ⅓ to ½ an octave from the prepubertal range.[27]

A dramatic example of hormonal laryngeal manipulation can be seen in the case of the *castrati*, young male singers in Italy who underwent prepubertal castration. This practice, though not common, was evident up through the early part of the 20th century. Conceptually, the preserved "angelic" child's vocal instrument could now be maintained and coupled to adult-sized pulmonary support and mechanics, in addition to the benefit of the experience from singing over the years.[28] In idiopathic hypogonadotropic hypogonadism (IHH), the absence of stimulus to the testes results in low testosterone levels and the failure of pubertal growth which involves the larynx and the rest of the body. These young men are left with high-pitched voices that are intermediate between males and females. When treated with exogenous androgens for 3 months, the mean F_0 for these patients was nearly equivalent to normal aged matched males.[29] In contrast, females with elevated androgen levels, such as in congenital adrenal hyperplasia have more masculine voices likely due to the same pathophysiology.[30]

CONCLUSION

Although the microstructure and function of the larynx continue to be defined by scientific investigation and clinical reflection, these fundamentals of laryngeal development provide the framework for our understanding of pediatric and adolescent laryngology. The clinical significance of subtly aberrant laryngeal development, for example, is not known or even widely considered. In other species the sexual selection and mate choice that is so dependent on birdsong, for example, places laryngeal function quite close to the fulcrum of evolutionary forces. In humans, this effect may have been suspected, but remains unestablished. The ability of the developing larynx to resist and repair injury will likely be better characterized in the forthcoming decades.

In summary, the scientific foundations and investigations in pediatric laryngology are in their infancy, much as the clinical discipline itself. However, appropriate foundations have been laid and the future is promising with respect to the tools, techniques, and interest in expanding this field.

REFERENCES

1. Baken RJ, Orlikoff RF. Voice measurement: is more better? *Logop Phoniatr Vocol.* 1997;22:147-151.
2. Sergeant D, Welch GF. Age-related changes in long-term average spectra of children's voices. *J Voice.* 2007, Jul 9; (Epub ahead of print).
3. Westermann G, Reck Miranda E. A new model of sensorimotor coupling in the development of speech. *Brain Lang.* 2004; 89(2):393-400.
4. Kalinowski J, Saltuklaroglu T. Choral speech: the amelioration of stuttering via imitation and the mirror neuronal system. *Neurosci Biobehav Re.* 27(4):339-347.
5. Saltuklaroglu T, Kalinowski J. How effective is therapy for childhood stuttering? Dissecting and reinterpreting the evidence in light of spontaneous recovery rates. *Lan Comm Dis.* 2005;40(3):359-374.
6. Williams JH, Massaro DW, Peel NJ, Bosseler A, Suddendorf T. Visual-auditory integration during speech imitation in autism. *Res Dev Dis.* 2004; 25(6):559-575.
7. Campisi P, Low A, Papsin B, Mount R, Cohen-Kerem R, Harrison R. Acoustic analysis of the voice in pediatric cochlear implant recipients: a longitudinal study. *Laryngoscope.* 2005;115(6):1046-1050.
8. Hocevar-Boltezar I, Vatovec J, Gros A, Zargi M. The influence of cochlear implantation on some voice parameters. *Int J Ped Otorhinolaryngol.* 2005;69(12):1635-1640.
9. Truong M, Milczuk H, Kerschner JE, Messner A. Pediatric vocal fold paralysis after cardiac surgery: rate of recovery and sequelae. *Otolaryngol Head Neck Surg.* In press.
10. Krival K, Kelchner LN, Weinrich B, et al. Vibratory source, vocal quality and fundamental frequency following pediatric laryngotracheal reconstruction. *Int J Pediatr Otorhinolaryngol.* 2007;71(8):1261-1269.
11. Hartnick CJ. Rehbar R. Prasad V. Development and maturation of the pediatric human vocal fold lamina propria. *Laryngoscope.* 2005;115(1):4-15.
12. Boseley ME. Hartnick CJ. Development of the human true vocal fold: depth of cell layers and quantifying cell types within the lamina propria. *Ann Otol Rhinol Laryngol.* 2006;115(10):784-788.
13. Duflo S, Thibeault SL, Li W, Shu XZ, Prestwich G. Effect of a synthetic extracellular matrix on vocal fold lamina propria gene expression in early wound healing. *Tissue Eng.* 2006;12(11):3201-3207
14. Pabon JPH, McAllister A, Sederholm E, Sundberg J. Dynamics and voice quality information in the computer phonetograms of children's voices. In: White P, ed. *Child Voice.* Stockholm: KTH Voice Research Centre, 2000;85-100.
15. Stathopoulos ET, Sapienza CM. Developmental changes in laryngeal and respiratory function with variations in sound pressure level. *J Speech Lang Hear Res.* 1997;40, 595-614.
16. Sergeant D, Welch GF. Age-related changes in long-term average spectra of children's voices. *J Voice.* 2007, Jul 9; (Epub ahead of print).
17. Kataoka R, Warren DW, Zajac DJ, Mayo R, Lutz RW. The relationship between spectral characteristics and perceived hypernasality in children. *J Acoust Soc Am.* 2001;109(5 pt1): 2181-2189.
18. Boseley ME, Cunningham MJ, Volk MS, Hartnick CJ. Validation of the Pediatric Voice-Related Quality-of-Life survey. *Arch Otolaryngol Neck Surg.* 2006;132(7):717-720.
19. Zur KB, Cotton S, Kelchner L, Baker S, Weinrich B, Lee L. Pediatric Voice Handicap Index (pVHI): a new tool for evaluating pediatric

dysphonia. *Int J Pediatr Otorhinolaryngol.* 2007;71(1):77–82.

20. Mirasola KL, Braun N, Blumin JH, Kerschner JE, Merati AL. Self-reported Voice-related quality of life in adolescents with paradoxical vocal fold dysfunction. *J Voice.* 2007; (Epub ahead of print).

21. Barr L, Thibeault SL, Muntz H, de Serres L. Quality of life in children with velopharyngeal insufficiency. *Arch Otolaryngol Head Neck Surg.* 2007;133(3):224-229.

22. Fitch W, Giedd J. Morphology and development of the human vocal tract: a study using magnetic resonance imaging. *J Acoust Soc Am.* 1999;106:1511-1522.

23. Kahane JC. Growth of the human prepubertal and pubertal larynx. *J Speech Hear Res.* 1982;25:446-455.

24. Newman SR, Butler J, Hammond EH, et al. Preliminary report on hormone receptors in the human vocal fold. *J Voice.* 2000;14:72.

25. Truong M, Damrose E. Endocrine disorders affecting the larynx. *Textbook of Laryngology.* San Diego, Calif: Plural. 2007;443-446.

26. Ferlito A. In:Ferlito A, ed. *Diseases of the Larynx.* London: Oxford; New York: Arnold; Copublished in the USA by Oxford University Press; 2000.

27. Pedersen M, Muller S, Krabbe S, Bennett P, Svenstrup B. Fundamental voice frequency in female puberty measured with electroglottography during continuous speech as a secondary sex characteristic. A comparison between voice, pubertal stages, oestrogens and androgens. *Int J Pediatr Otorhinolaryngol.* 1990;20:17-24.

28. Jenkins JS. The lost voice, a history of the castrato. *J Pediatr Endocrinol Metab.* 2000; 13(suppl 6):1503-1508.

29. Akcam T, Bolu E, Merati AL, et al. Voice changes after androgen therapy for hypogonadotrophic hypogonadism. *Laryngoscope.* 2004;114:1587-1591.

30. Furst-Recktenwald S, Dorr HG, Rosanowski F. Androglottia in a young female adolescent with congenital adrenal hyperplasia and 21-hydroxylase deficiency. *J Pedi Endocrinol.* 2000;13:959-962.

New Technologies: High-Speed Video, Videokymography, Optical Coherence Tomography, and 3D Holography

Ramon A. Franco, Jr.
Jennifer G. Andrus
Robert T. Sataloff

Because it is often impossible to obtain long, sustained utterances for stroboscopic evaluation in children, high-speed imaging may be of even greater importance for laryngologists treating this population than it is for those caring for adults. High-speed imaging allows the acquisition of a great deal of information from very short phonatory gestures. Even a cry of 2 seconds' duration may be sufficient to allow sophisticated evaluation of the vibratory margin using high-speed video or videokymography. These modalities and their potential clinical implications have been summarized in other literature,[1] and are reviewed here. Other evolving technologies include optical coherence tomography, a noninvasive technique that images the layered structures of the larynx, and holography, which allows a three-dimensional evaluation of the vocal folds. These modalities are also presented, as are comments on future directions of technology that will continue to influence the development of pediatric laryngology.

HIGH-SPEED VIDEO

The many investigators who used high-speed motion picture technology after it was introduced in 1960 by von Leden et al[2] showed that high-speed imaging provided extremely useful, detailed information about vocal fold function even under difficult circumstances such as aperiodic voices, dichotic phonation, and vocal fry. Actual motion pictures were recorded on film, processed at a separate session, and evaluated at still another sitting for patterns of vocal fold motion. It was an extraordinarily cumbersome process, but important to the current body of knowledge on vocal fold vibration. The next generation of high-speed technology allowed for recording information on videotape, which reduced processing time, but still required significant time for examination review. In order to try to reacquire this information in a more practical fashion, high-speed digital imaging was introduced in 1987.[3] Recently, equipment has been improved: high-speed digital video is now available commercially and is practical (although expensive) as an option with the Kay/Pentax Stroboscopy System (Fig 4–1, Video 4–1). Unlike strobo-

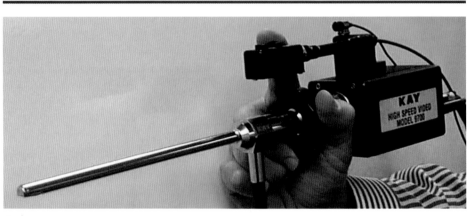

A

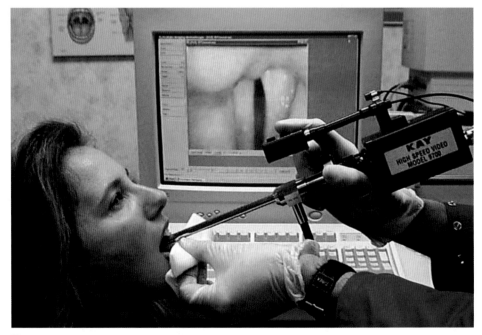

B

Fig 4–1. High-speed digital video. **A.** High-speed digital video camera. **B.** Sample high-speed digital video procedure. *(continues)*

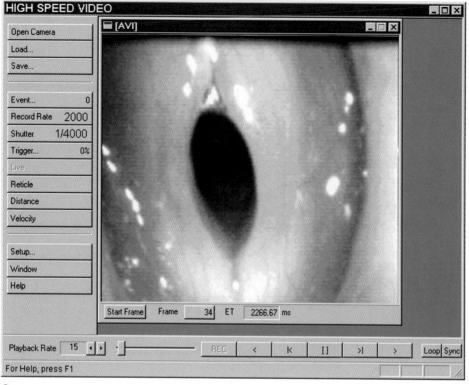

Fig 4–1. *(continued)* **C.** Sample monitor display of high-speed digital video on Kay/Pentax system. (Images courtesy of Kay/Pentax.)

videolaryngoscopy, images are in black and white, and no sound is linked with the images. At the camera's slower recording rate of about 2,000 frames per second, image resolution is reasonably good. At its upper limit of about 4,000 frames per second, additional information may be acquired, but the images become somewhat blurry. The amount of time during which images are captured is adjustable, but 2 seconds are usually sufficient. Images are played back at approximately 15 frames per second. Thus, a 2-second acquisition at 2,000 frames per second requires approximately 4.44 minutes to review. This limits the convenience of high-speed digital video for routine clin-

ical use, but it is manageable for special clinical problems such as evaluation of young children, and for research. In addition, a specific area can be identified on the initial video frame from the high-speed images and analyzed by computer software to generate a digital videokymogram (see section below on Videokymography).

Hess, Hertegard, Eysholdt, and other authors have reported on the usefulness of high-speed video.[4-6] Woo showed that digital high-speed video is useful in a variety of situations. He uses this method to study normal onset and offset of vocal fold oscillation; to analyze diplophonia; to study vocal fold tension, stiffness, mass, and other parameters in greater detail; and for other purposes.[7] High-speed video likely will play an increasing role in clinical practice, especially in pediatric laryngology, as more information is acquired and as equipment becomes less costly.

VIDEOKYMOGRAPHY

Videokymography (VKG) is a relatively new technology, introduced in 1984 by Gall.[8] It was not until 1996, however, that VKG was developed by Svec and Schutte into a system practical for clinical purposes.[9,10] A kymograph is an instrument that measures changes in pressure. VKG displays vibrations of the vocal folds and surrounding tissues in one image. Svec and Schutte's system is incorporated with the Kay equipment: a video camera with a continuous light source is used to register an image of the whole paired vocal folds, and allows identification of a single line of interest across the vocal folds for kymography. The line for VKG evaluation is always at the top of the whole vocal folds image. The camera records either the normal whole image, or the VKG image; and a foot switch controls the change from normal to high-speed VKG mode. The VKG images are therefore obtained sequential to the image of the entire vocal fold (Fig 4–2, Video 4–2). This requires that the examiner maintain the camera position relative to the vocal folds during both modes so that accurate correlations of the scanned line to the vocal fold can be made. This is one disadvantage of VKG: it scans only a single line on the vocal fold, rather than the entire vocal fold. So, the images illustrate only one point on the vocal fold, although they do so in considerable detail. Two-dimensional spatial resolution is lost, however, and like high-speed video, images are black and white and there is no coordination between the visual image and an auditory signal such as is obtained during strobovideolaryngoscopy.

Videokymography acquires nearly 8,000 frames per second. The images seen by the examiner are influenced by the fact that each video frame contains 512 lines, and video acquires 30 frames per second. VKG images are displayed on the monitor, with time dimension in the vertical axis. Time scrolls vertically at 144 line images per half frame. A monitor frame covers a time interval of 18.4 milliseconds. In the VKG system currently available as an option with the Kay/Pentax stroboscope, the camera can record vibrations of a single point along both vocal folds at a speed of 7,812.5 images per second, as compared with the 30 images per second recorded on standard videotape (a product of the 60 half-images acquired and fused per second). As mentioned above, videokymograms can also be generated from high-speed digital video. This is sometimes distinguished from VKG as digital kymography (DK). In DK, an area of interest on high-speed video can be identified and analyzed by computer software to generate a kymogram. DK essentially allows digital VKG to be obtained without losing spatial resolution or watching the entire video display. The information obtained is less detailed than that acquired from true VKG because of the difference in frames per second of acquisition (2,000 in DK via high-speed video, versus nearly 8,000 in VKG).

The clinical value of VKG was reported in 1998,[11] and its use has been increasing slowly. The author (R.T.S.) has found VKG to be a useful addition to strobovideolaryngoscopy in selected adult cases, as well as in children. It permits detailed evaluation

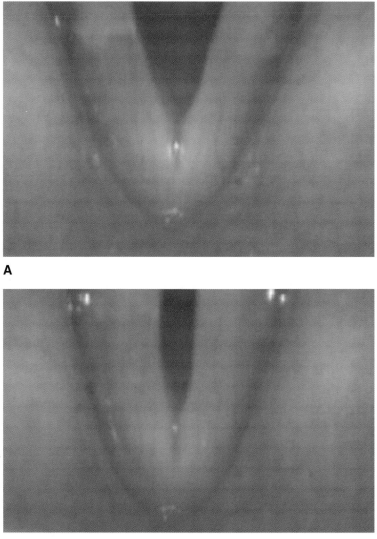

Fig 4–2. Videokymopgraphy is obtained using a high-speed digital video camera. Images of the whole vocal folds are obtained first (*A* and *B*) and a line of interest chosen for VKG scanning (*C* and *D*), in this case at the posterior glottis. **A.** Video still image—vocal folds open. **B.** Video still image—vocal folds closing. *(continues)*

of vibratory abnormalities that cannot be analyzed by strobovideolaryngoscopy, and allows assessment of patients with aperi-odic voice, which will not trip the strobe light to permit strobovideolaryngoscopy (Fig 4-3). VKG is useful in assessing the

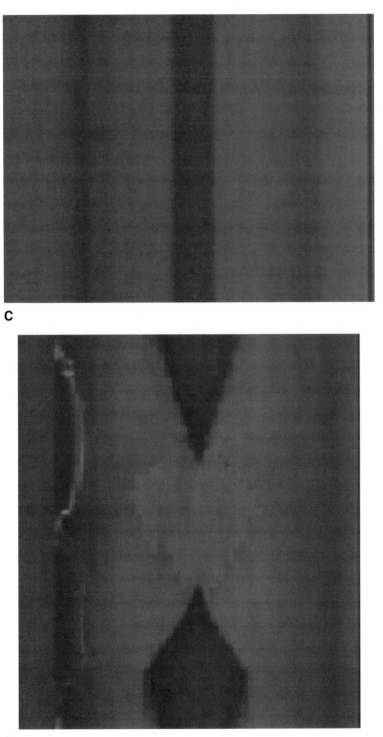

C

D

Fig 4–2. *(continued)* **C.** VKG—minimal vibration. **D.** VKG—vibration: opening/closing.

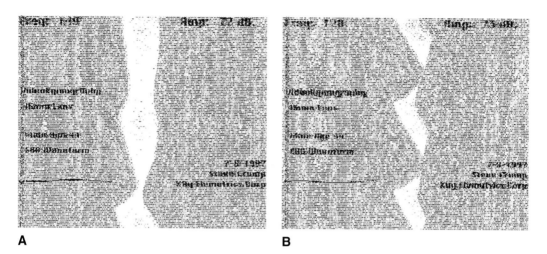

Fig 4–3. Videokymography. **A.** Vocal onset: note that the vocal folds are not vibrating at the top of the image, but that as time advances (moving down the image), the vocal folds begin to vibrate. **B.** Sustained phonation: note that each vocal fold is vibrating, but that they are not symmetric. This demonstrates phase-asymmetry and indicates a difference in vibratory function between the two sides, which can be accounted for by a mass lesion (benign or malignant), scar, unilateral paresis, or other pathology. More information from stroboscopy is required. (Images courtesy of Kay/Pentax.)

effects of scar and outcomes of surgical treatment of scar, the presence of subharmonic vibrations, double or triple vocal fold openings in a single glottal cycle, irregular vocal fold vibrations, and other abnormalities. Although each VKG image is limited to a single line along the vocal fold, VKG images can be acquired at multiple positions, thus providing a meaningful sample of vibratory detail throughout the length of the vocal fold. VKG lacks spatial resolution; however, when combined with strobovideolaryngoscopy, VKG obtains useful additional information. In some cases, even better information can be obtained with high-speed video; but videokymography equipment is substantially less expensive than high-speed video equipment.

Similar to strobovideolaryngoscopy, VKG interpretation requires an in-depth knowledge of the vocal fold vibratory cycle and comfort distinguishing between normal and pathologic findings (Fig 4–4). The advantage to VKG, however, is that differences between the right and left vocal folds at the specific point evaluated often appear more obvious than on strobovideolaryngoscopy, so that subtle asymmetries are more readily apparent. Recently, Svec, et al[12] reported the findings in 100 VKG images, extracted from 7000, from 45 patients with a wide range of voice disorders examined in sustained phonation. Laryngeal diagnoses included normal vocal folds, several benign masses/lesions including scar, vocal fold immobility, diffuse tumor, and a number of functional disorders. The vibratory patterns observed were divided into 10 feature categories, including traditional features evaluated on strobovideolaryngoscopy (ie, mucosal

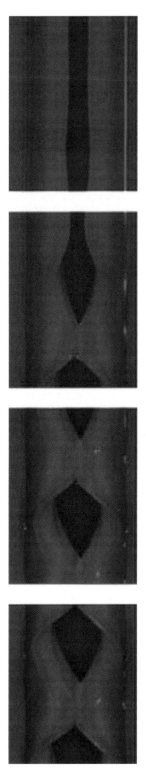

Fig 4–4. VKG series of normal vocal folds.

wave, and left-right asymmetry), and a number of features "obscured" or less well seen in strobovideolaryngoscopy (ie, cycle variability, absence of vocal fold vibration, lateral and medial peak shape, and others). Within each feature category, one or more specific vibration characteristic was identified. Stunning differences are easily seen in the VKG images presented, many of them measurable on the time and/or amplitude axis. Examples of these differences include total absence of vibration in one vocal fold versus the other due to presence of tumor; unequal amplitude of vocal fold vibration and phase asymmetry in vocal fold paralysis; and differences in opening and closing phases. The authors conclude that the variations in these features reflect different behavioral origins of different voice disorders. This work is the beginning of a classification system that will aid in the objective evaluation of voice disorders.

Recently, Larsson et al explored a combined high-speed, acoustic kymographic analysis package, concluding that combining such information appears promising for separating and specifying different voice qualities such as diplophonia and vocal tremor.[13] They believe that this will have both clinical and research value and speculate that combining such information should be helpful for improving the terminology used for different voice qualities.

The current body of knowledge on laryngeal VKG highlights the need for examiners to train in the interpretation of VKG to best judge the vibratory patterns this technology reveals, and to integrate this information with that yielded by strobovideolaryngoscopy. Together, the information derived from both modalities will help clinicians correlate voice quality with specific structural and vibratory characteristics of the vocal folds, aiding in medical and surgical treatment recommendations, as well as in tracking patient progress.

OPTICAL COHERENCE TOMOGRAPHY

Optical coherence tomography (OCT) is a new technology that is rapidly evolving. Developed in the late 1980s, and first reported in 1991,[14] it is considered the optic analogue to ultrasound, using light instead of sound to delineate specific tissue attributes in cross-sectional images. A noninvasive, noncontact modality, OCT involves shining infrared light on tissue and using interferometric methods to detect the light reflected back from the tissue and create an image. Specifically, a plate beam splitter is used to divide the light from the optical source into two beams, one directed to the tissue and the other to a reference mirror; the light reflected from both the tissue and the mirror is recombined and detected. If the lengths of the reference and sample pathways are within the coherence length of the light source, an interference pattern is formed. The reference beam can be adjusted in length, allowing detection of tissue properties at varying tissue depths, and thus used to create a depth profile (A-line). Multiple A-lines are acquired by scanning across the tissue sample and can be combined to form a 2-dimensional representation of the tissue (B-line), which is analogous to a vertical histologic section. OCT is limited by tissue turbidity, but detects light reflected up to 2-mm tissue depth, and has a tissue resolution of 10 μm,[15] and sometimes 9 μm.[16] The images created depict on a gray scale the different light reflection properties of issue, with white representing high tissue light absorption (or weak reflectivity), and black representing low light absorption (high reflectivity).

OCT has been applied clinically in areas where knowledge of tissue microstructure is important. It is most established in ophthalmology, being used to evaluate the eye for changes associated with macular holes,[17] glaucoma,[18] diabetic retinopathy,[19] in screening for corneal implants,[20] and for other ocular disorders.[21,22] OCT also has been used in dermatology, gastroenterology, urology, and gynecology, in all disciplines able to identify various layers within normal structures, and to distinguish normal, inflammatory, dysplastic, and malignant processes.[23-30] OCT has been used recently to study cardiovascular disease.[31,32] Applications of OCT in otolaryngology are still in their infancy, but growing rapidly. In 2000, Wong et al reported their initial studies imaging the rat cochlea.[33] Pitris et al and Bibas et al followed this with OCT imaging of cadaveric human temporal bones,[34,35] and OCT-assisted middle ear surgery has been performed since on a group of 10 patients.[36] Due to its layered microarchitecture, established by Hirano in the 1970s,[37,38] and considered a cornerstone in both the current understanding of voice production and the development of phonomicrosurgical techniques,[39-42] the larynx has drawn particular interest as a region for study using OCT.

The first clinical use of OCT in the larynx was reported in 1997,[43] describing OCT results in 15 patients with laryngeal lesions and establishing the potential value for OCT in the larynx. Subsequent studies have evaluated normal laryngeal structures, as well as laryngeal lesions and surrounding tissue, in ex vivo animal and human larynges,[15,44,45] as well as in human subjects.[16,46,47] The overwhelming consistent finding in these studies is that OCT is unique in its ability to image vocal fold microstructure, and that the layers demarcated correlate to those seen on corresponding histopathology sections. Specifically, the epithelium, basement membrane, and lamina propria can be seen well on OCT in normal larynges; and changes in these structures by vocal fold lesions can also be detected (ie, expansion of the epithelium in hyperkeratosis; disruption of the basement membrane by carcinoma; presence of a cyst in the lamina propria).[15,16,35,43,44,46,47] The most significant clinical implication of these findings to date is that, because images are obtained in real time, OCT can be used in vivo to guide biopsies of suspicious lesions, and resection of malignancies as margins between normal and abnormal tissue can be seen.[16,43,46] This is of paramount importance to management of true vocal fold lesions, as even small postsurgical defects can have enormous deleterious effects on the voice.

Although all published research on OCT to date involves adult subjects, the implications for pediatric laryngology are far reaching. First, OCT will have similar applications in the setting of phonomicrosurgical resection of lesions in the pediatric population. Although laryngeal malignancy is quite rare in children, and children with benign lesions such as polyps, nodules, and cysts are commonly managed medically with voice therapy, in cases where surgery is chosen, for example, in older adolescents who are serious singers and unable to advance due to vocal fold nodules, OCT may complement current surgical techniques to best preserve vocal fold structure and function. The management of recurrent respiratory papillomatosis (RRP), a virally mediated, benign but recalcitrant disease resulting in neoplasms limited to the epithelium, could be enhanced by OCT, whereby intraopertive OCT imaging could guide the surgeon's extent of resection and prevent violation of the lamina propria by ensuring preservation of the basement membrane. Second, OCT has tremendous potential to improve our current understanding of pediatric laryngeal development. Hirano established that the five-layered structure of the adult

vocal fold (epithelium, superficial lamina propria, middle lamina propria, deep lamina propria, and muscle), is absent in the newborn, consisting at birth of only the epithelium, a single layer of lamina propria, and muscle.[48] Hartnick[49] found in cadeveric pediatric larynges that a bilaminar lamina propria develops by age 2 months, and that the trilaminar structure is established by age seven. However, the time of transition from the two- to three-layerd lamina propria varied greatly (beginning anywhere from 11 months to 5 years); and the adult distribution of collagen and elastin throughout the three layers is not achieved until around age 13.[50] OCT in its current state does not distinguish the three layers of the lamina propria, although polarization-sensitive OCT (PS-OCT), which is more sensitive to oriented collagen fiber bundles,[47] may hold some promise in distinguishing these layers. Under rapid development, OCT has several new permutations, including optical frequency domain imaging (OFDI),[51,52] full-field optical coherence microscopy (FF-OCM),[53-55] and endoscopic reflectance confocal microscopy such as spectrally encoded confocal microscopy (SECM)[56,57] (Figs 4-5, 4-6, 4-7, and 4-8). These techniques offer different imaging capability in terms of depth of penetration, field of view, image resolution, and acquisition speed. A pilot study is underway to identifying the strengths and weaknesses of these technologies with regard to the in vivo evaluation of pediatric vocal folds. The results from initial trials in ex vivo porcine larynges[45] demonstrate that:

■ OFDI is a very fast imaging method and has a large penetration depth, potentially allowing visualization of all layers of the lamina propria, especially in its angle-resolved implementation. However, OFDI

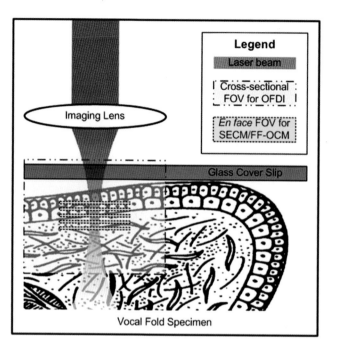

Fig 4–5. Schematic of advanced optical coherence tomography imaging methods showing their field of view (FOV) orientations and approximate relative size with respect to a vocal fold specimen. (Adapted from Boudoux et al, Preliminary Evaluation of Non-invasive Microscopic Imaging Techniques for the Study of Pediatric Vocal Fold Development. *J Voice*, in press.[45])

lacks the resolution at the cellular level. Implementation of OFDI through small, flexible catheters has been shown.

- FF-OCM provides comprehensive volumetric imaging with exquisite detail, but at a lesser penetration than OFDI, and more importantly, at imaging rates orders of magnitudes slower than OFDI, preventing for now its use in vivo
- SECM provides cellular imaging at a resolution approaching that of FF-OCM, at depth penetrations that allow visualization of the epithelium, basement membrane, and the upper layers of the lamina propria. SECM imaging rates are compatible with clinical motions and its implementation into a compact probe has been proven.

As this trial comes to completion, the ideal OCT technology for use in pediatric patients will be implemented via an in vivo probe with the goal of delineating the layers of the lamina propria in children of different ages and seeing how they change in individuals over time.

Finally, then, as the understanding of the three-layered lamina propria's development continues to advance, OCT may be

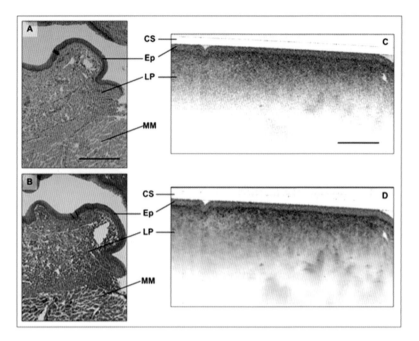

Fig 4–6. Histology (*A* and *B*) and OFDI cross-sections (*C* and *D*) of a porcine vocal fold sample. H&E (*A*) and trichrome (*B*) stains show transitions from an epithelium (*Ep*), a lamina propria (*LP*) and a muscularis mucosa (*MM*). OFDI imaging (*C*) and angle-resolved OFDI (*D*) image the epithelial layers and the lamina propria noninvasively through a cover slip (*CS*). Reduction of image granularity (*C*) through angle compounding (*D*) allows imaging of deeper structures. Scale bars for all images are 1 mm. Histology magnification 40×. (Adapted from Boudoux et al, Preliminary Evaluation of Non-invasive Microscopic Imaging Techniques for the Study of Pediatric Vocal Fold Development. *J Voice*, in press.[45])

used in the future to track this development in individual patients, and thus potentially guide clinical decision making (ie, success of voice therapy, recommendations for surgical intervention, and timing of surgery).

FUTURE DIRECTIONS

Although strobovideolaryngoscopy remains the cornerstone of voice evaluation in both the pediatric and adult populations, it is limited by its inability to capture aperiodic vocal fold vibrations, and by the subjective nature of clinicians' interpretation of it. The continued development of technologies able to overcome these limitations is critical to obtaining a full understanding of both normal and altered voice, as is the commitment to finding the best ways to evaluate pediatric voice disorders given the variations of laryngeal and global development in children over time.

Currently, videolaryngostroboscopy can be performed using either a rigid or flexible

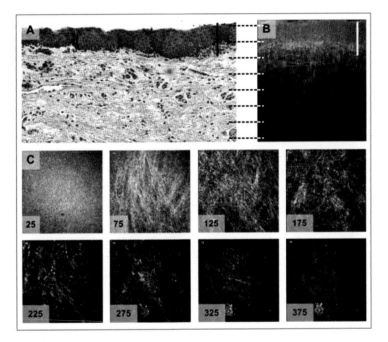

Fig 4–7. H&E histology (*A*), FF-OCM cross-section (*B*), and en face images (*C*) of porcine vocal fold. Cross-sectional reconstruction of FF-OCM images (*B*) of a porcine vocal fold sample allows for better correlation of en face images (*C*) with histology. Epithelial cells are observed up to 75 microns, after which details of a densely woven, signal-rich basement membrane can be observed. Contrast of deeper *en face* images (*C*) was individually adjusted to compensate for signal attenuation, allowing imaging of structures up to 375 microns. Imaging depths are indicated in microns and corresponding locations on cross-sectional images are indicated by the dashed lines. Scale bar for (*A*), (*B*), and (*C*) is 100 microns. Histology magnification 100×. (Adapted from Boudoux et al, Preliminary Evaluation of Non-invasive Microscopic Imaging Techniques for the Study of Pediatric Vocal Fold Development. *J Voice*, in press.[45])

endoscope. The latest generation of flexible endoscopes uses distal chip technology, offering significantly better resolution than the traditional fiberoptic endoscopes. Although distal-chip flexible scopes are a significant advance, they do not offer the illumination or magnification that rigid telescopes do. However, in time, we anticipate that smaller, higher resolution distal chips will be developed, such that excellent stroboscopic images will be attainable with flexible scopes, allowing patients to be assessed in the better physiologic phonatory position (as opposed to mouth open and tongue protruded as is necessary for rigid endoscopy).

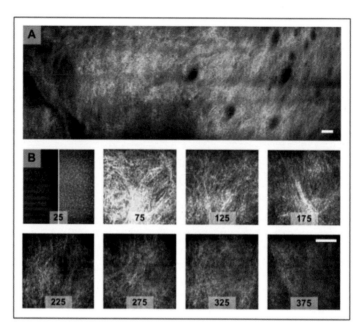

Fig 4–8. SECM mosaic reconstruction (*A*) and individual en face frames (*B*) of a porcine sample. Cellular membranes, cell nuclei and basement membrane fibers are visualized on the postprocessing mosaic reconstruction of adjacent images. Cellular and subcellular details can be appreciated in the series of en face scans taken at different depths (*B*) up to 375 microns. The two frames imaged at 25 microns show the appearance of epithelial nuclei after application of acetic acid (*right panel*). Depth is indicated in microns. Scale bars are 100 microns. Histology magnification 100×. (Adapted from Boudoux et al, Preliminary Evaluation of Non-invasive Microscopic Imaging Techniques for the Study of Pediatric Vocal Fold Development. *J Voice*, in press.[45])

Although high-speed video has evolved significantly over the years, evaluation of the data it generates, even digital, is cumbersome. We anticipate that in the future, after sufficient archiving of vocal fold images spanning the range of normal and abnormal, computer programs will be developed to link in real time to high-speed video cameras and to recognize patterns of vocal fold movement as well as calculate, based on the examination, certain vibratory characteristics such as opening and closing times, open and closed quotients, and so forth. Essentially, this would take away the separate step of having to analyze the data subsequent to the examination.

In 2006, Qiu and Schutte[58] introduced a new generation VKG system in which the normal and high-speed VKG mode operate simultaneously, with both images presented next to each other on the monitor screen. The scanned line along the vocal fold is determined by an optical beam splitter such that the VKG image is set to the center of the laryngoscopic image. This allows simultaneous recording of both images, so that if the laryngoscope position changes during the examination, the VKG image position changes with it. Additional advantages of the new system include that, unlike the original system, the kymogram produced is uninterrupted; the device is more sensitive and so requires less light and produces higher quality images; data do not require postprocessing for interpretation; and the system can synchronize the VKG images with audio signals. Although this system is not yet commercially available, it is playing an important role in voice research, and will likely be adapted for commercial use over time.

The applications of VKG, particularly in research, are also likely to expand over time. To date, most of the information gleaned from VKG has been during sustained phonation. Recall, however, that one of its biggest advantages is that it can record aperiodic vocal fold motion, which include vocal folds at vocal onset and offset, during cough, during inspiratory phonation, whisper, rest, and so forth. Undoubtedly more information on vocal fold function will be obtained as VKG is used to evaluate these conditions, as well as their equivalents in the pediatric larynx.

The reflectance-based optical microscopy techniques described here allow visualization of cellular detail and architecture in the porcine vocal fold. Further analysis of the pediatric vocal fold is required, however, as there seems to be a significant difference between porcine and human lamina propria in terms of its layered architecture (porcine lamina propria is not layered). The technical difficulties rendered by in vivo microscopy include the need for a small probe to fit through a suspension microlaryngoscopy, as children will often be unable to tolerate close inspection of their vocal folds while awake. An in vivo microscopy probe will therefore facilitate evaluation of the vocal folds in pediatric patients while under general anesthesia in the operating room, and this development is underway.[45] A second hurdle to overcome is the need for sufficient visual clarity to differentiate the hypocellular superficial lamina propria layer from more cellular layers, and to differentiate between the fine elastin fibers seen in the middle lamina propria from the thicker collagen fibers found within the deep lamina propria. Further imaging of human samples with these technologies should provide these answers, which are being sought prior to moving on to imaging of pediatric vocal folds in vivo.

3-D Holography

Holography has been used in the aerospace industry as well as by the military to detect minute deformations along the "smooth" curved surfaces of missiles, aircraft wings, and fuselages that may occur when they are subject to high airspeeds. Where, and to what extent such deformations occur—whether concavities or convexities—impact an object's aerodynamics, and therefore, efficiency. The same approach to these issues can be used to characterize vocal fold shape and surface deformations: fringe projection and holographic interferometric methodologies allow for acquisition of full-frame, real-time, three-dimensional images of the larynx that have direct applicability to clinical questions.[59] Unlike stroboscopy, the results from this type of evaluation lead to objective data that are quantifiable. As the technology evolves, mucosal wave values will be expressed in terms of micrometers of amplitude, thereby finally allowing the creation of normative data for mucosal wave.

The basic principle guiding this technology is that parallel lines will deform in predictable ways when projected onto a curved surface (Figs 4–9A and 4–9B). Through computer calculations, each frame recorded from a CCD camera can be processed to reveal the changes in the 'parallel' lines, telling the computer how the system is changing in time. Using the fringe projection technique micrometer resolution is possible, whereas with the use of holographic interferometry nanometer resolution is possible.

Regardless of technique used, the computer can color-code the vocal fold surface deformations so lower amplitude movements appear blue and larger than normal deformations are red. Once clinically applied,

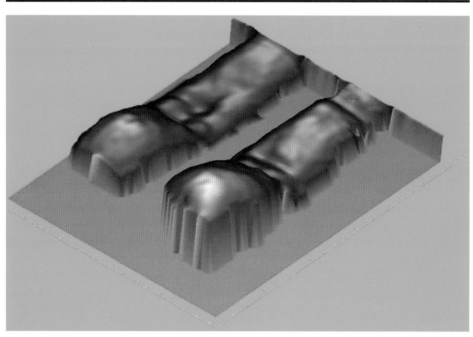

A

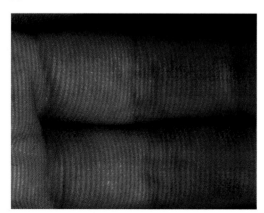

B

Fig 4–9. Representative shape measurements by fringe projection. **A.** Fringes projected onto a sample of interest; **B.** corresponding 3-D representation of the measured shape.

this would allow for rapid interpretation of hypo- and hyperdynamic vocal fold segments that may warn the surgeon of problem areas not well visualized with stroboscopy. The vocal folds could be represented in wire-frame and subtle surface changes could be identified. The three-dimensional information could be integrated with the now standard two-dimensional stroboscopic evaluation to add even more diagnostic information.

There are several technical challenges that need to be overcome to bring fringe projection and holographic interferometry from the bench to the clinical setting. At present, factors such as the proper wave-length of light, optimal illumination, and observation angles, and the use of surface preparations to increase the contrast are actively being investigated. The entire setup is being miniaturized to resemble a rigid endoscope, a tool familiar to most laryngol-ogists and speech pathologists.[59] A system that will work within a flexible endoscope is also envisioned.

VIDEOS IN THIS CHAPTER

Video 4–1. Endoscopic video images of vocal folds using Kay/Pentax system that demonstrates quiet breathing, and phonation. Note differences in detail of vibration seen on stroboscopy versus high-speed video. **A.** Strobovideolaryngoscopy normal voice. **B.** High-speed digital video normal voice: quiet breathing, vocal onset, sustained phonation, and vocal offset. **C.** High-speed digital video hoarse voice: quiet breathing, vocal onset, sustained phonation, vocal offset. (Video courtesy of Kay/Pentax.)

Video 4–2. Videokymography using Kay/Pentax system. Note that the image changes from high-speed video of the whole vocal folds to a VKG scanned line. Each change is made by the examiner with a foot pedal. The line scanned in VKG is at the top of the high-speed video image (in this case, at the posterior glottis). (Video courtesy of Kay/Pentax.)

REFERENCES

1. Sataloff RT. *Professional Voice: The Science and Art of Clinical Care*. 3rd ed. San Diego, Calif: Plural Publishing, Inc; 2005:374–375.
2. von Leden H, Moore P, Timcke R. Laryngeal vibrations: measurements of the glottic wave: part 3. *Arch Otolaryngol*. 1960;71: 16–35.
3. Honda R, Imagawa H, Hirose KS. Baer T, Sasaki C, Harris KS, eds. *Laryngeal Function in Phonation and Respiration*. San Diego, Calif: College-Hill Press; 1987:485–491.
4. Hess MM, Gross M. High-speed, light-inten-sified digital imaging of vocal fold vibrations in high optical resolution via indirect micro-layrngoscopy. *Ann Otol Rhinol Laryngol*. 1993;102:502–507.
5. Hertegard S, Lindestad PA. *Vocal Fold Vibra-tions Studied During Phonation with High-Speed Video Imaging*. Stockholm, Sweden: Karolinska Institute; 1994;9:33–40.
6. Eysholdt U, Tigges M, Wittenberg T, Proschel U. Direct evaluation of high-speed recordings of vocal fold vibrations. *Folia Phoniatr Logop*. 1996;48:163–170.
7. Colton RH, Woo P. Measuring vocal fold function. In: Rubin JS, Sataloff RT, Korovin GS, eds. *Diagnosis and Treatment of Voice Disorders*. 2nd ed. Clifton Park, NY: Delmar-Thomson Learning; 2003.
8. Gall V. Strip kymography of the glottis. *Arch Otorhinolaryngol*. 1984;240:287–293.

9. Svec JG, Schutte HK. Videokymography: High-speed line scanning of vocal fold vibration. *J Voice*. 1996;10:201-205.

10. Schutte HK, Svec JG, Stram F. Videokymography: research and clinical application of videokymography. *Log Phoniatr Vocol*. 1998;22:152-156.

11. Schutte HK, Svec JG, Stram F. First results of clinical application videokymography. *Laryngoscope*. 1998;108:1206-1210.

12. Svec JG, Stram F, Schutte HK. Videokymography in voice disorders: what to look for? *Ann Otol Rhinol Laryngol*. 2007;116:172-180.

13. Larsson H, Hertegard S, Lindestad PA, Hammarberg B. Vocal fold vibrations: high-speed imaging, kymography, and acoustic analysis: a preliminary report. *Laryngoscope*. 2000;110:2117-2122.

14. Huang D, Swanson EA, Lin CP, et al. Optical coherence tomography. *Science*. 1991;254:1178-1181.

15. Bibas AG, Podoleanu AG, Cucu RG, et al. 3-D optical coherence tomography of the laryngeal mucosa. *Clin Otolaryngol Allied Sci*. 2004;29:713-720.

16. Wong BJ, Jackson RP, Guo S, et al. In vivo optical coherence tomography of the human larynx: normative and benign pathology in 82 patients. *Laryngoscope*. 2005;115:1904-1911.

17. Hee MR, Puliafito CA, Wong C, et al. Optical coherence tomography of macular holes. *Opthalmology*. 1995;102:748-756.

18. Schuman JS, Hee MR, Arya AV, et al. Optical coherence tomography: a new tool for glaucoma diagnosis. *Curr Opin Ophthalmol*. 1995;6:89-95.

19. Goebel W, Kretzchmar-Gross T. Retinal thickening in diabetic retinopathy: a study using optical coherence tomography (OCT). *Retina*. 2002;22:759-767.

20. Neubauer AS, Priglinger SG, Thiel MJ, May CA, Welge-Lussen UC. Sterile structural imaging of donor cornea by optical coherence tomography. *Cornea*. 2002;21:490-494.

21. Hee MR, Puliafito CA, Wong C, et al. Optical coherence tomography of central serous chorioretinopathy. *Am J Ophthalmol*. 1995;120:65-74.

22. Uchino E, Uemura A, Ohba N. Initial stages of posterior vitreal detachment in healthy eyes of older persons evaluated by optical coherence tomography. *Arch Opthalmol*. 2001;119:1475-1479.

23. Gladkova ND, Petrova GA, Nikulin NK, et al. In vivo optical coherence tomography imaging of human skin: norm and pathology. *Skin Res Technol*. 2000;6:6-16.

24. Podoleanu AG, Rogers JA, Jackson DA, et al. Three dimensional OCT images from retina and skin. *Opt Expr*. 2000;7:292-298. Available from http://www.opticsexpress.org/abstract.cfm ?URI=OPEX-7-9-292

25. Welzel J. Optical coherence tomography in dermatology: a review. *Skin Res Technol*. 2001;7:1-9.

26. Bouma BE, Tearney GJ, Compton CC, Nishioka NS. High-resolution imaging of the human esophagus and stomach in vivo using optical coherence tomography. *Gastrointest Endosc*. 2000;51:467-474.

27. Zuccaro G, Gladkova N, Vargo J, et al. Optical coherence tomography of the esophagus and proximal stomach in health and disease. *Am J Gastroenterol*. 2001;96:2633-2639.

28. Tearney GJ, Brezinski ME, Southern JF, Bouma BE, Boppart SA, Fujimoto JG. Optical biopsy in human urologic tissue using optical coherence tomography. *J Urol*. 1997;157:1915-1919.

29. Zagaynova EV, Streltsova OS, Gladkova ND, et al. In vivo optical coherence tomography feasibility for bladder disease. *J Urol*. 2002;167:1492-1496.

30. Pitris C, Goodman A, Boppart SA, Libus JJ, Fujimoto JG, Brezinski ME. High-resolution imaging of gynecologic neoplasms using optical coherence tomography. *Obstet Gynecol*. 1999;93:135-139.

31. Patwari P, Weissman NJ, Boppart SA, et al. Assessment of coronary plaque with optical coherence tomography and high-frequency ultrasound. *Am J Cardiol*. 2000;85:641-644.

32. Kume T, Akasaka T, Kawamoto T, et al. Assessment of coronary arterial plaque by

optical coherence tomography. *Am J Cardiol.* 2006;97:1172-1175.

33. Wong BJ, de Boer JF, Park BH, Chen Z, Nelson JS. Optical coherence tomography of the rat cochlea. *J Biomed Opt.* 2000;5:367-370.

34. Pitris C, Saunders KT, Fujimoto JG, Brezinski ME. High-resolution imaging of the middle ear with optical coherence tomography: a feasibility study. *Arch Otolaryngol Head Neck Surg.* 2001;127:637-642.

35. Bibas A, Podolenau AGH, Cucu R, et al. Optical coherence tomography in otolaryngology: original results and review of the literature. *Proc SPIE.* 2003;5312:190-195.

36. Heermann R, Hauger C, Issing PR, Lenarz T. Application of optical coherence tomography (OCT) in middle ear surgery. *Laryngorhinootologie.* 2002;81:400-405.

37. Hirano M. Phonosurgery: basic and clinical investigations. *Otologia (Fukuoka).* 1975;21:239-442.

38. Hirano M. *Structure and Vibratory Behavior of the Vocal Folds.* Tokyo, Japan: University of Tokyo Press; 1977.

39. Sataloff RT, Spiegel JR, Heuer RJ, et al. Laryngeal mini-microflap: a new technique and reassessment of the microflap saga. *J Voice.* 1995;9:198-204.

40. Courey MS, Gardner GM, Stone RE, Ossoff RH. Endoscopic vocal fold microflap: a three-year experience. *Ann Otol Rhinol Laryngol.* 1995;104:267-273.

41. Courey MS, Garrett CG, Ossoff RH. Medial microflap for excision of benign vocal fold lesions. *Laryngoscope.* 1997;107:340-344.

42. Zeitels SM. Phonomicrosurgery I: principles and equipment. *Otolaryngol Clin North Am.* 2000;33:1047-1062.

43. Sergeev A, Gelikonov VG, Feldchtein F, et al. In vivo endoscopic OCT imaging of precancer and cancer states of human mucosa. *Opt Expr.* 1997;1:432-440.

44. Burns JA, Zeitels SM, Anderson RR, Kobler JB, Pierce MC, de Boer JF. Imaging the mucosa of the human vocal fold with optical coherence tomography. *Ann Otol Rhinol Laryngol.* 2005;114:671-676.

45. Boudoux C, Leuin SC, Oh WY, et al. Preliminary evaluation of non-invasive microscopic imaging techniques for the study of pediatric vocal fold development. *J Voice.* In press.

46. Shakhov AV, Terentjeva AB, Kamensky VA, et al. Optical coherence tomography monitoring for laser surgery of laryngeal carcinoma. *J Surg Oncol.* 2001;77:253-258.

47. Klein AM, Pierce MC, Zeitels SM, et al. Imaging the human vocal folds in vivo with optical coherence tomography: a preliminary experience. *Ann Otol Rhinol Laryngol.* 2006;115:277-284.

48. Sato K, Hirano M. Histologic investigation of the macula flava of the human newborn vocal fold. *Ann Otol Rhinol Laryngol.* 1995;104:556-562.

49. Boseley ME, Hartnick CJ. Development of the human true vocal fold: depth of cell layers and quantifying cell types within the lamina propria. *Ann Otol Rhinol Laryngol.* 2006;115:784-788.

50. Hartnick CJ, Rehbar R, Prasad V. Development and maturation of the pediatric human vocal fold lamina propria. *Laryngoscope.* 2005;115:4-15.

51. Yun SH, Tearney GJ, deBoer JF, Iftimia N, Bouma BE. High-speed optical frequency-domain imaging. *Opt Expr.* 2003;11:2953-2963.

52. Choma MA, Sarunic MV, Yang CH, Izatt JA. Sensitivity advantage of swept source and fourier domain optical coherence tomography. *Opt Expr.* 2003;11:2183-2189.

53. Beaurepaire E, Boccara AC, Lebec M, Blanchot L, Saint-Jalmes H. Full-field optical coherence tomography. *Opt Lett.* 1998:23244-23246.

54. Dubois A, Vabre L, Boccara AC, Beaurepaire E. High-resolution full-field optical coherence tomography with a linnik microscope. *Appl Opt.* 2002;41:805-812.

55. Oh WY, Bouma BE, Iftimia N, Yelin R, Tearney GJ. Spectrally-modulated full-field optical coherence microscopy for ultrahigh-resolution endoscopic imaging. *Opt Expr.* 2006;14:8675-8684.

56. Tearney GJ, Webb RH, Bouma BE. Spectrally encoded confocal microscopy. *Opt Lett.* 1998;23:1152-1154.

57. Boudoux C, Yun SH, Oh WY, et al. Rapid wavelength-swept spectrally encoded confocal microscopy. *Opt Expr.* 2005;13: 8214-8221.

58. Qiu Q, Schutte HK. A new generation videokymography for routine clinical vocal fold examination. *Laryngoscope.* 2006;116:1824-1828.

59. Franco RA, Jr, Furlong C, Hulli N. Development of an optoelectronic, high-speed, 3D shape measurement system for medical applications. *J Voice.* In press.

Evaluation of the Child with a Vocal Disorder

Paolo Campisi

INTRODUCTION

There are many inherent challenges in the evaluation of a child with a voice disorder. The attending physician must have a thorough understanding of pediatric vocal physiology and of factors that negatively influence the production of voice in children. Other challenges include gaining the trust and compliance of a young patient and having a mastery of endoscopy skills. This is a prerequisite to the application of technology and instrumentation that was originally designed for use in a compliant adult. Finally, access to equipment that is suitable for use in children is mandatory.

This chapter outlines the assessment protocol employed at the Centre for Paediatric Voice and Laryngeal Function, a voice laboratory dedicated to the study and care of pediatric voice disorders, at the Hospital for Sick Children, Toronto, Canada.

ASSESSMENT PROTOCOL

The Pediatric Voice History

Prior to evaluation in the voice laboratory, a standardized questionnaire is mailed to the patient and caregiver for completion. The completed questionnaire is reviewed by the attending pediatric otolaryngologist and speech-language pathologist to characterize the nature of the voice complaint, to identify risk factors for dysphonia, and to assess the impact of the voice complaint on the patient and family.[1] This approach allows for the efficient gathering of a large amount of information and provides the patient and caregiver ample opportunity to reflect on the voice problem and to provide accurate historical data.

The aim of the questionnaire is to retrieve demographic data, education and social history, voice use and voice problem history, past medical and developmental history, and voice related quality of life assessments. The questionnaire was designed in a check box format to facilitate completion by the patient and caregiver and facilitate review of the completed form by the physician and speech-language pathologist. In addition, the form was prepared in a "scannable" format to permit rapid and accurate integration into clinical and research databases. The standardized questionnaire is provided in Appendix 5.

The Directed Physical Examination

A physical examination of the head and neck is an important component of the assessment of pediatric voice disorders. There are many head and neck physical findings that may impact laryngeal function and vocal quality. For example, a middle ear effusion resulting in a conductive hearing loss may result in voice overuse and laryngeal tension as the child speaks loudly to compensate for the compromised auditory feedback. Adenotonsillar hypertrophy and anterior nasal obstruction may be responsible for a hyponasal resonance. In contrast, clefting and hypotonia of the soft palate may result in a hypernasal resonance which may be misinterpreted as a voice disorder. Neck masses, in particular thyroid lesions, may impinge on the recurrent laryngeal nerves resulting in a breathy and weak voice. Finally, facial dysmorphisms may be indicative of an underlying genetic syndrome associated with laryngeal abnormalities.

Perceptual and Objective Voice Assessments

Voice assessments are best performed by speech-language pathologists with specific training in voice disorders. Speech-language pathologists have the skills to screen young patients and discriminate dysphonia from common speech and language disorders such as articulation errors, oral motor dyspraxia, dysfluency, abnormal resonance, and higher function language difficulties. It is not uncommon for patients to be referred to the voice laboratory for problems that have been misinterpreted as voice disorders. As such, early screening is recommended to clarify the presenting complaint and provide appropriate and well-directed treatment.

Perceptual Voice Assessments

Ideally, voice assessments are performed perceptually and objectively (if specialized equipment is available). The perceptual assessment is primarily performed by a speech-language pathologist. Perceptual evaluations may be informal and descriptive or in accordance with several standardized testing formats. The most commonly used rating scales are the GRBAS (grade, roughness, breathiness, aesthenia, strain), Buffalo III Voice Profile, and CAPE-V (Consensus Auditory-Perceptual Evaluation of Voice).[2-4]

In young patients, the test stimuli are modified as not all children can fully cooperate with the evaluation. The clinician must make the exercise enjoyable and rewarding and may have to rely on limited voice samples (sustained vowels, syllable repetition, rote speech, reading, picture description, and general conversation) to complete the evaluation of voice quality. The perceptual assessment must also include an evaluation of breath support, secondary behaviors (cough, throat clearing, etc) and laryngeal muscle tension.[5]

Objective Voice Assessments

Perceptual voice assessments are invaluable and represent an indispensable tool used to characterize a voice disorder. However, the assessments are subjective and there may not be uniform agreement in opinion from one listener to the next. This limitation may confound evaluations of treatment efficacy if post-treatment evaluations are performed by a different listener. The physician and speech-language pathologist may also be subject to bias as they wish to demonstrate a noticeable improvement in their patients. These potential problems may be obviated with the use of computer-assisted voice analyses. Several software and hardware packages are available that are well tolerated and well suited to the evaluation of the young patient. Furthermore, pediatric normative data for several voice parameters are available.[6]

Computerized-voice assessments provide an objective evaluation of voice and a mechanism to sensitively monitor changes in voice over time. The efficacy of treatment, voice therapy, or surgery, can also be evaluated. At the Centre for Paediatric Voice and Laryngeal Function, computerized-voice assessments are routinely performed in all children at the initial evaluation and at subsequent visits. These assessments are performed with the Computerized Speech Laboratory (KayPentax Inc, Lincoln Park, New Jersey) which operates software packages such as the Multidimensional Voice Program, Real-Time Pitch, and Motor Speech programs (Fig 5–1). These programs provide a robust assessment of voice including fundamental frequency, pitch range, frequency and amplitude control, and speaking rates. There are several other hardware and software packages available that are less costly.

Endoscopy and Stroboscopy in Children

Technique

Any form of upper airway endoscopy in children is challenging. The endoscopist must be gentle, unrushed, and skillful with

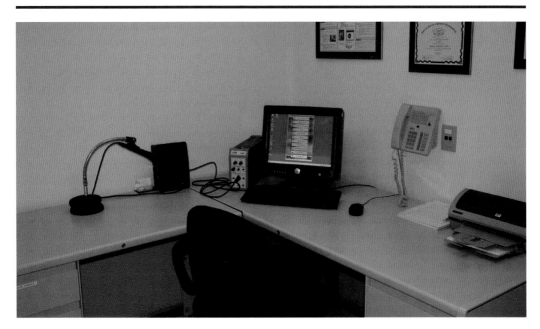

Fig 5–1. Computerized Speech Laboratory Model 4400 (KayPentax Inc, Lincoln Park, NJ).

children. Taking the time to explain the process and demystifying the equipment may facilitate an uneventful examination and minimize apprehension for future evaluations. In the very young or uncooperative child, a form of restraint may be necessary in spite of the pre-endoscopy preparation. In some instances, awake endoscopy is impossible and visualization of the larynx must take place in the operating theatre under general anesthesia.

Ideally, visualization of the larynx should be performed with both rigid and flexible endoscopes. Unfortunately, this is not possible in all young patients. As such, choice of endoscope should be based on the objectives of the evaluation. If the objective is to detect a structural abnormality (nodules, cysts, etc), rigid endoscopy will provide the best visual resolution. In contrast, if the objective is to detect abnormalities of function (vocal fold paralysis, supraglottic compression, etc), then flexible endoscopy is preferable as this modality is less disruptive to normal laryngeal posturing which permits the testing of numerous voice tasks. The availability of pediatric-sized digital flexible nasolaryngoscopes is highly anticipated as they will provide excellent visualization of structure and function.

In the very young or uncooperative child, restraint in a sitting position is maintained by the parent or nursing staff by placing one arm around the child's chest and arms and the other arm on the child's forehead. In the restrained child, flexible nasolaryngoscopy is the only possible endoscopic modality. Decongestion of the intranasal structures is rarely necessary.

In the cooperative child undergoing rigid laryngoscopy, careful attention must be paid to positioning. Patients are encouraged to sit with shoulders forward and head in a sniffing position. The tongue is held forward by the endoscopist using gauze. Lido-caine is applied to the oropharyx to minimize the gag reflex.

Equipment

A software package designed to acquire and store endoscopy images and video digitally is highly recommended for a pediatric practice (Fig 5–2). In children, many of the visualizations are brief and the ability to pause and play back video in slow motion is indispensable. The software packages also permit rapid recall of previous endoscopies for comparison and incorporate images into standardized reports in an automated fashion. This latter feature has greatly enhanced the quality of medical reports distributed to physicians and speech-language pathologists providing therapy in the community setting.

Rigid endoscopes are available in a variety of sizes ranging from 4 mm to 9 mm in diameter. The smaller rigid endoscopes provide excellent resolution and are very well tolerated by children. They are particularly useful in children with strong gag reflexes and tonsillar hypertrophy. Flexible fiberoptic endoscopes have been available in pediatric sizes for several years. The smaller fiberoptic endoscopes, however, have notoriously poor visual resolution. This limitation will be overcome in the near future as the next generation digital flexible endoscopes become readily available. The smallest commercially available digital flexible endoscope has a 3.1-mm diameter at the tip (VNL 1070K by KayPentax, Lincoln Park, New Jersey).

Stroboscopy provides a remarkable visualization of the mucosal wave of the vocal folds. However, the usefulness of stroboscopy in the very young and uncooperative patient is unclear. Stroboscopy is limited by the short duration of visualization in children, poor performance with small fiberop-

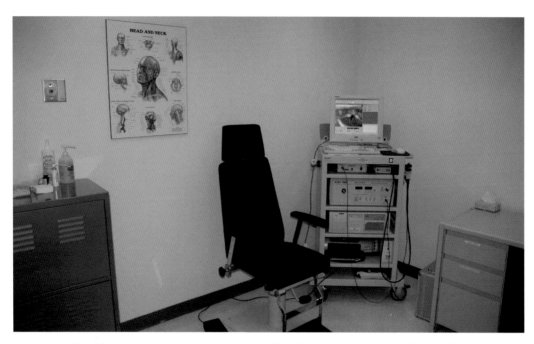

Fig 5–2. Laryngostroboscopy unit (KayPentax Inc, Lincoln Park, NJ).

tic endoscopes and occasional intolerance to the microphone that is strapped to the neck. Again, the introduction of digital flexible endoscopes may improve the usefulness of stroboscopy in this subgroup of patients.

Other Investigations and Consultations

Further investigations and consultations are requested as needed. The most common investigations requested include audiometry, pH probe studies, pulmonary function tests, and swallow assessments. As such, colleagues in gastroenterology, respiratory medicine, radiology, and occupational therapy are often involved in the care of voice patients.

Laryngeal electromyography (EMG) is not routinely performed in children as most will not tolerate the placement of transcutaneous electrodes into the laryngeal musculature. In neonates with equivocal vocal fold paralysis, laryngeal EMG is performed in the operating theatre under general anesthesia.

CONCLUSION

The assessment of pediatric voice disorders is challenging but rewarding. It requires a dedicated physician and speech-language pathologist, the use of specialized equipment, and a standardized assessment protocol that is tailored to children. Visual aids to help children and their parents understand normal vocal anatomy, the physiology of voice production, and examples of vocal pathology are strongly encouraged. An example of an educational poster used to educate children and their families is shown in Figure 5-3.

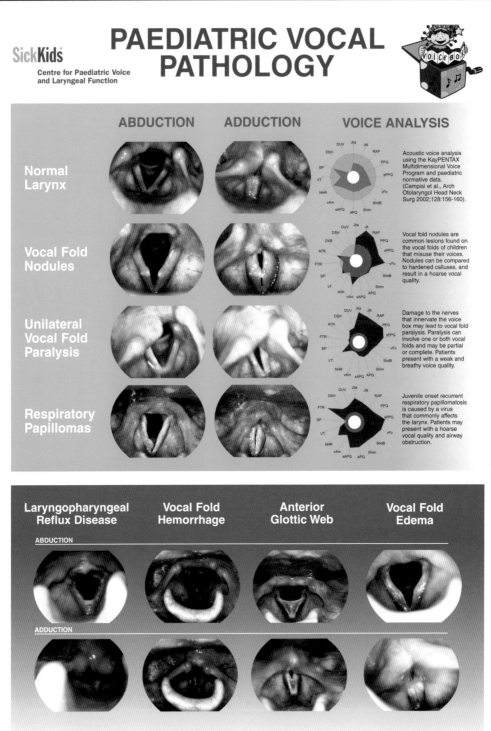

Fig 5–3. Educational poster of pediatric vocal pathology developed at the Centre for Paediatric Voice and Laryngeal Function.

REFERENCES

1. Hartnick CJ, Volk M, Cunningham M. Establishing normative voice-related quality of life scores within the pediatric otolaryngology population. *Arch Otolaryngol Head Neck Surg.* 2003;129:1090–1093.
2. Hirano M. *Clinical Examination of Voice.* Wien, NY: Springer-Verlag; 1981.
3. Wilson DK. *Voice Problems of Children.* 3rd ed. Baltimore, Md: Williams & Wilkins; 1987.
4. American Speech-Language-Hearing Association's (ASHA) Division 3: Voice and Voice Disorders. *Consensus Auditory-Perceptual Evaluation of Voice (CAPE-V).* Pittsburgh, Pa: American Speech-Language-Hearing Association; 2002.
5. Roy N, Ford CN, Bless DM. Muscle tension dysphonia and spasmodic dysphonia: the role of manual laryngeal tension reduction in diagnosis and management. *Ann Otol Rhinol Laryngol.* 1996;105:851–856.
6. Campisi P, Tewfik TL, Manoukian JJ, Schloss MD, Pelland-Blais E, Sadeghi N. Computer-assisted voice analysis: establishing a pediatric database. *Arch Otolaryngol Head Neck Surg.* 2002;128:156–160.

APPENDIX 5

HOSPITAL FOR SICK CHILDREN   82373 ■

Date: _____   Completed By: _____

Section A: Patient Information

Name: _____ Date of Birth: _____ Sex: ☐ Male ☐ Female Height___ Weight: ___

Address: _____ Telephone: _____

Language(s) spoken in the home: ☐ English   ☐ Other _____

Pediatrician: _____   Referred by: _____

Section B : Family History

2   Does your child have any brothers? If yes, are they older? ☐   Younger? ☐

3   Do they have any speech/language difficulties? If yes, describe_____ yes ☐   no ☐

4   Does your child have any sisters? If yes, are they older? ☐   Younger? ☐

5   Do they have any speech/language difficulties? If yes, describe_____ yes ☐   no ☐

6   Is there a history of speech, language, or voice problems in your family (including parents, aunts, uncles, etc) yes ☐   no ☐

Describe: _____

Does your child's voice sound like anyone else's in you family? Describe:_____ yes ☐   no ☐

Section C: Education and Social History

Preschool Child: Where does your child spend most of the day?

At home ☐   daycare/ nursery ☐   babysitter/nanny ☐   Other ☐ _____

School-Aged Child: Name of School: _____

Grade: JK ☐   K ☐   1 ☐   2 ☐   3 ☐   4 ☐   5 ☐   6 ☐   7 ☐   8 ☐   9 ☐   10 ☐   11 ☐   12 ☐   13 ☐

Address: _____ Teacher: _____

What type of program is your child in?   Half-day program ☐   Full day program ☐   Regular class placement ☐

Special class placement ☐   Receiving any remedial help ☐   Other ☐ Describe:_____

Describe your child's school performance: Excellent ☐   Good ☐   Fair ☐   Poor ☐

Is your child teased because of his/her voice difficulties?   yes ☐   no ☐

Section D: History Of The Voice Problem

Describe your child's voice problem. (fill in all that apply).

Hoarseness ☐   loss of voice ☐   breathiness ☐   voice breaks or cracks ☐   poor volume ☐
other ☐ _____

Does your child have any of the following problems (fill in all that apply)

throat pain ☐   swallowing ☐   throat dryness ☐   choking ☐   shortness of breath ☐   noisy breathing ☐

Describe your child's voice problem.

a) How did your child's voice problem begin   suddenly ☐   gradually ☐

b) How is it changing   better ☐   worse ☐   staying the same ☐

c) Is your child's problem constant or does it vary   constant ☐   varies ☐

d) If it varies, what is it dependent on   time of day ☐   season ☐   activity ☐   health status ☐

Has your child been previously evaluated or treated by any of the following

a) Ear, Nose and Throat Physician   No ☐   Yes ☐   describe

b) Speech-Language Pathologist   No ☐   Yes ☐   describe

Has your child ever received formal voice training (e.g., singing/vocal lessons) ? No ☐ ? Yes ☐, describe

Section E: Voice Use History

Below is a list of behaviours that sometimes influence voice quality. Please check how often you observe
these behaviours in your child.   **A = occasionally   B = frequently   C = most/all of the time**

	A	B	C		A	B	C
Throat clearing	☐	☐	☐	Caffeine consumption	☐	☐	☐
Crying	☐	☐	☐	"Non-stop" talking	☐	☐	☐
Whistling	☐	☐	☐	Use of inhalers	☐	☐	☐
"Funny voices", impersonations	☐	☐	☐	Smoking	☐	☐	☐
Yelling, shouting	☐	☐	☐	Coughing, croup	☐	☐	☐
Loud talking	☐	☐	☐	Singing	☐	☐	☐
Acting, performances	☐	☐	☐	Mouth breathing	☐	☐	☐

Section F : Medical History

Has your child ever had any of the following? (fill in all that apply)

☐ Asthma	☐ Thyroid problems	☐ Heart problems
☐ Nasal Regurgitation	☐ Frequent colds or throat infections	☐ Lethargy or fatigue
☐ Pain in ear	☐ Anorexia and/or bulimia	☐ Neurological problems
☐ Sinusitis	☐ Tics/involuntary movements	☐ Endocrine problems
☐ Reflux/"Heartburn"?	☐ Dry/sore throat	☐ Stress-related problems
☐ Jaw joint problems	☐ Vomiting	☐ Head injuries
☐ Post-nasal drip	☐ Feelings of depression/sadness	☐ Exposure to toxins, chemicals
☐ Weight loss	☐ Respiratory Problems(e.g.,wheezing)	☐ Other _____
☐ Seizures	☐ Exposure to cigarette smoke	

Has your child ever had surgery? (fill in all those that apply)

☐ Cardiac surgery	☐ Laryngoscopy	☐ Tracheostomy	☐ Tonsillectormy
☐ Thyroid surgery	☐ Bronchoscopy	☐ Adenoidectomy	
☐ Brain surgery	☐ Esophageal surgery	☐ Other head and heck surgery	

Has your child ever had any of the following tests?

a) Hearing test? No ☐ If Yes ☐ Describe: _____

b) Swallowing assessment? No ☐ If Yes ☐ Describe: _____

c) Gastro-intestinal evaluation? No ☐ If Yes ☐ Describe: _____

d) Allergy test? No ☐ If Yes ☐ Describe: _____

e) Neurological examination? No ☐ If Yes ☐ Describe: _____

f) Psychological or psycho-educational assessment? No ☐ If Yes ☐ Describe: _____

g) Genetics test? No ☐ If Yes ☐ Describe: _____

Does your child have any of the following?

a) Drug allergies No ☐ If Yes ☐ Describe: _____

b) Environmental allergies No ☐ If Yes ☐ Describe: _____

c) Food allergies No ☐ If Yes ☐ Describe: _____

Does your child take any medications? No ☐ If Yes ☐ Describe: _____

Does your child require prophylactic antibiotics prior to medical procedures (e.g., dental)? No ☐ If Yes ☐ Describe: _____

Section G: Developmental History and Speech/Language Information

Describe your child's speech and language skills. Please fill in any items that are a concern to you or your child:

☐ Late to talk	☐ Difficulty expressing ideas, sequencing events
☐ Stuttering or getting stuck while talking	☐ Hard to understand his/her speech
☐ Difficulty "pronouncing" sounds	☐ Difficulty hearing sounds or words
☐ Talking too fast	☐ Sounds "stuffy" as if he/she has a cold
☐ Sounds as if he/she is talking through the nose	☐ Difficulty understanding directions
☐ Other _____	

Please fill in any items that are currently a concern to you:

☐ Difficulty paying attention	☐ Difficulty with gross motor tasks (e.g., running, riding a bike)
☐ Always needing to be on the move	☐ Other _____
☐ Difficulty with fine motor tasks (e.g., colouring, cutting)	

The following items ask about activities that your child might do in a given day.

To what extent does your child's voice limit his or her ability to be understood in a noisy area?

☐ Limited a lot   ☐ Limited a little   ☐ Not limited at all

During the past 2 weeks, to what extent has your child's voice interfered with his or her normal social activities or with his or her school?

☐ Not at all   ☐ Slightly   ☐ Moderately   ☐ Quite a bit   ☐ Extremely

How often does your child have trouble with food or liquids "going down the wrong pipe" when he or she eats or drinks liquid and begins to cough after eating or drinking?

☐ All the time   ☐ Most of the time   ☐ Sometimes   ☐ Rarely   ☐ Never

Do you find your child "straining" when he or she speaks because of his or her voice problem?

☐ Not at all   ☐ Slightly   ☐ Moderately   ☐ Quite a bit   ☐ Extremely

Comments:

Thank you

Pediatric Laryngology: The Office and Operating Room Setup

Mark E. Boseley
Christopher J. Hartnick

INTRODUCTION

The field of pediatric laryngology has grown as the equipment and technology available to us has expanded. Where we were once limited by pediatric flexible fiberoptic laryngoscopes with poor optics, we now have distal-chip camera scopes with digital quality images displayed on a video monitor. Videostroboscopy is now possible using these scopes, a diagnostic tool that was often not used previously as it required the use of rigid telescopes that were not tolerated by pediatric patients. We are also now able to archive images and videos from both the office and operating room, making pre- and post-treatment evaluations more accurate than in the past. Furthermore, we are utilizing the services of our pulmonary and gastroenterology colleagues more and more in the care of these often complex patients with multiple medical problems. This has taken the form of pediatric aerodigestive clinics in several of our academic centers around the country. As this occurs, we have to be able to acquire digital images of both flexible bronchoscopies and esophagoscopies and archive them in some unified fashion to complement our rigid tracheobronchoscopies.

This chapter discusses both the office and operating room personnel and equipment important in the practice of pediatric laryngology. This is not intended to be an exhaustive list, but should provide a useful foundation if one is beginning a practice (or expanding one) to care for pediatric voice patients.

OFFICE-BASED PRACTICE

Personnel

Developing a pediatric laryngology clinic involves having at your disposal the appropriate personnel and equipment needed to diagnose and treat these patients. The personnel usually includes an otolaryngologist (usually pediatric otolaryngologist) who has an interest in caring for children with voice disorders. Another vital member of the team is the speech-language pathologist (SLP) who has a specific interest and training in treating pediatric patients. A clinic nurse is also invaluable for patient/parent teaching and helping with the care of the complex equipment that is utilized in the clinic.

Children with voice complaints often present with numerous aerodigestive symptoms. Medical histories can uncover such symptoms as chronic cough, wheezing, exercise intolerance, and feeding difficulties, in addition to the voice concern that brought them to your office. Prior experience suggests that these children were sent to other specialists, required multiple visits, and often involved poor communication between specialties. This problem can be alleviated by establishing a close working relationship with our pediatric pulmonary and gastroenterology colleagues. This may take the form of a formal aerodigestive workup or might simply involve an informal design where there is an open line of communication between the clinicians.

A visit to the aerodigestive clinic involves essentially three complete evaluations of the child. This is followed by a conference among the specialists involved and typically generates a detailed treatment plan before the patient leaves the office. Occasionally this plan involves an endoscopic evaluation in the operating room, where flexible bronchoscopy and flexible esophagoscopy can yield valuable information.

Equipment

We have included pictures and videos of the equipment outlined in this chapter in a CD compendium that accompanies the text. This chapter and subsequent chapters that have either photographs or videos that enhance the didactic portion the text have a second section where the images are explained in detail. This second section includes detailed information about list costs and catalog numbers if you are interested in purchasing any item discussed. We hope this will be a valuable tool for better understanding the equipment and techniques that are currently being utilized in the field of pediatric laryngology.

The diagnostic equipment available in the office has changed considerably over the past several years. The Kay Pentax Stroboscope Model 9100B is the latest in the line of videostroboscopic equipment allowing for digital quality imaging of the larynx, utilizing either a flexible rhinolaryngoscope or a 70-degree rigid peroral telescope. A 3.4-mm (Olympus) or 3.7-mm (Kay Pentax) flexible distal-tip-chip camera strobsocope can allow for full screen high-resolution images and stroboscopic observation of younger children's vocal folds (Fig 6–1). Alternatively, 2.7-mm and 3.0-mm angled rigid stroboscopes are available from Karl Storz (Fig 6–2).

Stroboscopy is not always possible in young children. This is not always due to their chronologic age, but may be more a function of their age-independent maturity. The skill and experience of the endoscopist is also important in this regard. Also, young

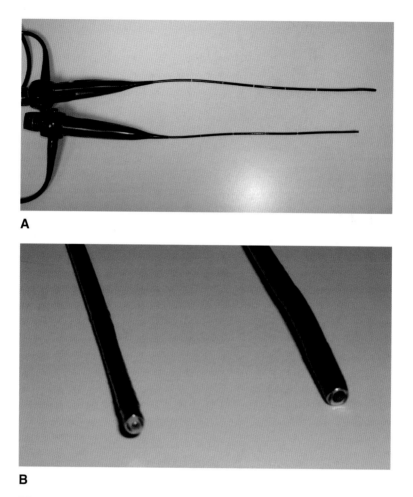

Fig 6–1. 3.4-mm (Olympus) and 3.7-mm (KayPentax) distal-tip-chip camera flexible rhinolaryngoscopes.

children are not always able to produce the asynchronous prolonged mucosal wave vibration needed to obtain stroboscopic images. Despite these potential hindrances, distal-chip camera technology allows for a more detailed evaluation of the vocal fold anatomy and of glottal aperture abnormalities even without the use of stroboscopy.

This new equipment can provide valuable information. One example of this is a flexible transnasal videostroboscopic examination on a 6-year-old child. The resolution of the digital video is much better than traditional flexible laryngoscopes and much easier accomplished than rigid peroral stroboscopy (Video 6-1, section 2). Examination for glottal insufficiency, as well as examination of the mucosal wave to identify overall pliability of the mucosa and points of stiffness, is now feasible. Mucosal wave abnormalities may also be useful in differentiating vocal fold pathologies. Additionally, acoustic measurements can be recorded and saved for future comparison.

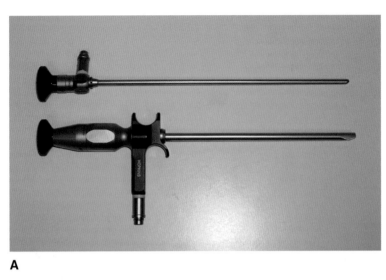

A

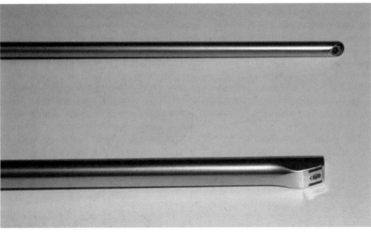

B

Fig 6–2. 70-degree pediatric rigid Hopkins rod strobscopes (Karl Storz Inc.).

Another office examination made both more practical, and perhaps more accessible by the new technology described above, is pediatric functional endoscopic evaluation of swallowing (FEES). FEES can be useful in the workup of children with swallowing difficulties or in those children whom you suspect may be aspirating. This is demonstrated by a 14-year-old girl who presents after skull base resection of a clival chordoma with signs of aspiration (Video 6–2, section 2).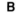

Archiving of digital images and videos in the office is very important for determining treatment outcomes. There are several programs that can be used for this purpose. We have experience with products from Karl Storz and NStream. Both were easy to use and we do not necessarily endorse one over the other. There are undoubtedly other programs that either are currently or soon will be on the market. The important message here is that archiving in both the operating room and the clinic setting is vital to assessing treatment outcomes in our voice patient population.

pended from either a Mayo or Mustard stand using the Benjamin suspension apparatus (Fig 6–4). Another laryngoscope that can be useful in the difficult-to-expose patient is the pediatric universal glottis-

OPERATING ROOM-BASED PRACTICE

Equipment

The operating room equipment that should be available to the pediatric laryngologist can be thought of in several distinct categories. These include tools for visualization, airway access instruments, microsurgical instruments, and video/picture capabilities with an archiving system. Each of these categories is described in detail.

Tools for Visualization

Most pediatric cases can be managed with the infant, adolescent, or adult Lindholm laryngoscopes (Fig 6-3) which can be sus-

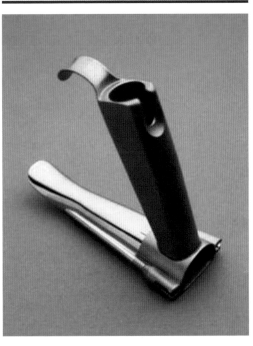

Fig 6–3. Lindholm laryngoscopes.

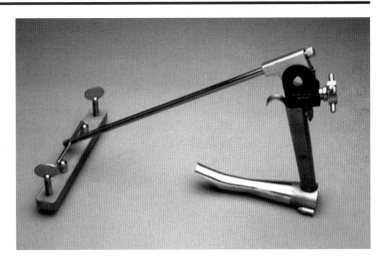

Fig 6–4. Benjamin suspension device which can rest on either a Mustard or Mayo stand.

cope with the gallows suspension device (Fig 6–5). This device takes advantage of torsion-fulcrum principles to achieve better exposure of the vocal folds.

All the aforementioned laryngoscopes may be used to visualize the larynx with a small endotracheal tube in place, or (as our preference) utilizing a tubeless spontaneous ventilation/apneic anesthetic technique. Magnification can be achieved with either a 4.0-mm Hopkins rod telescope with a camera attachment or with an operating microscope with a 400-mm lens. (We prefer the Leica M520S3 microscope although there are other microscopes that would suffice.) The latter is particularly useful when performing phonosurgical procedures that require bimanual manipulation. With these instruments and microscopes, close inspection of pediatric vocal folds is

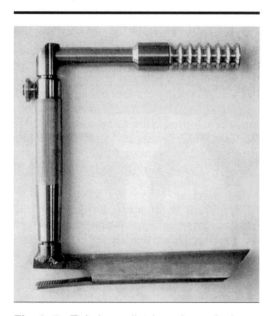

Fig 6–5. Zeitels pediatric universal glottoscope with gallows suspension. This instrument can be utilized when the Lindholm laryngoscopes are unable to give adequate visualization of the glottis.

possible. This often allows us to discriminate between lesions such as vocal nodules and cysts and allows for proper treatment and therapy plans to be developed (Fig 6–6). It is tantamount to realize that not all children will allow office visualization of their vocal folds, and that there is a time when operative endoscopy will be essential.

Tools for Airway Access

Although not always required, it is important that a variety of ventilating bronchoscopes are available and assembled to handle the difficult airway. A size 2.5 rigid bronchoscope with an inner diameter of 3.5 mm and an outer diameter of 4.2 mm with a 18-cm 1.9-mm Hopkins rod telescope is a scope that we have available for most of our infant airway cases. This is the smallest bronchoscope on the airway cart and should be able to be passed through most stenotic lesions that are encountered. If a tight distal airway stenosis is suspected, a modified endotracheal tube can be fashioned to get access to the distal airway (Fig 6–7). The point that must be emphasized is that a child with a suspected difficult airway **does not get muscle relaxants** until the airway is stabilized.

Microsurgical Instruments

The surgeon is only as good as the instruments that he or she has available. There is no place where this dictum is more true than when attempting to perform phonosurgical procedures. Developing microsurgical flaps between the vocal fold epithelium and superficial layer of the lamina propria requires great skill, but also necessitates the avail-

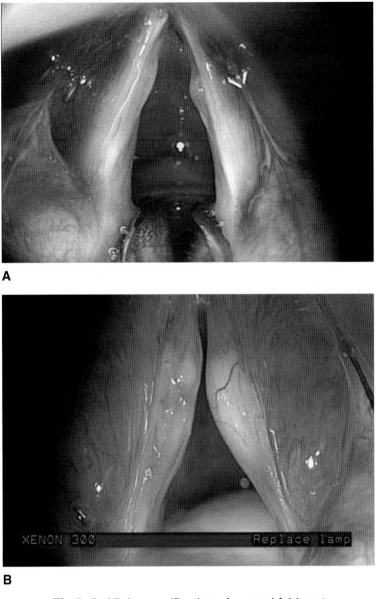

A

B

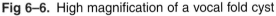

Fig 6–6. High magnification of a vocal fold cyst

ability of the proper instruments. These instruments should be analyzed routinely to be sure that they are sharp and of good working order. A typical microlaryngeal instrument set is pictured in Figure 6–8. The minimum requirements should be microscopic scissors (right, left, straight, and upbiting), atraumatic graspers such as the Sataloff forceps (right and left), a sickle knife, a microsurgical dissector, and set of laryngeal suctions. One-quarter-inch neurologic cotton pledgets soaked in oxymetazoline on a sponge carrier are often helpful to achieve hemostasis.

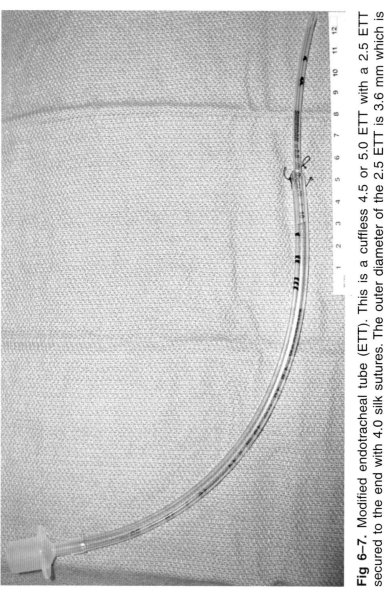

Fig 6–7. Modified endotracheal tube (ETT). This is a cuffless 4.5 or 5.0 ETT with a 2.5 ETT secured to the end with 4.0 silk sutures. The outer diameter of the 2.5 ETT is 3.6 mm which is smaller than the diameter of the 2.5 bronchoscope. This can be used to bypass a distal tracheal stenosis.

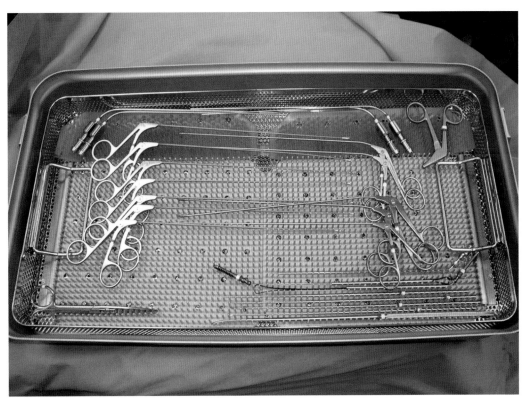

A

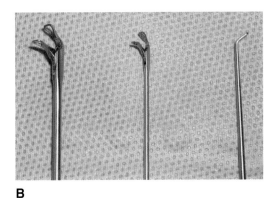

B

Fig 6–8. Example of a complete pediatric voice set for the operating room.

Archiving

Archiving images from the operating room are equally as important as in the office. This is extremely valuable for patients who make frequent trips to the operating room (ie, children following airway reconstruction and children with the diagnosis of juvenile onset recurrent respiratory papillomatosis). Photographs are also useful when discussing treatment plans with parents.

CONCLUSION

This chapter has described how to set up a pediatric voice clinic. It focused on those personnel and equipment that we find invaluable in the office and operating room. We have attempted to consolidate the list of equipment to make ordering these items much easier than searching through numerous catalogues (Appendix 6). We hope this information will be helpful to those of you considering starting or expanding a pediatric voice practice.

VIDEOS IN THIS CHAPTER

Video 6–1. The video demonstrates a 6-year-old child who presents with a history of dysphonia. The preoperative video is of a transnasal digital stroboscopic examination. The diagnosis of a unilateral vocal fold epithelial cyst was made. The cyst was removed in the operating room using a M520S3 microscope and microsurgical instruments. A lateral incision was made through the vocal fold epithelium and a microflap was raised over the cyst. The cyst was then removed and the overlying epithelium was carefully returned to its anatomically correct position. A second postoperative video of a transnasal digital stroboscopic examination demonstrates no glottal insufficiency and an improved voice

Video 6–2. The video is of a 14-year-old girl after a skull base resection of a clival chordoma. Her symptoms include new-onset dysphonia and aspiration. Transnasal digital stroboscopy demonstrates unilateral vocal fold immobility. The second video of a FEES evaluation shows evidence of aspiration. The final video is following an injection laryngoplasty and botulinum toxin injection to the cricopharyngeus. She has no glottal aperture defect and is no longer aspirating.

APPENDIX 6

Pediatric Vocal Fold Instrument Set*

Description	Company	Model #	# Required	List Price
Straight cup forceps (*straight*)	Karl Storz	8591A	1	$695.00
Curved cup forceps (*right*)	Karl Storz	8591C	1	$695.00
Curved cup forceps (*left*)	Karl Storz	8591D	1	$695.00
Alligator forceps (*right*)	Instrumentarium	L.70.925	1	$572.90
Alligator forceps (*left*)	Instrumentarium	L.70.926	1	$572.90
Small Sataloff forceps (*right*)	Instrumentarium	L.70.991	1	$776.40
Large Sataloff forceps (*right*)	Instrumentarium	L.70.191	1	$516.45
Large Sataloff forceps (*left*)	Instrumentarium	L.70.190	1	$516.45
Scissors (*angled up*)	Karl Storz	8594BM	1	$875.00
Scissors (*straight*)	Karl Storz	8594AM	1	$875.00
Scissors (*right*)	Karl Storz	8594DM	1	$875.00
Scissors (*left*)	Karl Storz	8594CM	1	$875.00
Universal knife handle	Pilling	506888	1	$391.06
Jako sponge carrier (26-cm)	Pilling	506751	2	$265.20 ea
Holinger laryngeal dissector	Pilling	506882	1	$153.00
Phono curved sickle knife	Pilling	506882	1	$229.50
Phono blunt probe elevator (60-degree)	Pilling	506832	1	$142.80
Zeitels vocal fold infusion needle	Endocraft	ZIN-100A	Box of 5	$500.00

*2007 list prices

VIDEO TOWER

Description	Company	Model #	# Required	List Price
Computer w/ DV/SDI	Karl Storz	22200011U102	1	$16,270.00
Flat panel monitor	Karl Storz	9319NR-A24	1	$8,920.00
3-chip camera	Karl Storz	22220130-3	1	$15,230.00
Sony printer	Karl Storz	9512C	1	$10,140.00
175-watt xenon light source	Karl Storz	201315-20	1	$3,075.00
Light cable	Karl Storz	495ND	1	$570.00
Cart	Karl Storz	9801T	1	$1,255.00

TELESCOPES

Description	Company	Model #	# Required	List Price
Hopkins II 0-degree (4-mm × 18-cm)	Karl Storz	7230AA	1	$3,980.00
Hopkins II 0-degree (2.7-mm × 18-cm)	Karl Storz	7219AA	1	$4,425.00
Hopkins II 0-degree (1.9-mm × 18-cm)	Karl Storz	10017AA	1	$4,660.00
Hopkins II 70-degree (4-mm × 18-cm)	Karl Storz	7230CWA	1	$4,110.00
Hopkins II 70-degree (4-mm × 15-cm)	Karl Storz	7228CA	1	$3,795.00
Hopkins II 70-degree (3-mm × 14-cm)	Karl Storz	7220CA	1	$3,570.00
Hopkins II 70-degree (2.7-mm × 18-cm)	Karl Storz	7219CA	1	$4,425.00
Hopkins II 120-degree (4-mm × 18-cm)	Karl Storz	7230EA	1	$3,980.00

LARYNGOSCOPES

Description	Company	Model #	# Required	List Price
Infant Lindholm	Karl Storz	8587 P	1	$1,645.00
Light carrier	Karl Storz	8587 PF	1	$515.00
Child Lindholm	Karl Storz	8587 N	1	$1,645.00
Adult Linholm	Karl Storz	8587 A	1	$1,645.00
Light carrier	Karl Storz	8587 GF	1	$515.00
Pediatric universal glottiscope	Endocraft	UMG-100A	1	$3,900.00
Light cable for universal glottiscope	Endocraft	UMG-100 LC	1	$450.00
Gallows suspension	Endocraft	ZVG-100A	1	$3900.00
Benjamin suspension & chest support	Karl Storz	8574 KW	1	$1,470.00

BRONCHOSCOPES AND ACCESSORIES

Description	Company	I.D.	O.D.	Model #	# Required	List Price
2.5 × 20 cm	Karl Storz	3.5 mm	4.2 mm	10339F	1	$875.00
3.0 × 20 cm	Karl Storz	4.3 mm	5.0 mm	10339D	1	$875.00
3.5 × 20 cm	Karl Storz	5.0 mm	5.7 mm	10339CD	1	$875.00
3.5 × 30 cm	Karl Storz	5.0 mm	5.7 mm	10339DD	1	$875.00
4.0 × 30 cm	Karl Storz	6.0 mm	6.7 mm	10339C	1	$875.00
4.5 × 30 cm	Karl Storz	6.6 mm	7.3 mm	10339BB	1	$875.00
5.0 × 30 cm	Karl Storz	7.2 mm	7.7 mm	10339B	1	$875.00
6.0 × 30 cm	Karl Storz	7.5 mm	8.2 mm	10339A	1	$875.00

Description	Company	Model #	# Required	List Price
Prism light defelector	Karl Storz	10101FA	1	$445.00
Glass plug window	Karl Storz	10338M	1	$80.00
Rubber telescope guide	Karl Storz	10338N	1	$65.00
Adapter for respirator	Karl Storz	10924D	1	$15.00

OFFICE EQUIPMENT

Fiberoptic Scopes (flexible and rigid)

Description	Company	Model #	# Required	List Price
ENF-V2 flexible video rhinolaryngoscope with video system (3.4-mm diameter)	Olympus	K230000229	1	$26,350.00
ENF-XP flexible fiberoptic rhinolaryngoscope (2.2-mm diameter)	Olympus	1111900	1	$8,820.00
ENF-GP flexible fiberoptic rhinolaryngoscope (3.6-mm diameter)	Olympus	1113308	1	$6,325.00
Rigid endoscope (70-degrees, 10-mm diameter)	Kay pentax	9106	1	$4,195.00

Videostroboscopic Equipment

Description	Company	Model #	# Required	List Price
Rhinolaryngeal stroboscope	Kay pentax	9100B	1	$15,995.00
Camera, 3-CCD	Kay pentax	9106	1	$4,195.00
22-37-mm zoom lens coupler	Kay pentax	9118	1	$1,375.00
Digital video capture module	Kay pentax	9200C	1	$16,995.00
Color printer	Kay pentax	9264C	1	$325.00
Electroglottograph	Kay pentax	6103	1	$1,995.00
Cart	Kay pentax	9271	1	$1,995.00
Setup/training	Kay pentax	9198	1	$995.00

The Speech Pathologist's Role in the Evaluation of a Child with a Voice Disorder

Shirley Gherson
Barbara M. Wilson Arboleda

INTRODUCTION

Voice disorders in the pediatric population are as varied as those in the adult population, but present special considerations for the voice evaluation team. Chronic hoarseness in children can stem from functional, structural, or neurologic bases. Reflux, asthma, allergies, and medication side effects may be complicating factors even among very young children. Recent advances in neonatal intensive care, although life saving, often present a series of traumas to the airway and voicing mechanism.[1,2] A child's voice disorder may be congenital, acquired after a period of normal voicing, or may present from the earliest stages of communication. Congenital problems include: laryngeal papilloma, glottic web, paralysis, vocal fold sulcus, laryngomalacia, and subglottic stenosis.[3,4] Acquired voice problems include use-related injuries, trauma, and those secondary to intubation.

The diversity of etiology, presentation, and perception of voice disorders among children is a complicating factor in discerning the presence of a voice disorder and in making management decisions. Vast variability in prevalence rate has been reported. Most often quoted is 6 to 9%, but some authors report prevalence as high as 38%.[5-7] One study revealed vocal fold nodules in almost 17% of a large cohort of children, regardless of voicing or functional status.[8] Comparison across studies is complicated by the differing criteria applied to each study. For example, parent and physician questionnaires tend to report a lower incidence than clinic or speech-language pathologist evaluation.[9] Overlooking the presence of a pediatric voice disorder may lead to undertreatment. In one study by Powell,[10] 82 children out of 203 identified with a voice disorder continued to demonstrate symptoms in a 4-year follow-up. By nature, children with congenital abnormalities of the larynx and those who have had surgical intervention to the airway will have a higher incidence of voice disorders. In one study by Zalzal, cited by Baker,[2] 15 of 16 children status postlaryngotracheal reconstruction were considered to be dysphonic by the voice clinician.

Differences in prevalence based on gender are different between the adult and the pediatric voice populations. In the school-aged population, more males present with use-related voice disorders.[5,7,8] This is reversed for adults, where over two-thirds of patients diagnosed with vocal fold nodules are female.[8,11]

Parents are not always certain what represents typical variation versus disordered voicing. In particular, parents may not be tuned in to their child's voice if hoarseness has been present since birth. One study in which a voice screening was administered to over 7,000 children revealed a disparity between clinician reporting of atypical voice versus parents' reporting of atypical voice.[5] Young children are not able to express functional limitations and parents may not understand the implications a voice disorder will have on their children as they grow. For this reason, parents will be heavily reliant upon the judgment of the voice evaluation team to understand prognosis and propose treatment solutions.

The voice evaluation may also be a portion of a larger review of the child's speech, language, and developmental skills. One study found that over half of children with voice disorders had a concomitant articulation disorder and language disorders were found in over 40% of the children in the study.[12] Children who have gone through periods of intubation or tracheostomies are at high risk for language and speech delays due to prolonged periods of aphonia.[1]

All of the above considerations make the voice evaluation team pivotal in the care of a child with a voice disorder. Undiagnosed voice disorders can result in difficulties in school and later in life. The team, in consultation with parents and teachers, will be required to present an argument for treatment based at times on current functional limitations, but also at times based on presumed functional limitations that will present if the disorder is allowed to continue to run its course. These recommendations must be clinically correlated and prioritized appropriately among other, sometimes complex, medical conditions. A thorough voice evaluation will not only tell us about the quality and function of the voice, but can also provide us with a guide for how we might remediate the problem with therapy.

The purpose of this chapter is to provide a guideline for understanding the unique factors at play in the evaluation of a child with a voice disorder and to provide a framework for structuring the evaluation and eliciting the vocal behaviors needed for decision making.

CHILDREN VERSUS ADULTS— A COMPARISON

Guidelines and protocols for use in the pediatric realm are extremely limited. Most of the protocols for voice diagnostics have been written for adults. Most of the textbooks are also based on the adult model. In this section, we present several broad areas of consideration when approaching evaluation of a child with a voice disorder.

Anatomy and Physiology

A complete description of the anatomic and physiologic differences between children and adults can be found elsewhere in this book. Therefore, we offer only a brief summary here.

The infant larynx sits high in the neck with the lower border of the cricoid cartilage reportedly resting around the level of C2 to C4.[13,14] The shape of the pediatric larynx is also different from that of adults, with the thyroid cartilage taking on a more semicircular shape[13,15] and the epiglottis more likely to be omega-shaped.[15] A greater percentage of the glottis is cartilaginous in children than in adults, with the ratio of the membranous to the cartilaginous portion progressing from 1.5 in the newborn to 5.5 in the adult male.[13] There is no differentiation of the vocal ligament until near 4 years of age[13-15] and the low calcification of laryngeal cartilages leaves the entire larynx more flexible than that of an adult.[15] An examination of the thyrohyoid space reveals that the hyoid bone overlaps the edge of the thyroid cartilage of the larynx, reducing the thyrohyoid space to a narrow seam.[15,16] Of particular importance in the management of airway issues is the size of the larynx in relation to the tracheobronchial tree, which is comparatively larger in infants than adults.[16]

One organizing factor in considering the differences between the child larynx and the adult larynx is the prioritization of food and the airway over other functions in early life. The position and shape of the mechanism at birth supports rapid alternation between swallowing and breathing.

Voice Norms

Given the vast anatomic and physical changes that take place in the vocal mechanism between birth and adulthood, it stands to reason that acoustic, aerodynamic, and perceptual parameters will be different between the two groups. Nonetheless, no reliable set of norms has been specifically developed for the pediatric population. Small sample sizes and differences in voice elicitation techniques make current studies difficult to interpret.

Acoustic measures will be impacted by children's high fundamental and formant frequencies due to their vocal tract being shorter and smaller in diameter than adults'.[17] Tables 7-1 and 7-2 present normative acoustic and maximum phonation time measures for children. Separate normative values for jitter and shimmer have not been presented, but Leeper[7] did find increased jitter among children with vocal fold nodules when compared to matched peers without vocal fold lesions. Campisi and colleagues[18] determined that the acoustic profiles of prepubescent boys and girls were similar and that children with vocal fold nodules did have consistently increased perturbation measures. Of note, however, Boltezar[19] discovered increased instability overall in vowel production among children, in particular in boys. Therefore, perturbation measures must be interpreted with caution in the pediatric population. Repeated measures and female settings for vowel production tasks will minimize the impact of this instability and compensate for the fact that acoustic analysis programs are more likely to make mistakes in interpreting signals with a high fundamental frequency.[17] Nonetheless, Boltezar[19] cautions that no one voice analysis parameter used in his study was capable of discerning normal variation from pathology.

Increased fundamental and formant frequency values in children can make spectrograms difficult to interpret as high fundamental frequency creates less defined formants. This may be aided by setting a wider filter in order to read the formants more accurately.[17]

Table 7–1. Acoustic Normative Measures of Children

Average Fundamental Frequency: Speech			
Age/Sex	*Norm*	*SD/Range*	*Source*
7 yr/F	294	—	Fairbanks, Wiley, & Lassman (1949)[45]
7 yr/M	281	—	
8 yr/F	297	—	
8 yr/M	288	—	
8 yr 2 m/F	235	221–258	Bennet (1983)[46]
8 yr 2 m/M	234	204–270	
9 yr 2 m/F	228	215–239	
9 yr 2 m/M	226	198–263	
10 yr 2 m/F	228	215–239	
10 yr 2 m/M	224	208–259	
11 yr 2 m/F	221	200–244	
11 yr 2 m/M	216	195–259	
10 to 12 yr/F	237.5	198–271	Horii (1983)[47]
10 to 12 yr/M	226.5	192–269	
Average Fundamental Frequency: Sustained Vowels			
Age/Sex	*Norm*	*SD/Range*	*Source*
3 yr	298	30.8	Eguchi & Hirsh (1969)[48]
4 yr	286	20.9	
5 yr	289	46.3	
6 yr	271.2	27.9	
7 yr	262.5	38.5	
8 yr	261	31.1	
9 yr	262.5	35.9	
10 yr	261.9	32.9	
11 yr/F	252.5	42.5	
11 yr/M	244.2	24.4	
12 yr/F	248.6	19.2	
12 yr/M	243.2	26.8	
13 yr/F	239.8	19.6	
13 yr/M	221.1	66.4	

Table 7–1. *continued*

Perturbation Measures: Sustained /a/			
Acoustic Measure	*Norm*	*SD*	*Source*
Jitter %	1.24	0.07	Campisi (2002)[18]
Relative Average Perturbation	0.75	0.04	
Shimmer %	3.35	0.12	
NHR*	0.11	0.002	

Intensity Measures (dB SPL) with SD: Sustained /a/				
Age/Sex	*Soft*	*Medium*	*Loud*	*Source*
4 yr/F	73.79 (2.30)	80.82 (3.44)	91.04 (5.54)	Stathopolous & Sapienza (1993)[21]
4 yr/M	73.12 (3.88)	82.49 (3.68)	89.91 (4.80)	
8 yr/F	74.58 (3.68)	81.14 (4.66)	90.01 (9.05)	
8 yr/M	73.66 (2.62)	80.8 (3.41)	91.34 (8.09)	

Speech: Norms from Fairbanks, Wiley, and Lassman (1949). Normal children reading a 52-word passage embedded in a longer reading passage.

Bennet (1983). 15 boys and 10 girls measured over a period of 3 years, reading "There is a sheet of paper in my coat pocket." Horii (1983). 36 10- to 12-year-old children reading the Rainbow Passage and the Zoo Passage

Sustained Vowels: Norms from Eguchi and Hirsh (1969). Average fundamental frequency of 6 vowels produced 5 times. Five subjects in each age group.

Perturbation Measures: Norms from Campisi (2002). 100 children (50 girls and 50 boys) sustaining 'ah' three times at a comfortable pitch. Multi-Dimensional Voice Program (MDVP) in conjunction with Computerized Speech Lab (CSL) was used for acoustic analysis.

Intensity Measures: Norms from Stathopolous and Sapienza (1993). Twenty 4-year-olds and 20 8-year-olds produced three trials of syllable trains on /pa/ at soft, comfortable, and loud vocal intensity levels.

Table 7–2. Normative Ranges in MPT Measures in Children

Age/Sex	*Norm (range)*	*Source*
3–5 yr	6–10 seconds	Finnegan (1984)[49]
6–9 yr	14–17 seconds	
10–12 yr	15–22 seconds	

Finnegan (1984). 286 normal children, ages 3 to 17, were instructed to sustain the vowel /a/ for as long as possible for 14 trials.

When looking at volume dynamics, Stothopoulus[20] noted that children increase pitch more dramatically when asked to get louder as compared to adults because their vocal folds are smaller and more easily influenced by increases in subglottic pressure.

Aerodynamic measurements will be impacted by respiratory differences between children and adults. Table 7–3 presents normative subglottic measures for children. Stathopoulos and Sapienza[21] found children generate lung pressures 50 to 100% greater than adults. In association with this, rib cage excursion can be twice that of adults due to their smaller capacity and the need to move their rib cages more to achieve the same lung volume displacement. Compared to adults, children work harder to use their voices. They use a higher subglottic pressure and have shorter maximum phonation time.[13] Children use a high percentage of rib cage contribution to breathing, versus abdominal contribution when compared to

adults.[20] Baker[2] cautions us that true vocal fold vibration is necessary for the accurate measurement of a number of aerodynamic parameters, including measurement of open quotient, speech quotient and maximum flow declination rate. He proposes that average airflow rate in children who have undergone laryngeal-tracheal reconstruction, although more variable overall, is more accurate when assessing a child with true vocal fold vibration.

Given the complications and artifacts involved in the acoustic and aerodynamic assessment of children, the perceptual rating of voice remains a key component in determination of the severity of the functional voice limitation. For children, we may rate voice using a traditional GRBAS[22] scale or the CAPE-V.[23] The necessity of children to take more frequent breaths and use greater rib cage movement during speech must be taken into account during the perceptual evaluation.

Table 7–3. Average Subglottal Pressures

Average Subglottal Pressure (H_2O) at Varying Intensity with SD			
	Soft	**Medium**	**Loud**	**Source**
4 yr/F	5.37 (1.62)	8.46 (2.05)	14.55 (3.22)	Stathopolous & Sapienza (1993)[21]
4 yr/M	5.6 (2.49)	8.75 (4.15)	13.83 (4.44)	
8 yr/F	6.21 (1.57)	8.24 (2.11)	11.98 (3.11)	
8 yr/M	5.97 (2.23)	7.95 (2.03)	11.75 (3.47)	
Average Subglottal Pressure (H_2O) at Varying Pitches with SD			
	Low	**Comfortable**	**High**	**Source**
6 yr–10 yr 11 m	8.72 (2.91)	9.29 (2.97)	9.86 (3.16)	Weinrich et al (2005)[50]

Stathopolous and Sapienza (1993). Twenty 4-year olds and 20 8-year olds produced three trials of syllable trains on /pa/ at soft, comfortable, and loud vocal intensity levels.

Weinrich, Salz, and Hughes (2005). 75 children between the ages of 6 and 10 years 11 months were asked to produce a sustained /a/ at low, comfortable, and high pitches.

Cognition and General Speech and Language Development

Special consideration must be given to the child's level of cognitive development during the evaluation process. Age alone should not be the sole determinant of cognitive expectations. Rather, the child's functional cognitive level will guide the clinician in terms of the vocabulary he or she uses and the manner in which he or she elicits evaluation tasks.

Very young children may be shy around new people. Therefore, directing your initial introduction to the parent rather than the child may be helpful in allowing the child to get comfortable in the evaluation environment.

Children also tend to be concretely oriented. Cues that rest firmly in the five senses, such as seeing, feeling, and hearing will be more successful than abstract cues in eliciting the behaviors you are looking for. Young children, in particular, may be approached with games or play to elicit vocal behaviors.

Evaluation of the voice should also account for the possibility of concurrent speech, language, and developmental delays.[12] There is some evidence to show that sensory motor or other oral motor deficits may coincide with voice disorders in children.[12]

Behaviors

Andrews[24] listed "high risk factors" with regard to interpersonal behaviors, such as talking too much, ignoring feedback, ignoring differences between people and situations, ignoring the needs and interests of others, and aggressive behavior. Akif Kilic[8] suggested that boys who get vocal fold nodules are those who are active and who scream. Green[25] compared a group of children with vocal fold nodules to matched normal peers in terms of their parents' responses to the Walker Problem Behavior Identification Checklist. Those with vocal fold nodules rated significantly higher, in particular on the Acting Out scale and as a group were found to be distractible and immature with less stable peer relations.

Special Diagnoses

Advances in neonatal care have resulted in an increase in the number of children who have undergone sometimes numerous, invasive medical procedures at a very young age. It is currently estimated that approximately 12% of babies are born at less than 37 weeks gestation.[6] Although vocal fold nodules are the most common diagnosis for school-age children, very young children presenting with disorders of the laryngeal mechanism are more likely to have subglottic stenosis, laryngomalacia or vocal fold paralysis.[26]

Knowledge of the specific anatomic and physiologic changes caused by these disorders is crucial in evaluating these medically fragile children. Detailed discussions can be found elsewhere in this text.

Considerations for Functional Impairment

Numerous children who are known to have dysphonia do not receive treatment for the disorder. This is often the result of a misunderstanding of or lack of knowledge regarding the long-term consequences of nontreatment. Conversely, parents of children who have struggled with life-threatening airway issues may consider dysphonic voicing to be a minor nuisance in comparison.[2]

Nonetheless, a voice disorder can have a significant impact on a child's ability to participate in daily activities. Ruddy[27] suggests that children with voice disorders may display decreased classroom participation that will negatively impact learning by decreasing their opportunity to benefit from instructor feedback and practice time. Among activities that are potentially negatively impacted by the presence of a voice disorder are peer interaction, teacher evaluation of the student, extracurricular activities (such as music or cheerleading), interviewing, and internship opportunities.[2,27]

Some parents and pediatricians believe that children will grow out of their voice disorder. Instead, a chronic voice disorder may prompt the child to develop maladaptive compensations that become habituated and more difficult to modify as the child grows to adulthood.[27] This is particularly important considering the large number of professions that require high-level spoken communication skills.

THE SPEECH-LANGUAGE PATHOLOGIST'S ROLE IN PEDIATRIC VOICE EVALUATION

Voice evaluations may be done in conjunction with the otolaryngologist, at a specialized clinic, in a hospital, or school setting. Referrals sources include parents, doctors, teachers, and school-based speech-language pathologists. Speech-language pathologists are often called on to address the nonmedical aspects of dysfunctional voice. With a strong background in the anatomy and physiology of the larynx, feeding and swallowing, cognition, and speech, speech-language pathologists are well equipped to assess behavioral issues that may be contributing

to the voice disorder and subsequently establish an effective treatment program targeting these behaviors. The speech-language pathologist's holistic understanding of the communication process and the anatomic and physiologic underpinnings allows him or her to treat the whole child in an integrated manner.

Medically complex children often have a history of emergency surgical intervention to preserve the airway, which by its nature does not consider the functional limitations imposed on the child once healing has taken place. In some cases, the speech-language pathologist may provide education to medical personnel regarding the benefits of speech therapy intervention in establishing a functional voice in the absence of a structurally normal voicing mechanism.

THE EVALUATION PROCESS

Multidisciplinary Teams

The evaluation of a child with a voice disorder is best accomplished in a multidisciplinary team that includes an otolaryngologist, a speech-language pathologist, the child's pediatrician, the child's parents, the school nurse, and perhaps specialists (eg, pulmonologist, gastroenterologist, neurologist, allergist). The speech-language pathologist often serves as the liaison between the parents, the school, and the medical team. Throughout the evaluation process the speech-language pathologist will gather and clinically correlate information from the various medical specialties and communicate this plainly to the parents and school. Important new information gleaned from the interview process may, in turn, be relayed to the physician.

From Recognition to Diagnosis

Recognition of a voice disorder and the need for evaluation may originate from a variety of sources, including the child's parent, pediatrician, teacher, or school-based speech-language pathologist. Once the need for evaluation has been identified, the child's first stop is usually to their pediatrician, who will refer the child to a pediatric otolaryngologist. The otolaryngologist will then refer appropriate children to the speech-language pathologist for evaluation. At this point in the process, evaluations from other specialists, such as allergists or gastroenterologists, will be obtained as necessary.

The Pediatric Voice History

Basic History

Many components of a basic history for pediatric voice disorders are similar to those of the adult case history. These will include details regarding the onset of the dysphonia, the progression of symptoms, variability of voice, typical daily voice activities, psychosocial milieu (who lives at home, sibling structure), medications, allergies, surgical history, medical conditions, and vocal hygiene factors (hydration, vocal misuse, environmental exposure to inhaled irritants such as secondhand smoke, and reflux). Even when the child has had extensive medical intervention, a review of the medical history with the parent is important as it may reveal updated information or information that was previously forgotten by the parent. Table 7–4 presents a detailed review of history elements. Appendix 7 is a sample pediatric case history form.

Cultural considerations regarding family communication and the role of the child in the family and social structure may affect the manner in which evaluation tasks are conducted. Gaining an understanding of these factors prior to or during the initial interview with the child's parent or caregiver will aid in acquiring the most accurate evaluation information possible. Some examples of this may include children who are raised to respond to but not initiate communication with adults or a child in the social service system who lacks trust in the integrity of the intentions of adults.

Unique considerations for the pediatric population include: the details of the child's birth history, general development across domains (physical, cognitive, social/pragmatic, and communication—including articulation, vocabulary development, receptive language, and fluency).

Medically Complex Children

A history of airway complications and congenital conditions or acquired injuries will be particularly important for medically complex children. Examples of medically complex diagnoses include: laryngeal stenosis, papillomatosis, laryngomalacia, laryngeal web, craniofacial syndromes, infantile intubation injuries, vocal fold paralysis, and tracheostomy. A thorough understanding of these pediatric voice etiologies will be important in guiding the direction of your evaluation.

Specific Evaluation Tasks

Children have a shorter attention span than adults and tend to be more distractible. Directing the child in such a way as to collect the voice measures needed can be challenging. In this section, we outline specific voice evaluation tasks that may comprise a

Table 7–4. Pediatric Voice History

Onset	Congenital may include surgery after birth for airway obstruction or a malformation of the anatomy (eg, sulci, web)
	Acquired may include trauma (eg, external injury or intubation), use-related injury (eg, nodules, polyps)
	Was onset sudden or gradual?
	Has the child always been hoarse (eg, even when crying) or did the dysphonia begin with a certain event (medical or circumstantial) or under certain conditions?
Progression of Symptoms	Is the dysphonia progressing from intermittent to constant?
	Is the dysphonia improving overall or becoming worse over time?
Variability of Voice	Are there certain conditions under which the dysphonia worsens (eg, after school, with certain friends, during certain seasons, time of day, after eating certain foods)
Developmental History	Was the child born premature (at how many weeks)? Were there other complications in the birthing process?
	Is the child seeing any other therapists (eg, physical therapist, occupational therapist, psychotherapist)?
Speech-Language History	Are there other speech-language delays (articulation disorder, receptive/expressive language, learning disabilities, global delays)? Is the child dysfluent?
Typical Daily Voice Activities	This question will help the speech-language pathologist to determine not only what behaviors may be maintaining the dysphonia, but what the child's functional needs are in his/her community.
	How often does the child use loud voice, scream, make character voices?
	What are the child's extracurricular activities (eg, sports, acting, singing)?
	Has the child had to stop any activities because of her voice problems?
Psychosocial Milieu	Who lives at home with the child? What communication style is used within the family (eg, constantly talking over each other versus quiet group activities)?
	Is anyone at home hard of hearing?
	How is the child's relationship with their siblings (Is there animosity or competition? Do they fight?)
	Is this child very talkative or does the child have an aggressive personality?
	Does the child have many friends? Is the child left out of group activities with other children due to his/her poor intelligibility or "funny sounding" voice?

Table 7–4. *continued*

Medications	Consider whether or not the child's medications may be impacting the dysphonia (eg, drying medications, medications that affect the child's energy level or affect).
	Special consideration should be given to asthma medications, which may contribute to hoarseness or laryngeal candidiasis.
Allergies	Have the child's allergies been properly diagnosed and treated?
	Is the child a chronic mouth-breather due to allergic congestion?
	Are allergies long-standing or recent?
	Are food allergies present? To what extent are these controlled?
Surgical History	Consider the impact of surgeries such as tracheal or laryngeal reconstruction, cardiac surgery, oromaxillary facial reconstruction.
Other Medical Conditions	These may include developmental disorders, chromosomal disorders, cerebral palsy, apraxia, seizures. These conditions may impact the child's cognitive level and ability to participate in therapy as well as suggest certain modifications that may be necessary to the therapy program.
Vocal Hygiene Factors	How much water does the child drink?
	Does the child have reflux (eg, mini-throw-ups, repeat taste after dinner, soreness in the back of his or her throat)?

typical voice evaluation for a dysphonic child and provide ideas for how to obtain each measure as accurately and quickly as possible.

General Tips

Tips to improve child participation:

1. Do not present yourself too aggressively to younger children. Begin by speaking casually with the parent, addressing the child directly when the child has had the opportunity to adjust to the new environment.

2. As in early intervention, a young child may be more apt to carry out a task when accompanied by a favorite toy. Involve the parents by asking them to bring a favorite toy or book for discussion.

3. Take your time; allow the child to process what is going on.

4. For younger children, provide concrete instructions.

5. Never jump into the task without explaining first.

6. Make use of play in demonstrating the task using a child's favorite toy or puppet first. This may open them to performing the task themselves or engaging in imaginative play, taking on the persona of a puppet. This is often less threatening and more fun.

7. When recording the child, Visi-Pitch can offer a pleasing visual aid in guiding the child through maximum phonation time, pitch glides, and connected speech tasks.

8. Always repeat tasks several times (if possible) as performance may vary greatly.

Oral-Motor Assessment

The oral-motor assessment evaluates the strength, speed, coordination, and range of motion of the oral-facial mechanism as well as to inspect for structural deviations that could be interacting with or exacerbating the child's vocal symptoms. A screening of the cranial nerves, in as far as the child can comply with this, is useful in determining whether the child's voice disorder is related to a more broad reaching neurologic condition.[28] A thorough oral-motor assessment will help to rule out a motor speech disorder such as developmental apraxia of speech or dysarthria. There are three areas of particular interest to this assessment: oral structure, oral movement skills (lips, tongue, jaw), and motor speech function (articulation in single words, connected speech, and diadochokinesis).[29]

It is not uncommon to find that fluency and articulation disorders coincide with a voice disorder.[30] Articulation skills should be screened with regard to age-related articulatory processes and delayed phonological patterns. If one suspects a lingering articulation disorder that is not currently being treated, a quick screening test may be in order, for example the Fluharty preschool speech and language screening test.[31]

Speech Sample and Perceptual Assessment

In this task, we are interested in several domains. These include the child's vocal characteristics, learning style, temperament, motivation, and social interaction with their caregiver.[32] The speech-language pathologist may use a simple GRBAS scale[22] (Grade, Roughness, Breathiness, Asthenia, Strain) or the CAPE-V[23] (Consensus Auditory Perceptual Evaluation of Voice) to rate aspects of the child's voice quality such as roughness, breathiness, strain, phonation breaks and the presence of hard glottal attacks. Also, during this conversational task, one may observe the child's alertness, attention, muscle tone, and overall emotional stability.[32] Difficulty attending, poor emotional stability, and erratic social interaction may be symptomatic of more in-depth behavioral problems that may be driving or adding to the severity of the voice disorder.[25]

One easy way to elicit this task is to observe parent-child interaction during free play. If the child attends the evaluation with a sibling, the speech-language pathologist can document whether sibling relationship factors stimulate more stressful vocal patterns. If the child is reluctant to participate in free play in an unfamiliar environment, a structured activity such as book reading may engage the child in discussion of the characters and story line. Monologue can be encouraged by asking the child to retell the story you have just read. Use of picture description or open-ended questions (best for older children) such as "Tell me what you like to do in the summer time?" may also elicit longer utterances.

Rate of speech may be calculated from the speech sample as a simple count of syllables per minute.

Tension and Breath Patterns

As mentioned previously, children naturally take more frequent breaths with larger rib cage excursion. Nonetheless, truly uncoordinated breathing patterns may still be observed. In particular, one must attend to clavicular breathing, shallow or inadequate breath replenishment, and extraneous muscular effort in the strap muscles of the neck upon inhalation. Respiratory incoordination will impact speech patterns as well, including choppy/short sentences or running out of air at the ends of phrases.

Some of the information you need may be gleaned from parents, who may be important informants in reporting how much the child "works" to phonate at the end of the day and if they push through increasing hoarseness. To directly observe the child's respiratory patterns, you may try having the child count or say the alphabet and measure syllables per breath. Does the child have to push their breath to reach the end of the phrase? Does the child's breath pattern change as the child progresses through the numbers or letters?

Pitch and Volume Range

Pitch and volume measures are important in mapping out the parameters of vocal flexibility. Many times children with voice problems may exhibit increased instability at the extremes of their range where vocal quality is more easily disrupted by changes in biodynamic quality of vocal folds. As pitch and volume are the major building blocks of spoken inflection, vocal inflexibility can negatively impact intelligibility and speech naturalness. Volume irregularities may also be indicative of the state of the vocal folds. For example, some children with voice problems have difficulty producing soft voicing and use increased volume in compensation for poor glottal valving.[14]

As young children do not have an abstract understanding of pitch and volume control, cues to obtain these measures should be concrete and related to sounds with which they are familiar. Modeling and frequent praise for attempts is important in this realm.[33]

Pitch Flexibility. High and low pitch may be obtained with visual aids such as the Visi-Pitch with which the child can use his or her voice to draw a hill on the screen. If you have no access to this type of equip-ment, simpler means may include having the child trace his or her finger up and down a hill on a piece of paper while vocalizing. Moya Andrews[34] uses an image of stairs on which the child can move his or her voice up to the "attic" of a house and then down to the "basement." In addition, she describes using an animal in order to "climb" to the top and bottom of the stairs for maximal high and maximal low pitches.[34]

Volume Flexibility. Volume, like pitch, may be approached through the use of metaphors such as animals. Large animals elicit a louder voice; small animals elicit a softer voice.[35] One may also utilize prompts that elicit naturalistic behavior, such as "a voice you would use in the library" or "the voice you would use on the playground." Cognitive cues[36] like "shhh don't wake the baby" or "hey there!" are another route to naturalistic volume variation.

Inflection. Observation of volume and pitch use during conversation may be revealing as well. Inflection may be assessed during collection of the speech sample.

Maximum Phonation Time

This measure will provide the speech-language pathologist with important information regarding the efficiency of coordination between the respiratory and phonatory systems. Maximum phonation time may be difficult to attain depending on the cognitive level of the child.

A stuffed animal may be used to demonstrate the task, with the child repeating.[34] Tracing the path of an object from start to finish, such as a "walking" stuffed animal or a toy truck or car driving across the floor makes the task request more concrete. Use of an object getting to it's destination, tracing the path of an object from start to finish, or stretching a Slinky across a table or floor all suggest prolongation. As maximum phonation time is an unfamiliar task for most children, multiple trials will lead to more accurate results.

Recording Acoustic and Aerodynamic Measures

When recording acoustic measures, it is ideal to have a headgear-mounted microphone to avoid the effect of body shifting and maintain consistency of mouth to microphone distance. For very young children, use of a table microphone or a lapel microphone allows for gross method of recording the child's voice (but is not sensitive enough for research purposes).

Aerodynamic measures must be collected using a Rothenberg mask. Use of this equipment requires proper sizing. In addition, some children may experience anxiety associated with the placement of the mask and the need to create a seal around the nose and mouth.[37]

Stimulability Tasks

The child's response to stimulability tasks will provide the therapist with information regarding the child's ability to participate in direct therapy methods and which task types elicit the best voicing. Stimulability techniques may focus on decreasing muscular tension, improving airflow, or improving vocal quality. These may include decreasing or increasing rate, increasing attention to resonance, exaggerating articulation, negative practice, or imitation of therapist.[14]

Quality of Life Survey

A Quality of Life (QOL) questionnaire reveals information about the way in which a voice disorder is affecting a patient's life.

It is typically used as a supplementary tool in the context of a complete evaluation. Although several questionnaires have been developed and widely used to measure QOL in adults (Voice Handicap Index,[38] Voice Outcome Survey,[39] Voice-Related Quality of Life[40]), questionnaires for children, in regard to voice, remain somewhat underdeveloped.[41] Each of the adult questionnaires has been modified to address pediatric voice concerns. These include the Pediatric Voice Outcome Survey (PVOS),[42] the Pediatric Voice-Related Quality of Life questionnaire (PV-RQOL),[43] and the pediatric Voice Handicap Index (pVHI).[44]

The PVOS is a 4-item parent-proxy questionnaire that rates the overall severity of the child's speaking voice, level of strain, and limitations faced by the child in social and noisy environments. The PVOS is simple to administer and to complete and sensitive to changes in voice-related quality of life; however, it is thought to be somewhat limited in scope. The PV-RQOL is a 10-item parent-proxy questionnaire that was designed to measure both social-emotional and physical functioning aspects of voice problems. More recently, the pVHI is a 23-item parent proxy questionnaire was developed by Zur et al.[44] This tool focuses on the functional, physical, and emotional impacts of a voice disorder on a child's daily activities. Both the PV-RQOL and the pVHI are broader in scope than the PVOS and therefore thought to be more sensitive to subtle changes in voice QOL over time.

Stroboscopic Examination

Most children being evaluated for a voice disorder will experience some anxiety surrounding the stroboscopic examination. Children with complex medical conditions, in particular, may have a history of invasive and painful procedures. For this reason, the environment in which the stroboscopic examination will be conducted should be calming and the examiner should not appear to be rushed.

The examiner may wish to conduct a brief "show and tell" session with an anxious child, allowing the child to touch the instrument or put it to their tongue in order to acclimate to the feeling and increase the child's feeling of control over the environment. Some children may be motivated by the promise of seeing the photographs after the examination is complete. Younger children may be more comfortable supported on their parent's lap. Regardless of the manner in which the child is prepared for stroboscopy, the examination should be completed as quickly as possible.[14]

Discussion with Parent

Discussion with the parent begins with the initial interview and continues through the review of the findings and generation of the treatment plan.

During the initial interview, the therapist should praise the parent for things they have already done to improve their child's voice, even if those attempts were small or ultimately unhelpful. This establishes an internal locus of control within the family network and encourages the family taking future steps to help the child through the intervention process.

At the completion of the evaluation, the therapist should discuss the plan of intervention and answer any questions. The parent should understand what is happening and why and have the opportunity to participate in the formulation of the treatment plan. Interventions should be discussed in terms of the family's daily life schedule. The therapist may need to help the family problem solve for creation of practice time.

The conclusion of the evaluation may be a good time to introduce simple guidelines for vocal hygiene or to present a "voice tracker" sheet on which they can keep track of potentially harmful vocal behaviors.

CASE STUDIES

Case 1: A Child with Vocal Abuse

Comprehensive History

Emily was a 7–year-old second grader and well adjusted socially and academically. Her mother noted that Emily's voice had been "hoarse and husky" since she was able to talk, but found that in the past 6 to 7 months her voice quality had become much more "gravelly" and hoarse. Symptoms included persistent hoarseness, difficulty getting loud, frequent pitch breaks, frequent voice loss (especially after increased or aggressive voice use or at the end of the day), and vocal fatigue with strain. Additional medical history was significant for Hashimoto's disease (hypothyroidism) and juvenile arthritis.

The otolaryngologic report indicated Emily had a right vocal fold cyst with a left vocal fold reactive nodule. In addition, there were indications of laryngopharyngeal reflux (edema and erythema surrounding the arytenoids). Closure patterns revealed an hourglass shape. Emily had not been sick or suffering from allergies when her voice worsened.

Emily's mother described her as a very loud and verbal child who talked constantly at home and in school. She was the "leader of the pack" often raising her voice to be heard above others and gaining attention through grunting or squealing. Her mother reported that Emily would often yell in anger when fighting with her older sister, yell in excitement when playing with her friends, and engage in a guttural grunting sound when playing or refusing to do something. She noted that by the end of the day, Emily talked in a whisper, or pushed her voice to a much louder volume; "There's no middle ground." Her vocal symptoms were mild to moderately disruptive and lowered her overall intelligibility. When asked, Emily noted that her voice was not a problem; however, her mother found Emily's frequent voice loss to be worrying as people were having more difficulty understanding her. Emily drank 2 to 3 glasses of water per day and had 1 glass of chocolate milk per day.

Speech Sample and Perceptual Measures

During the interview and in spontaneous conversation, Emily was noted to talk relatively fast with a markedly monotone intonation pattern. Her voice was consistently too low for her and nearly all of her phrases ended in vocal fry. Emily's voice quality was noted to be consistently severely hoarse and breathy with frequent voice breaks and delayed voiced onset. Resonance was severely reduced, although during maximum phonation, voice quality was markedly better at the beginning of her production and deteriorated by the end of the tone.

Tension and Breathing Patterns

During conversation and in more structured tasks, Emily appeared to be straining most visibly in her strap muscles and also in her shoulders and jaw. Respiratory behaviors during conversation and reading included shallow, audible, and seemingly effortful inhalation initiated with her chest and shoulders raised. Once having taken a breath,

Emily often spoke too long on one breath, pushing past her resting expiratory level in attempts to force out the rest of the phrase.

Pitch and Volume Range

Emily's pitch was consistently too low for her age and sex. In addition, pitch flexibility or intonation was also noticeably reduced, lending to a monotone pattern which often dropped off into vocal fry. She had difficulty controlling her volume during loud and soft tasks. In loud tasks, voicing was effortful, and often felt uncomfortable to her. In softer tasks, voicing was moderately inconsistent and she had difficulty sustaining easy, soft voicing and frequently vacillated between aphonic intervals and louder abrupt onset phonation.

Acoustic Measures:

1. Pitch Range = 238 to 440 Hz (A#3 – A4 = 11 ST)
2. Loudness Range = 64 to 119 dB SPL
3. Average fundamental frequency (taken on sustained "ah") = 277 Hz
4. Loudness (during reading of Rainbow Passage) = 67 dB SPL
5. Perturbation Measures (taken on sustained "ah"): jitter (1.6%) and shimmer (4.9%)
6. MPT = 4.0

Aerodynamic Measures:

Emily exhibited increased subglottal air pressure in both comfortable and loud phonation (taken with the pneumotachometer using inverse filtering on "pae-pae-pae" repetitions).

Quality of Life Survey

Both Emily and her mother filled out a QOL survey, which revealed a difference in perceived difficulty in the efficiency of voice use. Emily's mother's rating was much higher, indicating more functional limitations; whereas Emily's ratings were low. When this was discussed during the evaluation, both Emily and her mother came to an agreement that her vocal quality was beginning to get in the way of playing with friends and speaking up in class.

Impressions

When taking acoustic measures, an analysis of a sustained "ah" in her speaking pitch revealed increased pitch and volume perturbation (jitter and shimmer %). Her fundamental frequency was too low for her age and sex. Her volume during reading (Rainbow Passage) was slightly above normal dB SPL. Further vocal testing revealed a markedly limited maximum phonation time and pitch range. When asked to sustain the quietest voice possible, Emily had difficulty getting below 64 dB SPL, a volume considered to be more akin to conversational voice.

Emily presents with a typical profile of a patient with a diagnosis of vocal fold masses. Her videoendoscopic evaluation findings of poor vocal fold closure coincides with perceptual measures of increased breathiness and acoustic findings of reduced maximum phonation time. In addition, a large vocal fold cyst, in Emily's case, may explain reduced vocal loudness and pitch dynamics, lowered pitch (due to increased vocal fold mass), and increased hoarseness (which coincides with high perturbation measures of jitter and shimmer).

Trial Therapy

When Emily was asked to breathe easily before each trial of sustained phonation on "ah," her vocal quality became clearer and more resonant, although breathiness was still present. She was then introduced to the concepts of "easy" versus "strained" voicing. Easy voice was characterized as smooth and relaxed with somewhat increased airflow; strained voicing was described as gravelly and tense. Initially, Emily relied on frequent models from the therapist. She quickly identified when the therapist used strained versus easy voicing and benefited from negative practice. This helped her to gain a better understanding of the effects of deliberately increased tension on her own voice quality. Easy voicing was then carried into humming with continued focus on smooth quality and relaxed sense of production. This was initiated with vowels and then slowly carried into *m*-initial words and phrases. Emily was attentive to tasks and noticed the difference in levels of effort when using an easy voice versus strained. Emily's "smooth" voice revealed reduced vocal strain and increased breathiness.

Treatment Plan

Emily was referred for voice therapy in order to decrease vocal strain and improve vocal function. Although surgical excision would be an appropriate option for an adult presenting with Emily's profile, a child of this age cannot be expected to maintain absolute voice rest throughout the post-surgical period. Due to the danger of scarring associated with noncompliance with postsurgical voice rest, this option will have to be postponed until Emily reaches a more mature age.

Case 2: A Child with a History of Intubation

Comprehensive History:

Jeff was a 3½-year-old boy with a history of premature birth followed by several weeks of intubation. He had a history of pulmonary compromise as well as laryngomalacia. He had global delays in expressive and receptive language and fine and gross motor skills. Jeff had received early intervention and at that time was noted to have a pronounced raspy voice quality to his cry which became more noticeable when he began talking.

Jeff was seen by a pediatric otolaryngologist who performed a brochoscopy with examination of his vocal folds. This examination revealed marked bilateral vocal fold sulci. Closure and mucosal wave could not be evaluated due to the nature of bronchoscopy (Jeff was under general anesthesia).

His mother complained that friends and family found his speech to be extremely difficult to understand and complained of a low-pitched, gravelly, "froggy" voice quality when Jeff became excited or during play. She reported that when Jeff was more relaxed, or when singing, his voice was much higher and softer. This contrast was also noted by his preschool teachers.

Speech Sample and Perceptual Evaluation

Jeff's vocal quality was severely hoarse, breathy, and strained with frequent periods of an abnormally low-pitched, monotone, rough voice quality. Notably, there were moments of voicing that revealed increased breathiness, reduced volume, and a higher pitch more appropriate to a boy his age and size. This was also apparent when he sang a song with his mother.

Tension and Breath Patterns

Visible strain was noted in his upper torso and in the strap muscles of his neck during all voicing tasks. This was much more prominent during loud voicing or when Jeff became excited. Breathing patterns included shallow breathing. Utterances were relatively short during the evaluation, therefore true documentation of breathing during longer phrases was not available. By parent report, his breathing was more labored when excited.

Pitch and Volume Range

During conversational speech, volume was either extremely loud or too soft. Observation of pitch control revealed a somewhat high, soft quality of voice during relaxed moments of speech and abnormally low speech when excited. During the course of a conversation with his mother, pitch and volume were highly variable depending on context and subject matter.

Acoustic Measures

1. Pitch Range = unattainable due to poor participation
2. Loudness Range = unattainable due to poor participation
3. Average fundamental frequency (taken on sustained "ah") = 168 Hz
4. Perturbation Measures (taken on sustained "ah"): jitter (0.73%) and shimmer (7.74%)
5. MPT = 5.3
6. s/z ratio = 0.78

Aerodynamic Measures

Aerodynamics taken with the Rothenberg mask were unachievable due to Jeff's increased activity levels and cognitive level.

Quality of Life Survey

A parent-proxy QOL questionnaire revealed considerable limitations at home and during preschool. Jeff's preschool teacher found it difficult to understand him and interaction with other children was also limited given his low intelligibility. In addition, Jeff was becoming aware of his voice limitations. He was starting to display behavioral indicators of frustration at his inability to be understood by other children, teachers, and family members. His mother became visibly upset when describing the fact that other children often avoided playing with him due to his voice quality and the way in which he became frustrated during communicative exchanges to the point where he simply abandoned the attempt.

Impressions

Pitch and volume control was poor, which contributed to low intelligibility. Articulation delays added to this. Acoustic measures revealed extremely high measures of shimmer and jitter and abnormally low fundamental frequency. Perceptual assessment revealed severely limited frequency and intensity range. Acoustic measures coincided well with perceptual measures and further defined the severity of Jeff's dysphonia.

Jeff's use of false vocal fold vibration as a vocal quality when excited is not uncommon in children who have significant difficulty achieving vocal fold closure prior to language development. It is a strong compensatory strategy used to effectively access increased volume. True vocal fold vibration, in this case, would only yield a soft, breathy vocal quality. In Jeff's case, the use of false vocal fold vibration correlates with perceptual measures of abnormally low, hoarse, monotone, and strained vocal quality. Moments of higher pitch and breathy, weak vocal quality is likely the result of true vocal fold vibration, but may have been too weak for his functional environment. The poor closure pattern created by the bilateral vocal fold sulci would encourage the use of false vocal fold phonation to solve this problem.

Trial Therapy

Trial therapy revealed a higher more stable sound quality with inhalation phonation and increased involvement in therapy activities using musical instruments. For example, when Jeff sang songs with slower rhythms while beating on a drum, his voice quality became more stable.

Treatment Plan

Young children under the age of 5 are best involved in therapy using child-directed techniques as well as implementing small changes in daily routines and places. It was clear that in trial therapy, Jeff had a propensity for playing musical instruments and singing. This was used as the basis for further exploration and treatment at home. Jeff was already receiving speech therapy services for delayed articulation. A phone conference with the voice specialist and the current therapist was planned for integrating several voice activities (musical in nature) into his regular therapy sessions. The goals were to begin increasing Jeff's vocal repertoire and comfort with adapting to different vocal pitches using the easier, but slightly softer voice. With continued focus on building coordination between respiration, phonation, and resonance, overall vocal strength should continue to grow.

Case 3: The Medically Complex Child

Comprehensive History

Molly was a 10-year-old girl with a medically complex background. She was born 3 months premature. Seven chest tubes were placed at birth and she underwent numerous surgical procedures for airway compromise (including laryngomalacia and subglottic stenosis). Laryngeal surgeries included an initial tracheotomy (in infancy) and laryngeal reconstruction using a rib graft at 5 years of age, which resulted in granulation tissue formation. She underwent a revision laryngeal reconstruction with tracheotomy and an arytenoid trim several months later as a result of these complications. One year later, she underwent tube placement (airway stent) to maintain airway patency.

Molly had been diagnosed with reflux and was put on a trial of Protonix in the past which did not appear to be helpful (as per Molly's mom). Additional medical history includes adenoidectomy and tonsillectomy. Molly had significant global delays including fine and gross motor development and language and articulation (verbal apraxia). She was receiving speech-language services at school 4 times per week in addition to occupational and physical therapy. A recent stroboscopic examination revealed bilateral vocal fold scarring, limited motion of the left arytenoid cartilage, and severe supraglottal constriction during phonation, which limited visualization of vocal fold vibratory characteristics.

Perceptual Assessment and Speech Sample

Voicing during conversation was noted to be severely hoarse, harsh, gravelly, and raspy in quality. Frequent aphonic breaks, low volume, and frequent use of inhalation false vocal fold phonation were also noted. Voice quality during inhalation phonation was predominantly low pitched and somewhat louder, causing erratic shifts in volume and pitch. In turn, this disrupted articulation and intelligibility. Articulation revealed backed consonants and stopping of sibilants. Overall speech intelligibility was extremely poor.

Tension and Breath Patterns

Respiration was uncoordinated, extremely effortful, audible, and shallow. Visibly low tone was noted in Molly's torso. Respiration patterns during conversation revealed poor breath replenishment with use of inhalation phonation with engagement of the false vocal folds during conversation. Phrase length was particularly long, because Molly used a strategy of inhalation phonation to continue voicing after her breath was depleted. Visible tension sites were noted in the jaw, neck, shoulders, and chest.

Pitch and Volume Range

During spontaneous speech and structured speech tasks, pitch was noted to be consistently too low for Molly's age and size. Pitch variation during speech was also noted to be severely restricted leading to a monotone quality. Volume range was reduced. Although she could attain softer and louder voicing, keeping volume stable for longer than several seconds was difficult.

Acoustic Measures

1. Pitch Range = 149 to 246 Hz (D3 – B3 = 9 ST)
2. Loudness Range = 48 to 97 dB SPL
3. Average fundamental frequency (taken on sustained "ah") = 182 Hz
4. Loudness (during reading of Rainbow Passage) = 51 dB SPL
5. Perturbation Measures (taken on sustained "ah"): jitter (20%) and shimmer (21%)
6. MPT = 5.0

Aerodynamic Measures

Molly demonstrated extremely high airflow and subglottal pressure at both conversational and loud phonation.

Quality of Life Survey

A QOL questionnaire revealed difficulty academically and socially. In school, teachers had difficulty understanding her and she was often reluctant to participate in class. She was required to use an amplifier in the classroom to be heard. In addition, she had limited interaction with her peers during play and in the classroom due to poor intelligibility. Molly was showing signs of embarrassment and social stigma due to the sound of her voice.

Impressions

Respiratory and phonatory coordination was disrupted in several ways; vocal fold closure was inadequate, and expiratory pressure was not sufficient to meet the needs of vocal fold vibration. The use of inhalation phonation in children who are status postlaryngotracheal reconstruction has been documented several times in the literature.[1,2] Molly's weak inspiration was insufficient to generate enough force on exhalation to meet the needs of phonation, particularly in the context of having such a stiff vocal mechanism. Therefore, she used her false vocal folds in the context of inhalation phonation to generate greater volume during conversation.

Trial Therapy

In Molly's case, inhalation phonation engaged false vocal fold phonation instead of true vocal fold phonation. This resulted in an extremely low, hoarse voice quality that did not match Molly's age and gender. Intelligibility was significantly negatively impacted by intermittent inhalation phonation, which also appeared to affect articulation. Molly demonstrated little ability to generate the oral pressure needed for plosives and many of her forward consonants were backed. Abdominal effort released false vocal fold tension, but resulted in weak voice production due to Molly's low muscle tone. A combination of louder volume and increased abdominal support was slightly easier for Molly to manage and resulted in a consistent voice. Negative practice was employed to help Molly distinguish between inhalation phonation and exhalation phonation.

Treatment Plan

Molly was referred for voice therapy in order to improve her overall intelligibility and voice quality to better match her age and sex. Given that trial therapy revealed a more appropriate vocal quality with exhaled phonation, a treatment program designed to strengthen respiratory and phonatory coordination and improve articulation was implemented. Respiratory strength was addressed by starting Molly on a resistance training program based on the Expiratory Muscle Strength Training program (EMST) developed by Christine Sapienza, Ph.D. Articulation exercises were geared towards increasing Molly's overall attention to plosives and oral movements.

Case 4: The Child with Laryngeal Candidiasis

Comprehensive History

Gary is a 10-year-old boy who complained of chronic hoarseness, lowered pitch, decreased volume, decreased stamina, frequent coughing, and throat clearing. Gary had a long-standing chronic cough. He was diagnosed with asthma the year before and placed on Advair. His mother noted that Gary's voice symptoms began 4 to 5 months previous to his voice evaluation and 2 weeks after starting Singulair. Medical history was otherwise unremarkable.

A stroboscopic examination revealed bilateral nodules on the mid-third of the vocal folds, bilateral medial surface scarring, bilateral medial and superior surface varices, bilateral erythema, laryngopharyngeal reflux, periarytenoid and posterior cricoid edema, and vocal hyperfunction. Results were consistent with a probable fungal infection. During the evaluation, Gary reported that his voice was slowly improving since starting to take Fluconozol and Zantac, and initiating behavioral and dietary precautions for reflux.

Gary and his parents denied any vocally abusive activities (screaming/yelling, incessant talking, creating guttural sounds). Due to his dysphonia, Gary stopped singing in the school choir and at home on the recommendation of his choir teacher. He felt it strained his voice to sing for even short periods of time.

Perceptual Assessment and Speech Sample

Gary was consistently severely hoarse and strained; consistently moderately breathy with intermittent throat clearing, and pitch and phonation breaks. Vocal pitch was adequate, however, vocal loudness was intermittently too soft. He also exhibited consistently severely decreased oral resonance.

Tension and Breath Patterns

Gary demonstrated shallow breath replenishment with increased visible tension noted in the shoulders, chest, neck, and jaw. Respiratory coordination was noted to be poor with occasional audible inspiration.

Pitch and Volume Range

These measures were within normal limits with the exception of quiet voicing. This would be expected, given the edema and erythema noted on examination.

Acoustic Measurements

1. Pitch Range = 171 to 617 Hz (F3 – D#5 = 22 ST)
2. Loudness Range = 65 to 94 dB SPL
3. Average fundamental frequency (taken on sustained "ah") = 243 Hz
4. Loudness (during reading of Rainbow Passage) = 67 dB SPL
5. Perturbation Measures (taken on sustained "ah"): jitter (1.8%) and shimmer (6.3%)
6. MPT = 12.0

Aerodynamic Measurements

Increased airflow, and increased subglottal pressure for both conversational and loud voicing.

Quality of Life Survey

Gary was unable to sing with ease; he felt extremely frustrated by his vocal quality and restricted volume range (especially when playing sports or with his friends).

Impressions

Gary was a typically developing child with no history of voice problems prior to this most recent incident. A fungal infection brings about increased edema and erythema of the vocal fold tissue. This leaves the phonatory system much more susceptible to vocal fold injury with use. Gary became increasingly dysphonic as his laryngeal infection progressed. As a result of the vocal fold changes caused by the infection, there was greater pressure required to initiate phonation, which resulted in a change in his voicing patterns for both speech and singing.

Trial Therapy

Increased attention to oral resonance through sustained hums with decreased tension during production, resulted in improved voice quality. Carryover into words and phrases revealed decreased breathiness and hoarseness, and diminished laryngeal strain (as evidenced by decreased visible tension). Gary was quick to learn therapy techniques and found his resonant voice to be much easier to use.

Treatment Plan

Continue using resonance-based therapy techniques in order to reduce compensatory behaviors and restore vocal function.

CONCLUSION

Evaluation of pediatric voice disorders is complicated by the vast physical and cognitive differences between children and adults. The majority of research on voice disorders to date has been conducted on adults and is not necessarily applicable to the pediatric population. Special considerations regarding the high survival rate of premature babies and the multiple airway issues that can present also require specialized knowledge. A thorough pediatric voice evaluation may involve input from multiple medical specialties, the child's parents, and school personnel. Evaluation tasks will be similar to those

presented in an adult evaluation; however, they may need to be adapted to the needs of various age groups. At times some measures may be unattainable. The therapy plan is a natural progression from the observations made during the evaluation and will be tailored to each child's specific needs.

REFERENCES

1. Smith ME, Marsh JH, Cotton RT, Myer CM, 3rd. Voice problems after pediatric laryngotracheal reconstruction: videolaryngostroboscopic, acoustic, and perceptual assessment. *Int J Ped Otorhinolaryngol.* 1993; 25(1-3):173-181.

2. Baker S, Kelchner L, Weinrich B, et al. Pediatric laryngotracheal stenosis and airway reconstruction: a review of voice outcomes, assessment, and treatment issues. *J Voice.* 2006;20(4):631-641.

3. Harvey GL. Treatment of voice disorders in medically complex children. *Lang Speech Hearing Serv Schools.* 1994;27:282-291.

4. Gray SD, Smith ME, Schneider H. Voice disorders in children. *Ped Clin North Am.* 1996;43(6):1357-1384.

5. Carding PN, Roulstone S, Northstone K, Team AS. The prevalence of childhood dysphonia: a cross-sectional study. *J Voice.* 2006;20(4):623-630.

6. Lee L, Stemple, JC, Glaze, L, Kelchner, LN. Quick screen for voice and supplementary documents for identifying pediatric voice disorders. *Lang Speech Hear Serv Schools.* 2004;35:308-319.

7. Leeper L. Diagnostic examination of children with voice disorders: a low-cost solution. *Lang Speech Hear Serv Schools.* 1992;23: 353-360.

8. Akif Kilic M, Okur E, Yildirim I, Guzelsoy S. The prevalence of vocal fold nodules in school age children. *Int J Ped Otorhinolaryngol.* 2004;68(4):409-412.

9. McKinnon DHM, Reilly S. The prevalence of stuttering, voice, and speech-sound disorders in primary school students in Australia. *Lang Speech Hear Serv Schools.* 2007;38:5–15.

10. Powell M, Filter MD, Williams B. A longitudinal study of the prevalence of voice disorders in children from a rural school division. *J Comm Dis.* 1989;22(5):375–382.

11. Roy N, Bless DM. Personality traits and psychological factors in voice pathology: a foundation for future research. *J Speech, Lang Hear Res.* 2000;43(3):737–748.

12. St. Louis KO, Hansen GR, Buch JL, Oliver TL. Voice deviations in coexisting communication disorders. *Lang Speech Hear Serv Schools.* 1992;23:82–87.

13. Smith ME, Gray SD. Developmental laryngeal and phonatory anatomy and physiology. *Perspect Voice Voice Dis.* 2002;12.

14. Hersan R, Behlau M. Behavioral management of pediatric dysphonia. *Otolaryngol Clin North Am.* 2000;33(5):1097–1110.

15. Sapienza CM, Ruddy BH, Baker S. Laryngeal structure and function in the pediatric larynx: clinical applications. *Lang Speech Hear Serv Schools.* 2004;35:299–307.

16. Elluru RG. Reconstruction techniques for the treatment of anatomical upper respiratory tract anomolies in children. *Perspect Voice Voice Dis.* 2006;15(3):3–10.

17. Shrivastav R. Acoustic analysis of children's voices. *Perspect Voice Voice Dis.* 2002;12(1):11–12.

18. Campisi P, Tewfik TL, Manoukian JJ, Schloss MD, Pelland-Blais E, Sadeghi N. Computer-assisted voice analysis: establishing a pediatric database. *Arch Otolaryngol Head Neck Surg.* 2002;128(2):156–160.

19. Boltezar IH, Burger ZR, Zargi M. Instability of voice in adolescence: pathologic condition or normal developmental variation? *J Pediatr.* 1997;130(2):185–190.

20. Stathopoulos ET. Consideration of children's voices: understanding age-related processes. *Perspect Voice Voice Dis.* 2002;12(1):8–10.

21. Stathopoulos ET, Sapienza C. Respiratory and laryngeal measures of children during vocal intensity variation. *J Acoust Soc Am.* 1993;94(5):2531–2543.

22. Hirano M. *Clinical Examination of Voice.* New York, NY: Springer-Verlag Wein; 1981.

23. Association TAS-L-H. *Consensus Auditory-Perceptual Evaluation of Voice.* Retrieved May 14, 2007 from: http://www.asha.org/NR/rdonlyres/79EE699E-DAEE-4E2C-A69E-C11BDE6B1D67/_0/CAPEVform.pdf .

24. Andrews M. *Voice Therapy for Children.* San Diego,Calif: Singular Publishing Group 1986.

25. Green G. Psycho-behavioral characteristics of children with vocal nodules: WPBIC ratings. *J Speech Hear Dis.* 1989;54(3):306–312.

26. Saniga RD, Carlin MF. Vocal abuse behaviors in young children. *Lang Speech Hear Serv Schools.* 1993;24:79–83.

27. Ruddy BH, Sapienza CM. Treating voice disorders in the school-based setting: working within the framework of IDEA. *Lang Speech Hear Serv Schools.* 2004;35:327–332.

28. Witzel MA, Riski J. *The Oral Mechanism Examination for Children and Young Adults: Craniofacial and Oral Evaluation.* Rockland, MD: American Speech-Language Hearing Association. 2003.

29. McCauley R, Strand E. Assessment of children's oral and speech motor skills: a review. Retrieved March 4, 2007 from: http://www.asha.org/NR/rdonlyres/48052BC4-6AC7-4BD6-82AF-0899858D4F90/_0/985Handout.ppt .

30. McAllister A. Voice disorders in children with oral motor dysfunction: perceptual evaluation pre and post oral motor therapy. *Logo Phoniatri Vocolo.* 2003;28(3):117–125.

31. Fluharty NB. *Fluharty-2 Preschool Speech and Language Screening Test.* Austin, Tex: Pro-Ed; 2001.

32. Batshaw ML. *Children with Disabilities.* 5th ed. Baltimore, Md: Paul H. Brookes Publishing Co. 1997.

33. Verdolini K. *Pediatric LMRVT.* Paper presented at: Pittsburgh Voice Conference, 2006; Pittsburgh, Pa.

34. Andrews M. *Voice Treatment for Children and Adolescents.* 2nd ed. San Diego, Calif: Singular Thompson Learning; 2002.

35. Champley EH, Adrews ML. The elicitation of vocal responses from preschool children. *Lang Speech Hear Serv Schools.* 1993;24:146-150.

36. Bohnenkamp TA, Andrews M, Shrivastav R, Summers A. Changes in children's voices: the effect of cognitive cues. *J Voice.* 2002;16(4):530-543.

37. Shrivastav R. Acoustic analysis of children's voices. *Perspect Voice Voice Dis.* 2002;12(1):11-12.

38. Jacobson BH, Johnson A, Grywalski C, et al. The Voice Handicap Index (VHI): development and validation. *Am J Speech-Lang Pathol.* 1997;6:66-70.

39. Gliklich RE, Glovsky RM, Montgomery, WW. Validation of a voice outcome survey for unilateral vocal cord paralysis. *Otolaryngol Head Neck Surg.* 1999;120(2):153-158.

40. Hogikyan ND, Sethuraman G. Validation of an instrument to measure voice-related quality of life (V-RQOL). *J Voice.* 1999;13(4):557-569.

41. Zur KB, Cotton S, Kelchner L, Baker S, Weinrich B, Lee L. Pediatric Voice Handicap Index (pVHI): a new tool for evaluating pediatric dysphonia. *Int J Pediatr Otorhinolaryngol.* 2007;71(1):77-82.

42. Hartnick CJ. Validation of a pediatric voice quality-of-life instrument: the pediatric voice outcome survey. *Arch Otolaryngol Head Neck Surg.* 2002;128(8):919-922.

43. Boseley ME, Cunningham MJ, Volk MS, Hartnick CJ. Validation of the Pediatric Voice-Related Quality-of-Life survey. *Arch Otolaryngol Head Neck Surg.* 2006;132(7):717-720.

44. Zur KB, Cotton S, Kelchner L, Baker S, Weinrich B, Lee L. Pediatric Voice Handicap Index (pVHI): a new tool for evaluating pediatric dysphonia. *Int J Ped Otorhinolaryngol.* 2007;71(1):77-82.

45. Fairbanks G, Wiley JH, Lassman FM. An acoustical study of vocal pitch in seven- and eight-year-old boys. *Child Develop.* 1949;20(2):63-69.

46. Bennet S. A 3-year longitudinal study of school-aged children's fundamental frequencies. *J Speech Hear Res.* 1983;26:137-142.

47. Horii Y. Automatic analysis of voice fundamental frequency and intensity using a VisiPitch. *J Speech Hear Res.* 1983;25:467-471.

48. Eguchi S, Hirsh IJ. Development of speech sounds in children. *Acta Oto Laryngolo Suppl.* 1969;257:1-51.

49. Finnegan DE. Maximum phonation time for children with normal voices. *Folia Phoniatr.* 1985;37:209-215.

50. Weinrich B, Salz B, Hughes M. Aerodynamic measurements: normative data for children ages 6:0 to 10:11 years. *J Voice.* 2006;19(3):326-329.

APPENDIX 7

Pediatric Case History Form

Date: _____ Person filling out this form (include relation): _____

Patient Name: _____ Date of Birth: _____ Sex: M F
            First   M. I.   Last

Address:

Contact #: Home (____)_____   Work (____)_____

          E-mail: _____

School and Grade: _____

Background Information

1. Briefly describe your child's voice problem and what you believe is its cause:

2. When was the voice problem first noticed? Was it sudden or gradual?

3. Describe any events or conditions which you associate with the onset of the problem (eg, cold, increased voice use, yelling, injury)?

4. Over time, has the problem changed (eg, better, worse, stayed the same)?

5. Has your child had voice problems in the past?

6. Does someone else in your family have a similar problem? If so, who?

7. Is your child's voice worse during certain seasons? Or at a certain time of day (eg, upon awakening, after school)

8. Are there any situations in which your child's voice is better or seems to improve?

9. **Vocal Symptoms (check all that apply)**
   _____ **NONE**
   _____ hoarse voice quality   _____ effortful/strained speaking
   _____ raspy/scratchy voice quality _____ voice tires easily
   _____ weak/breathy voice quality   _____ nasal voice quality
   _____ voice too low   _____ stuffed nose quality
   _____ voice too high   _____ trouble speaking loud or soft
   _____ other: _____

10. Voice Use: Does your child engage in these behaviors?

Screaming/yelling (in anger):	Rarely	Sometimes	Constantly
Yelling/Cheering (sports, games, play):	Rarely	Sometimes	Constantly
Talking loudly:	Rarely	Sometimes	Constantly
Talking over noise:	Rarely	Sometimes	Constantly
Aggressive crying/Tantrums:	Rarely	Sometimes	Constantly
Coughing:	Rarely	Sometimes	Constantly
Throat clearing:	Rarely	Sometimes	Constantly
Singing:	Rarely	Sometimes	Constantly
Talking on the phone or cell:	Rarely	Sometimes	Constantly
Making noises during play (animals, cars):	Rarely	Sometimes	Constantly

11. Has your child ever received voice therapy? If so, please list when, where, and for how long.

Other Symptoms/Circumstances

12. Check the following symptoms or circumstances that apply to your child:

_____ **NONE**
_____ frequent sore throats   _____ hoarseness first thing in the morning
_____ chronic cough/throat clearing _____ night coughing that interrupts sleep
_____ bad breath/"smelly" burps   _____ regurgitation or "mini throw-ups"
_____ antacid use   _____ anxiety/depression
_____ other (specify: _____)

13. Does your child frequently eat or drink:

_____ Sweets/candy
_____ Orange juice/lemonade
_____ Very spicy foods
_____ Heavily fried foods
_____ Large meals
_____ Late at night
_____ On the run

14. Estimate the combined daily servings of: water _____ soda _____ chocolate _____ coffee/tea _____

Medical History

15. Please check any medical conditions:

_____ **NONE**
_____ Gastroesophageal reflux   _____ Ear infections
_____ Bronchitis/pneumonia   _____ Diabetes
_____ Asthma   _____ Seizures
_____ Sinus problems   _____ Cancer
_____ Cleft palate   _____ Tracheostoma (when: _____)
_____ ADD and/or Hyperactivity   _____ Injury to head/neck/chest
_____ Medically diagnosed
      depression/anxiety

16. Please list any surgical or medical procedures your child has had (include date and place performed)

17. Please list all medications (prescription and over-the-counter) that your child has taken or is currently taking:

18. List all allergies (eg, dust, animals, foods, medications) and include treatments:

19. Does your child have any diagnosed speech-language learning difficulties?

20. Does your child receive therapeutic/education services? If so list type of therapy and frequency:

Laryngeal Electromyography in Pediatric Patients

Al Hillel

The understanding of laryngeal disorders has been greatly advanced in recent years with the increasing use of laryngeal electromyography (LEMG). LEMG is the only test that can define the underlying neurophysiology of abnormal laryngeal function. Although vocal fold mobility can be assessed and described by video studies, paralysis and paresis can only be assessed by LEMG.

In the adult population diagnostic LEMG can be performed in almost all patients. Limited topical anesthetic, or even no anesthetic, is required. No sedation is needed. Patients are asked to perform various tasks during LEMG, and the patient's ability to cooperate with the examiner greatly enhances the quality of the information acquired during testing. A detailed LEMG can provide information about the degree of injury, the age of injury, the ongoing or stable nature of an injury, and the prognosis for recovery. The ability of a patient to tolerate needle insertion quietly and to perform various tasks when requested are both necessary requirements for a thorough LEMG study.

The pediatric population presents unique challenges for the laryngeal electromyographer. Children are generally frightened of needles, do not tolerate painful tests, and often are limited in their ability to cooperate with test procedures, especially if they are uncomfortable and performed by an unfamiliar adult.

This chapter attempts to address the complexities of LEMG in children. A brief description of LEMG is presented in order to outline the procedure as well as the patient tasks required.

LEMG

Electromyography is the study of the electrical activity of muscles. Based on the results of the recordings, many aspects of the condition of the muscle and the motor nerve can be deduced. Three general types of electromyography are commonly used.

Diagnostic electromyography closely examines the types of electrical waveforms while the muscle is at rest, mildly contracting, and maximally contracting.[1-4] Fine wire EMG uses indwelling hooked-wire electrodes to examine many muscles simultaneously to determine the degree and timing of participation of each muscle during a specific task.[5,6] Repetitive stimulation and nerve conduction velocity tests record the electrical activity in the muscle when the motor nerve is triggered by a nerve stimulator.[7,8]

To achieve accurate and in-depth results, all types of electromyography require the skills of an experienced electromyographer and, with laryngeal electromyography, require the skills of an otolaryngologist comfortable with laryngeal anatomy and management of airway issues. It is most important to understand that electromyography and, in particular, LEMG, is most effective when the clinical information from a thorough evaluation and exam is well known to both the electromyographer and otolaryngologist. It is a fallacy to regard electromyography as simply an isolated "test" that can report "test results."

Conceptually, LEMG should be considered an examination rather than a prescribed procedure.[9] A chest radiograph is a fairly standard procedure with an expected "product" that can be interpreted by standard criteria. However, with an ultrasound examination, the examiner needs to know what he is looking for, and needs to conduct the test until a result can be seen and interpreted. In this analogy, LEMG is closer to ultrasound. When the examiners know the clinical history and know what they are looking for, they can then examine the patient with EMG and can continue the testing until results are obtained. Also, the examiners have the option of changing test techniques as the testing proceeds.

Generally, the most useful type of electromyography in laryngeal evaluation is diagnostic EMG. Diagnostic EMG is usually performed with an insulated monopolar electrode that allows the examiner to search for the muscle by directing the needle. The position of the needle in the muscle can often be confirmed by a simple vocal task (confirmation test).[10] Once the needle is in the muscle, the examiner can sample multiple sites to look for the presence of a variety of waveforms.

A complete presentation of the possible findings with diagnostic EMG is not the purpose of this chapter, but a brief description of the terminology and of the types of results found with LEMG serves as a guide to some of the following discussions.

When the needle is inserted in a muscle at rest, it usually stimulates the motor units to fire briefly. The presence of this "insertional activity" is a sign that muscle fibers are present. The degree of the insertional activity is a clue about the state of the muscle. If there is brisk insertional activity, then one can assume that there is little fibrosis, and if further testing reveals no voluntary or stimulable activity, then this muscle might be a good candidate for reinnervation. If there is minimal or no insertional activity, then the muscle might be completely fibrosed. Insertional activity should be seen as a clue, and is one of the findings that can help develop an interpretation of LEMG.

With the needle in place in the muscle, the patient is instructed in a task to activate the muscle (generally an "eee" or a "sniff"). This response is called voluntary recruitment and is a sign of how well the patient can control the activity of the muscle. The pattern of voluntary recruitment can also give an indication whether the deficit is due to a peripheral nerve injury or a central nervous system process. The timing of the recruitment during a variety of tasks can also provide clues regarding the presence of synkinesis that can sometimes present as immobility on fiberoptic laryngoscopy.

With the muscle at rest, the needle is moved slowly through the muscle looking for diagnostic waveforms or motor unit action potentials (MUAPs). During voluntary recruitment, the MUAPs are also examined, and most EMG machines are able to capture individual motor units during the test. The types of MUAPs found offer clues about the age of a nerve injury, the maturity of the injury, whether the injury is ongoing, stable or recovering, and a general prognosis for further recovery.

The clinical interpretation with LEMG is based on the "normal" MUAP (Fig 8-1)

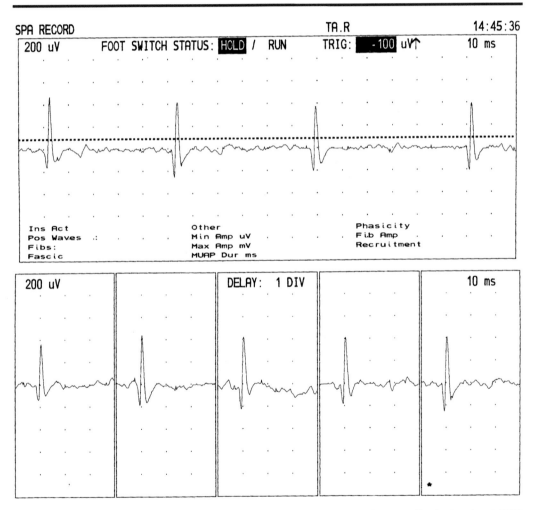

Fig 8–1. A normal motor unit from the TA muscle. Note that the amplitude is about 700 millivolts (200 mV/division) and the duration is about 7 milliseconds (10 ms/division).

which is the electrical signal generated by the muscle fibers controlled by one nerve fiber. A fibrillation potential (Fig 8–2) is a sign of ongoing denervation whereas a polyphasic potential (Fig 8–3) is a sign of ongoing regeneration. A large MUAP (Fig 8–4) is a matured polyphasic potential and signifies an older peripheral nerve injury that is now stable. When the patient is asked to phonate (voluntary recruitment), a full pat-

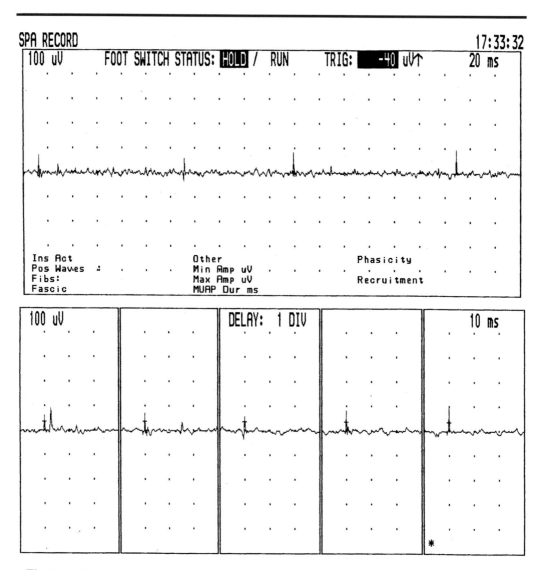

Fig 8–2. Fibrillations potentials. Note that the duration of this waveform is about 1 ms.

tern with many MUAPs is seen (Fig 8-5). The finding of few MUAPs firing fast (Fig 8-6) suggests that very few MUAPs are present and that they are being driven by the central nervous system to compensate by firing quickly. The presence of many MUAPs firing slowly (Fig 8-7) indicates that the initiating signal is at a deficit and is a sign of a central nervous system disorder.

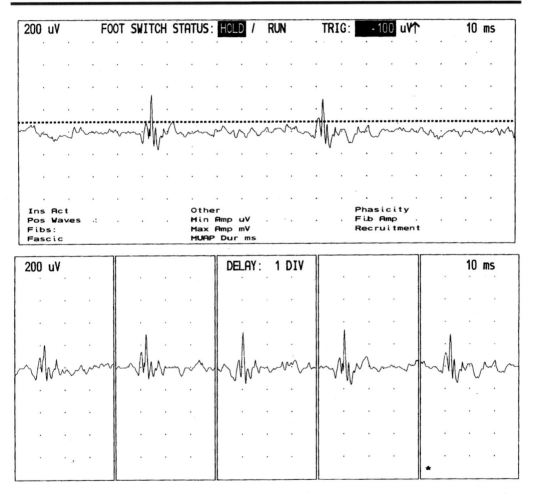

Fig 8–3. Polyphasic potentials. Note that there are at least 5 "turns" in the tracing, and that the duration is prolonged at about 12 ms.

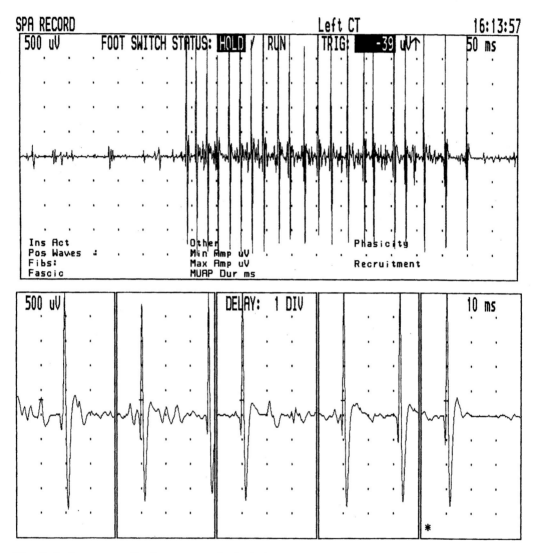

Fig 8–4. Large amplitude motor unit depicting an old but stable peripheral nerve injury. The amplitude is about 4 mV (200 mV/division) with under 2 mV being the normal range. Note that the waveform is triphasic and that the duration of the waveform is about 7 ms.

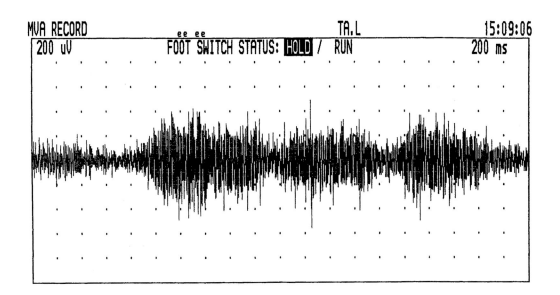

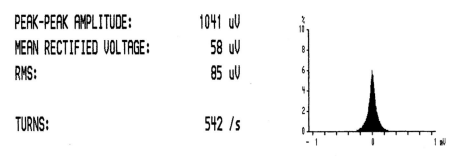

Fig 8–5. Normal recruitment pattern during the phonation task of "eee,eee,eee" (/i,i,i/). Note the dense recruitment representing the firing of many motor units.

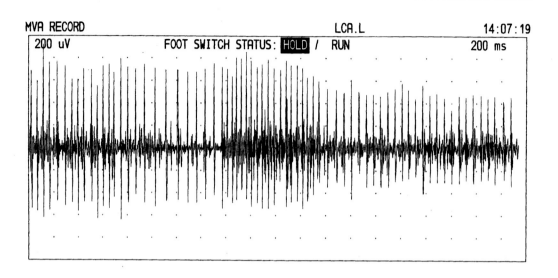

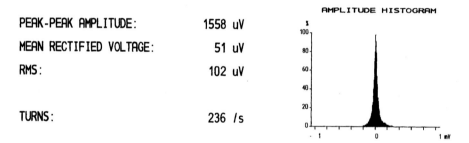

PEAK-PEAK AMPLITUDE:	1558 uV
MEAN RECTIFIED VOLTAGE:	51 uV
RMS:	102 uV
TURNS:	236 /s

Fig 8–6. Few motor units firing fast indicating evidence of a peripheral nerve injury. Note that the recruitment pattern is less dense than in Figure 8–5. Also note that in contrast to Figure 8–5, individual motor units can be seen and are repetitive at a rate indicating fast firing. This condition is known as "few motor units firing fast."

CLINICAL INTERPRETATION OF LEMG

LEMG, as previously mentioned, is most useful when used with clinical history and physical examination. In many cases, LEMG can confirm a suspected diagnosis. In other cases, it can help the clinician decide among a number of reasonable treatment options. In some cases, the LEMG can be very direc- tive toward a clinical treatment pathway. Many of the benefits of LEMG are seen primarily in adults who can undergo a test while awake that allows an in-depth examination. These benefits are often less clear in the pediatric population due to the limitations of testing awake children.

The most classic use of LEMG is in the evaluation of unilateral vocal cord immobility.[11,12] Generally, the timing of the LEMG is just prior to intervention. If the clinical

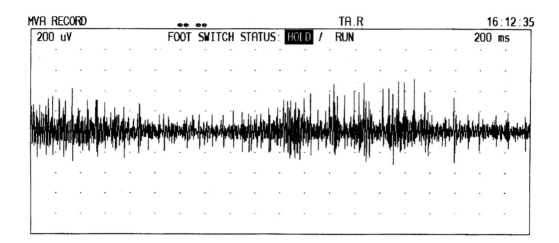

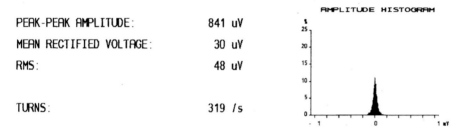

PEAK-PEAK AMPLITUDE:	841 uV
MEAN RECTIFIED VOLTAGE:	30 uV
RMS:	48 uV
TURNS:	319 /s

Fig 8–7. Many motor units firing slowly indicating concern for a central deficit. Note that the recruitment pattern is not as full as in Figure 8–5, and that the motor units do not seem to be rapidly repetitive as in Figure 8–5. This condition is characterized as "many motor units firing slowly."

decision is to wait the traditional one year to allow for spontaneous recovery, then the time to perform the LEMG is at one year, prior to surgical intervention. A partially innervated vocal fold, or a synkinnetic vocal fold, might be best treated with laryngeal framework surgery. If many polyphasic potentials are seen (a sign of ongoing recovery), it might be reasonable to delay treatment in the hopes of further spontaneous improvement. If little or no voluntary activity is seen (indicating a dense nerve injury), then a reinnervation procedure might be the ideal choice.

If early intervention is considered, due to the needs of the patient, whether temporary improvement is sought by injection medialization or permanent intervention is considered with framework medialization, then a LEMG should be considered. If there are vigorous signs of ongoing recovery, then the patient might choose to wait a little bit longer. If no clear signs of imminent recovery are seen, both the patient and surgeon might feel clearer in the decision to intervene.

Another valuable use of LEMG that can provide definitive clinical direction is with the patient who is suspected of having had an arytenoid dislocation. Classically, these patients have a general anesthetic with an attempt to "relocate" the arytenoid, often with forceful maneuvers. Unfortunately, rarely do these patients have the opportunity to have an LEMG prior to the decision to undergo this procedure. Many, or most, of these patients actually have a paralysis that presents with an arytenoid that is tipped forward, mimicking a dislocation. An LEMG that demonstrates paralysis would allow the patient to avoid a surgical procedure.

LEMG is also very valuable in the evaluation of patients who present with bilateral vocal fold immobility. In many cases, especially those who present without an iatrogenic etiology, the underlying disorder is cricoarytenoid joint fixation. The evaluation of the cricoarytenoid joint (CAJ) under general anesthetic is often difficult, and in this author's opinion, is one of the most underrated assessments undertaken during laryngoscopy. An accurate assessment requires deep paralysis, careful position of the laryngoscope so CAJ mobility is not impaired, and firm manual fixation of laryngeal movement during palpation of the CAJs. In addition, the examiner must be careful to avoid confusion between CAJ fixation and interarytenoid scarring. A suspicion of CAJ fixation can be greatly reinforced with an LEMG that demonstrates laryngeal innervation adequate to suggest vocal fold movement in the absence of CAJ fixation.

PATIENT SELECTION

In a cooperative patient, the LEMG results, along with the patient's history and physical examination, can guide the physician to a good understanding of the underlying pathophysiology, and in many cases can significantly influence recommendations for treatment options. To a certain degree, the "quality" of the LEMG is often based on the extent of the patient's ability to remain quiet during the waveform study, and their ability to perform assigned tasks on cue. Sedation is rarely used, and if needed is usually very mild. In the adult population, some test sessions are very limited due to patient anxiety whereas some test sessions are extraordinarily thorough due to the patient being calm during the examination. Almost all adult patients are able to tolerate LEMG well.

LEMG in the pediatric population is usually rather limited due to patient tolerance. LEMG is not a test that can be done without a patient's willingness to undergo the procedure. Standard awake-LEMG is rarely accomplished in children under 10 years old. A few children between 10 and 12 can be coaxed to have the procedure, but the LEMG usually needs to be halted after one or two needle insertions. Very little can be accomplished once the patient becomes anxious. Often children 13 and older will cooperate with at least a limited LEMG study if they are carefully prepared.

As LEMG is performed by a team of specialists, it is unusual for the physicians to know the child very well before the test. Whereas adults are accustomed to examination by strangers, children usually will not be able to cooperate with a painful procedure by someone they do not know. Our experience has led us to defer the LEMG to the second or third visit, and to spend a lot of time with the child before the test. Whereas an adult LEMG might take 20 minutes from the time the patient enters the room, an hour or more is typical for a limited awake-test in a child.

In an adult LEMG, there is great benefit to being somewhat systematic in the procedure. Examining the unaffected side is usually performed first to get familiar with the individual anatomy, and to get a baseline result. In an LEMG for a child, the procedure should be changed to examine the critical area first as study of only one or two areas might occur before the test is terminated.

Due to the difficulty of performing awake-LEMG in children, other options can be tried. Sedation can be used but confirmation tests to ensure accurate needle placement cannot be performed. Light sedation usually allows the examiner to begin the procedure easily, but usually results in a terminated study once the needle insertions begin.

Deep sedation with the help of an anesthesiologist is usually successful in allowing needle insertion, but the patient then is not able to initiate voluntary tasks. Some limited information can be obtained with needle insertion and by moving the needle through the muscle to look for abnormal MUAPs.

Another option for LEMG in children is in the operating room. In this scenario, the child is given a general anesthetic. Direct laryngoscopy is performed and either endoscopic or percutaneous wire electrodes are placed in the vocal cords (TA or thyroarytenoid muscle). With greater difficulty, fine wires can also be placed in the posterior cricoarytenoid (PCA) muscles. With the laryngoscope still in place, the anesthetic is stopped, and the vocal folds are observed by stimulating a cough to look at the TAs, or by obstructing the airway to stimulate abduction and the PCA muscles. Generally, the information gathered in this type of LEMG is limited to a gross evaluation of recruitment. The hooked-wire technique does not allow the electrode to be moved to sample different areas in the muscle.

Another indication for testing in the operating room, both in adults and children, is bilateral vocal fold immobility because of the concern that the LEMG could trigger an airway crisis. In our early experiences, we did electrode placement under a light general anesthetic and recorded responses as the patient awakened. However, as noted above, the results in these cases were difficult to interpret. Currently, if there is a concern about the airway, we do a limited awake-LEMG by testing just the LCA muscles to avoid the risk of vocal fold edema caused by needle insertions in the TA muscles.

INTERPRETATION OF LEMG IN CHILDREN

The limitations of voluntary needle studies in children make interpretation of LEMG difficult. As previously mentioned, LEMG is valuable in conjunction with the history and physical findings. The goal of an LEMG is to provide information that can further the understanding of the pathophysiology of the underlying disorder. The brief recordings that can be obtained in children are often not in depth enough to adequately sample diagnostic MUAPs. The gross recruitment gathered with hooked-wire electrodes as a child awakens from a general anesthetic does provide clues regarding the innervation of the muscles. However, when we compared the LEMGs obtained in a similar fashion in adults with the eventual clinical outcomes, we concluded that the gross recruitment sampled as patients awoke from anesthetic, although a positive sign of innervation, did not predict meaningful voluntary recruitment postoperatively. For the most part, we have abandoned this type of testing.

CASE REPORTS

Case 1

A 10-year-old girl presented in our clinic with a diagnosis of bilateral vocal fold paralysis since a colon interposition for esophageal reconstruction after a lye ingestion. The patient had a limited airway since the surgery, even after a posterior cricoid split with interposition graft 2 months prior to her visit. Laryngoscopy demonstrated a 1-mm glottic gap at rest with paradoxic movement during a sniff. A diagnosis of laryngeal synkinesis was considered but it was felt that she was too young for an LEMG. Empirically, an injection of 0.5 units of botulinum toxin to the LCA muscles was performed with EMG guidance under moderate sedation.

The patient returned to clinic 4 weeks later noting an improved airway and a breathy voice. On laryngeal exam, the glottic gap was 5 to 6 mm on inspiration with slight paradoxing. Over the next 3 years she had 8 more injections of botulinum toxin without sedation. She maintained a good airway until the last two injections. At that time, she was 13 years old and agreed to have awake-larygneal EMG testing to evaluate her presumed diagnosis of laryngeal synkinesis.

The LEMG results demonstrated bilateral innervation of the LCA muscles. The muscles were active during phonation and had less than 10% activity during inspiration. The PCA muscles were not tested due to stridor and patient tolerance. No evidence of abductor synkinesis was noted.

Further evaluation was undertaken in the operating room. Under sedation, an LEMG was attempted. Fine wire electrodes were placed in the TA muscles, the LCA, and PCA muscles. The TAs demonstrated an estimated 70 to 100% recruitment with a cough,

the LCAs demonstrated reduced numbers of motor units firing fast, and the PCAs demonstrated large amplitude motor units but limited recruitment when the patient was stimulated to sniff. Again, no clear synkinesis was demonstrated and the innervation was felt to be adequate for good vocal fold movement.

Based on the LEMG results, a direct laryngoscopy was performed. Palpation of the cricoarytenoid joints showed a fixed joint on the right and a stiff joint on the left. These findings, along with the results of the LEMGs, led us to be confident that she would not likely benefit from any further botulinum toxin, and a right vocal cordotomy was performed.

The patient did well postoperatively, and 7 years later gave birth with a normal vaginal delivery without airway issues.

A review of this case raises a number of questions. It is not clear why the patient had 2 years of improved airway with botulinum toxin. Clearly, at the time the botulinum toxin stopped working, LEMG showed that the patient did not have synkinesis. It would have been interesting if she had been able to have an LEMG at initial presentation. The lack of vocal fold movement seen in clinic, along with the good recruitment seen in the intraoperative LEMG, predicted the finding of cricoarytenoid joint fixation which was confirmed during direct laryngoscopy. Although the finding of fixed joints alone would have been a good indication for cordotomy, the finding of innervation without movement offered confirmation of the clinical decision.

Case 2

A 12-year-old boy presented to our clinic with a history of inspiratory stridor. The patient was noted to have wheezing, shortness of breath, and poor exercise tolerance since birth. Examination showed a healthy appearing boy with inspiratory stridor and a barking cough. Laryngeal exam revealed essentially no abduction of either vocal fold, with slight adduction noted with phonation. The glottic gap was estimated at 1.5 mm.

His history included a reference to bilateral vocal fold paralysis and some type of nerve procedure to his larynx at age 7 which, by report, was felt to be unsuccessful. These records were not available.

The family history was notable for two preceding generations with inspiratory stridor. The patient's mother carried a diagnosis of bilateral vocal fold paralysis, diaphragmatic paralysis, heart failure, short stature, and diffuse muscle weakness. A tracheotomy maintained her airway. The grandmother was also reported as having bilateral vocal fold paralysis, short stature, and lower extremity weakness.

The patient had a formal neurologic evaluation which noted definite weakness in the small hand muscles, some absent deep tendon reflexes in the arms, and short stature. These findings, along with the history of bilateral vocal fold paralysis led to the conclusion that he suffered the familial disorder of his mother and grandmother.

The patient was taken to the OR to perform a laryngeal EMG under controlled conditions in the event the procedure triggered an airway crisis. Under anesthesia, fine wire electrodes were placed in both TA muscles, the IA, and the right PCA. EMG activity was monitored as the patient awakened. During early awakening, motor units in the TA muscles were noted to be firing fast (about 25 Hz), but when the endotracheal tube was clamped, periodic bursts in the TA muscles and right PCA appeared to be normal. The IA muscle had occasional motor unit potentials but had less activity than the other muscles.

Based on these findings, an examination under anesthesia was performed. A band was found between the arytenoids that appeared to restrict arytenoid movement. The band was cut and increased arytenoid mobility was noted. Due to vocal fold edema from the procedure, a tracheostomy was performed.

Three weeks after the procedure, examination showed a 2 to 3-mm glottic opening with good adduction. Six weeks after the procedure the glottic gap was estimated at 4 mm. The tracheostomy tube was removed. Five months after the surgery, the glottic gap was estimated at 3 mm and bilateral adduction/abduction was noted. At 9 months after his procedure, the glottic gap was estimated at 3.5 mm and complete glottic closure was achieved during phonation. The patient was able to run over a mile but did have some difficulty when wrestling in gym class.

The last visit by the patient was 3 years after the procedure. At that time he indicated that he continued to run and play basketball. He noted noisy breathing with significant activity. Examination showed that he had an estimated glottic gap of 2.5 to 3 mm on a sniff, which increased to about 5 mm on deep inspiration. Paradoxing of vocal fold movement was not noted during breathing tasks but was noted during deep inspiration while laughing.

The case shows the value of LEMG, even within the constraints of the setting of a general anesthetic. The LEMG results demonstrated that, in spite of the long history of assumed vocal fold paralysis, bilateral vocal fold innervation was present. Based on these results, further evaluation led to the interarytenoid lysis with a successful result of mobile, although limited, vocal fold function and the avoidance of a permanent tracheostomy.

Case 3

A 12-year-old boy presented to our clinic 2 years after a tracheal transection suffered from a water ski tow rope as he was crossing the wake in a personal watercraft. He had a tracheostomy for 5 months after the accident. Examination showed no left vocal fold movement and minimal right vocal fold movement.

The patient was taken to the operating room for an LEMG under controlled conditions. The left TA showed markedly reduced numbers of motor units firing fast (50 Hz). The right TA appeared normal. The left PCA showed rare motor units, whereas the right PCA showed decreased numbers of motor units with a few polyphasic potentials. Based on these results, an anterior/posterior cricoid split with interposition rib graft was performed with the hope that the residual innervation would be enough to allow for glottic closure.

When the laryngeal stent was removed, the rib graft was noted to have failed. Four months later, with the tracheostomy tube plugged, the airway was estimated at 2 to 3 mm with some movement of the right vocal fold and the tracheostomy tube was removed. Ten months after the procedure the patient had some increasing shortness of breath but was still active, noting stridor when running beyond two bases in baseball.

At 3 years after his surgery, the patient, now 15 years old, reported a poor airway. The patient was again taken to the OR for an LEMG. The left TA showed reduced motor unit action potentials active with phonation and with a sniff. The left PCA showed reduced numbers of large amplitude motor units active with a sniff. The right TA and right PCA did not demonstrate any crisp recruitment. In the hopes that the left side had enough innervation to allow for vocal fold movement, an anterior/posterior cricoid split with interposition rib graft was performed. Again the rib graft failed. Over the next months the patient did not tolerated decannulation, and a conservative left cordotomy was performed. The cordotomy was enlarged 4 months later and the tracheostomy was later removed.

The patient was last seen 4 years after his cordotomy at age 21. He reported that his voice was serviceable for his needs. He was able to run a mile and snowboard without difficulty unless the hill was steep with moguls. Audibly, he had a breathy voice with low volume with a large component of false fold phonation. His cordotomy remained open and there was no paradoxic movement with rapid respiration.

This case shows that the intraoperative LEMGs were used to make the decisions to proceed with anterior/posterior cricoid splits with the belief that the innervation was adequate to allow for glottic closure during phonation and swallowing. The outcomes of these surgeries are difficult to evaluate due to the failure of the rib grafts. In retrospect, when looking at the LEMG results, it is not convincing that the amount of innervation seen would have been adequate to achieve the movement needed. It is also notable that the two LEMGs performed 3 years apart did not have the same results. An awake-LEMG with controlled voluntary recruitment might have demonstrated less convincing signs of innervation than the results obtained during the "bursts" seen in the patient when his endotracheal tube was clamped. The re-sults of this case, as well as a number of similar cases in adults with bilateral immobility, have led us to abandon concern of airway compromise as a key indication for intraoperative LEMG testing. Instead, we now do a limited awake-LEMG of the LCA muscles.

CONCLUSION

LEMG is a valuable tool to evaluate the abnormal larynx. LEMG is the only test that can confirm a suspected paresis or paralysis. All other evaluations, at best, can only strongly suggest a neurologic etiology for the dysmobility or immobility. In many instances, LEMG can be helpful in deciding the best treatment course for a patient. Admittedly, in the pediatric population, LEMG has the limitation imposed by the difficulty of performing the test in child.

Overall, laryngologists, both in the adult and the pediatric populations, are forced to make treatment choices with a limited understanding of the pathophysiology of patients' disorders. Although in many cases, an LEMG can contribute to the understanding of a disorder, and in some cases clearly direct the clinician, LEMG should be considered in all cases of disordered mobility in the larynx. Our understanding of the neurophysiology in these patients, even in those cases that are not influenced by the LEMG results, will make us better clinicians, and over the time of our careers, will further our ability to make wise choices and devise improved treatment options.

See Appendix for a description of a novel technique available to enable operative LEMG in children with vocal fold immobility.

REFERENCES

1. Faaborg-Andersen K. *Electromyography of Laryngeal Muscles in Humans: Technics and Results.* Vol. 3. Basel: S. Karger. 1965: 1–71.
2. Golseth JG. Diagnostic contributions of the electromyogram. *Calif Med.* 1950;73(4): 355–357.
3. Golseth JG. Electromyographic examination in the office. *Calif Med.* 1957;87(5): 298–300.
4. Faaborg-Andersen K, Buchthal F. Action potentials from internal laryngeal muscles during phonation. *Nature.* 1956;177: 340–341.
5. Hirano M, Ohala J. Use of hooked-wire electrodes for electromyography of the intrinsic laryngeal muscles. *J Speech Hear Sci.* 1969; 12:363–373.
6. Hillel AD. The study of laryngeal muscle activity in normal human subjects and in patients with laryngeal dystonia using multiple fine-wire electromyography. *Laryngoscope.* 2001;111(4 pt 2 suppl 97):1–47.
7. Petyz F, Rasmussen H, Buchtal F. Conduction time and velocity in human recurrent laryngeal nerve. *Dan Med Bull.* 1965;12: 125–127.
8. Atkins J. An electromyographic study of recurrent laryngeal nerve conduction and its clinical applications. *Laryngoscope.* 1973;83(5):796–807.
9. Sulica L, Blitzer A. Electromyography and the immobile vocal fold. *Otolaryngol Clin North Am.* 2004;37(1):59–74.
10. Hirose H, Gay T., Strome M. Electrode insertion techniques for laryngeal electromyography. *J Acoust Soc Am.* 1971;50: 1449–1450.
11. Hiroto I, Hirano M, Tomita H. Electromyographic investigation of human vocal cord paralysis. *Ann Otol.* 1968;77:296–304.
12. Kotby MN, Haugen LK. Clinical application of electromyography in vocal fold mobility disorders. *Acta Otolaryngol.* 1970;70: 28–437.

Voice Quality of Life Instruments

Mark E. Boseley
Christopher J. Hartnick

CORE INFORMATION

1. Validity—face, criterion, and discriminant validity are defined.
2. Reliability—test-retest reliability and internal consistency are defined.
3. The Voice Outcomes Survey (VOS) and Pediatric Voice Outcomes Survey (PVOS) are described.
4. The Voice-Related Quality of Life (V-RQOL) and the Pediatric Voice-Related Quality of Life (PV-RQOL) are described.
5. The Voice Handicap Index (VHI) and Pediatric Voice Handicap Index (pVHI) are described.
6. Conclusion—voice quality of life instruments are important in voice outcomes research and the PV-RQOL seems to offer the most information for the least amount of required time.

INTRODUCTION

One of the difficulties that we have faced in treating children with voice disorders is that we have lacked quantitative data to assess the results of our treatments. Normative acoustic measurements have been published utilizing computer assisted voice analysis software. However, until recently, there was no tool available to determine how this would affect a child's quality of life. The need for such instruments has spurned interest in clinicometrics and psychometrics, which provide the methods to construct and evaluate quality of life surveys. This chapter briefly describes the steps in validating these tools. We also discuss the validated pediatric voice surveys that currently exist and their adult counterparts.

VALIDITY

Before an instrument can be used in a clinical setting, it must first be proven to be valid and reliable. Validity is typically described in terms of face validity, criterion validity, and discriminant validity. The first of these can be explained simply as whether the survey is deemed valid by a group of experts in the field. Criterion validity is then tested by comparing the scores from the instrument with other well-established means of testing. Validating a voice survey in this fashion would involve comparing test scores to results obtained from acoustic measurements and other valid voice instruments that were obtained from the same group of subjects. Discriminant validity describes the ability of a survey to discriminate between two groups of individuals. In the case of patients with voice disorders, the instrument should be able to discriminate patients with voice concerns from those who have no voice concerns.

Reliability must also be tested before a quality of life instrument can be utilized in the office. The two most common means employed to test reliability are test-retest reliability and internal consistency. Test-retest reliability usually involves having a patient complete the instrument twice in a 2-week interval. There is no treatment given during that period of time. Ideally, the answers would be the same on both surveys, thus a change in score could only be explained by the treatment rendered. Internal consistency is tested by sequentially eliminating questions on the survey to determine if the remaining questions are more reliable without the deleted item. This is typically reported as a Cronbach's alpha value with a score >0.55 deemed acceptable.[1]

Until recently, there were no validated voice-specific quality of life surveys for the pediatric population. Fortunately, our adult laryngology colleagues have created several voice instruments that have been used for adult patients. However, these instruments were not, until recently, validated for use in the pediatric population. The three most commonly utilized of these are the Voice Outcome Survey (VOS), the Voice-Related Quality of Life Survey (V-RQOL), and the Voice Handicap Index (VHI). The Pediatric Voice Outcome Survey (PVOS), the Pediatric Voice-Related Quality of Life Survey (PV-RQOL), and the Pediatric Voice Handicap Index (pVHI) are the parent-proxy instrument counterparts that may now be utilized in the general pediatric population. The Pediatric Voice Outcome Survey (PVOS) has also been validated for use in pediatric patients with velopharyngeal insufficiency.

VOS/PVOS

The Voice Outcomes Survey (VOS) was initially validated as a tool to assess voice outcomes following surgery for unilateral vocal fold paralysis. The VOS (Fig 9–1) is a 5-item instrument that was found to be valid, reliable, and responsive to change in a group of patients who had undergone an Isshiki thyroplasty. The brevity of the VOS has both advantages and disadvantages. Although it is easy to administer and to score, the VOS is unable to discern subcategories such as physical and emotional components that contribute to one's quality of life.[2]

The Pediatric Voice Outcome Survey (PVOS) was developed as a modification of the VOS to be given to a parent-proxy of a child. This was first validated by comparing two groups of pediatric patients. These groups consisted of children who previously had a tracheotomy that had subsequently

Voice Outcomes Survey (VOS)

1. In general, how would you say your speaking voice is:
   - ☐ Excellent
   - ☐ Good
   - ☐ Adequate
   - ☐ Poor or inadequate
   - ☐ I have no voice

The following items ask about activities that your child might do in a given day.

2. To what extent does your voice limit your ability to be understood in a noisy area?
   - ☐ Limited a lot
   - ☐ Limited a little
   - ☐ Not limited at all

3. During the past 2 weeks, to what extent has your voice interfered with your normal social activities or your work?
   - ☐ Not at all
   - ☐ Slightly
   - ☐ Moderately
   - ☐ Quite a bit
   - ☐ Extremely

4. How often do you have with your food or liquids going "down the wrong pipe" when you eat or find yourself coughing after eating or drinking?
   - ☐ All the time
   - ☐ Most of the time
   - ☐ Sometimes
   - ☐ Rarely
   - ☐ Never

5. Do you find yourself "straining" when you speak because of your voice problem?
   - ☐ Not at all
   - ☐ A little bit
   - ☐ Moderately
   - ☐ Quite a bit
   - ☐ Extremely

Fig 9–1. Voice Outcomes Survey (VOS)

been decannulated and a group of children who remained tracheotomy dependent.[1] The final version of the PVOS consisted of 4 questions (Fig 9-2), with one question being dropped after determining the inter-nal consistency was improved when it was excluded (question 4 on the VOS).

Normative data were later obtained for the PVOS by administering the survey to a group of 385 parents of children and ado-

---

Pediatric Voice Outcomes Survey (PVOS)

1. In general, how would you say your child's speaking voice is:
   - ☐ Excellent (25 pts)
   - ☐ Good (18.75 pts)
   - ☐ Adequate (12.5 pts)
   - ☐ Poor or inadequate (6.25 pts)
   - ☐ My child has no voice (0 pts)

The following items ask about activities that your child might do in a given day.

2. To what extent does your child's voice limit his or her ability to be understood in a noisy area?
   - ☐ Limited a lot (0 pts)
   - ☐ Limited a little (12.5 pts)
   - ☐ Not limited at all (25 pts)

3. During the past 2 weeks, to what extent has your child's voice interfered with his or her normal social activities or with his or her school?
   - ☐ Not at all (25 pts)
   - ☐ Slightly (18.75 pts)
   - ☐ Moderately (12.5 pts)
   - ☐ Quite a bit (6.25 pts)
   - ☐ Extremely (0 pts)

4. Do you find your child "straining" when he or she speaks because of his or her voice problem?
   - ☐ Not at all (25 pts)
   - ☐ A little bit (18.75 pts)
   - ☐ Moderately (12.5 pts)
   - ☐ Quite a bit (6.25 pts)
   - ☐ Extremely (0 pts)

Fig 9–2. Pediatric Voice Outcomes Survey (PVOS).

lescents; most of whom presented to the pediatric otolaryngologist for reasons other than their voice. The mean score obtained was 80.5 ± 19.9.[3] The PVOS was also validated for use in determining the functional impact of surgery to correct velopharyngeal insufficiency. The PVOS scores in that study were 38.3 ± 12 prior to surgery and 72.3 ± 22.7 after surgical intervention in a group of 12 patients which was a statistically significant change.[4]

Using the PVOS

Scores on the PVOS range from 0 to 100 points with higher scores indicating a relative better quality of life. The questions and point values are found in Figure 9–2.

V-RQOL/PV-RQOL

The Voice-Related Quality of Life Survey (V-RQOL) is a 10-item instrument that was validated in a group of 109 adult voice patients. There are also two subdomains within the V-RQOL which consist of scores for physical functioning and social-emotional components of quality of life. This survey was shown to be responsive to change in voice in patients who had treatment for their disorder. The V-RQOL has an advantage over the VOS in that it provides more information to the clinician at very little cost in terms of time required to complete and score.[5]

The Pediatric Voice-Related Quality of Life (PV-RQOL) instrument is the parent-proxy form that was validated in a group of 120 parents of children with a variety of otolaryngologic problems (Fig 9–3).[6] This instrument contained all of the 10 questions that are on the V-RQOL; simply reworded

for parent administration (ie, instead of "do you have . . . " the question was changed to "my child has . . . "). The PV-QROL was shown to have excellent internal consistency and had a high correlation to scores on the previously validated PVOS (criterion validity). The instrument was also able to discriminate between patients who had a voice change during treatment (adenoidectomy patients) and those who had procedures that should not have affected their voice (discriminant validity).[6]

Using the PV-RQOL

The PV-RQOL has 10 questions that each has scores from 0 to 10 points (10 points = no problem, 0 points = problem is "as bad as it can be"). Thus the raw scores can range from 0 to 100 points with higher scores indicating a better quality of life. There are also 2 subdomains within the PV-RQOL. The social-emotional score is determined by adding the scores from questions 4, 5, 8, and 10. The physical functioning score is calculated by adding the scores of questions 1, 2, 3, 6, 7, and 9. The questions and point values for responses are given in Figure 9–3.

VHI/PVHI

The Voice Handicap Index (VHI) is the other commonly cited adult vocal quality of life instrument. The VHI was validated in 1997 and consists of 30 questions, equally distributed in 3 subdomains (10 questions each in functional, physical, and emotional categories).[7] These additional questions were added to prior instruments in an attempt to better differentiate between the different areas in a person's life that a voice

Pediatric Voice-Related Quality of Life Survey (PV-RQOL)

Please answer these questions based upon what your child's voice (your own voice if you are the teenage respondent) has been like over the past 2 weeks. Considering both how severe the problem is when you get, and how frequently it happens, please rate each item below on how "bad" it is (that is, the amount of each problem that you have). Use the following rating scale:

    1 = None, not a problem (10 pts)
    2 = A small amount (7.5 pts)
    3 = A moderate amount (5 pts)
    4 = A lot (2.5 pts)
    5 = Problem is "as bad as it can be" (0 pts)
    6 = Not applicable

Because of my child's voice, how much of a problem is this?

1. My child has trouble speaking loudly or being heard in noisy situations.
    1   2   3   4   5   6

2. My child runs out of air and needs to take frequent breaths when talking.
    1   2   3   4   5   6

3. My child sometimes does not know what will come out when s/he begins speaking.
    1   2   3   4   5   6

4. My child is sometimes anxious or frustrated (because of his or her voice).
    1   2   3   4   5   6

5. My child sometimes gets depressed (because of his or her voice).
    1   2   3   4   5   6

6. My child has trouble using the telephone or speaking with friends in person.
    1   2   3   4   5   6

7. My child has trouble doing his or job schoolwork (because of his or her voice).
    1   2   3   4   5   6

8. My child avoids going out socially (because of his or her voice).
    1   2   3   4   5   6

9. My child has to repeat himself/herself to be understood.
    1   2   3   4   5   6

10. My child has become less outgoing (because of his or her voice).
    1   2   3   4   5   6

Fig 9–3. Pediatric Voice-Related Quality of Life Survey (PV-RQOL).

disorder can affect. The necessary tradeoff is the additional time burden required. Scores for each question range from 0 to 4 points (0 = never, 4 = always). The scores range from 0 to 120 points with higher scores representing worse perceived quality of life.[7]

Two variations of the VHI have recently been added to our armamentarium. The VHI-10 is a 10-item variation of the VHI that has been shown to correlate well with the scores obtained from the VHI.[8] The pediatric VHI (pVHI) is a 23-item parent-proxy version of the original VHI.[9] The pVHI was validated in a group of 45 nonvoice pediatric patients. Scores were compared to visual analogue scale and 10 open-ended questions regarding the impact of the child's voice quality on his or her overall communication, development, education, and social and family life. Normative scores were 1.47 for the functional, 0.20 for the physical, and 0.18 for the emotional components. The pVHI was then administered to children before and after laryngeal reconstruction. A correlation matrix comparing the overall pVHI scores with the subscores showed moderate correlation. Also, the visual analogue scores where compared to the pVHI scores and revealed moderate correlation. Furthermore, test-retest reliability was moderately high.[9]

Using the pVHI

The pVHI has 23 questions that each has scores from 0 to 4 points (0 points = no problem, 4 points = always a problem). Thus, the raw scores can range from 0 to 92 points with higher scores indicating a worse quality of life. There are also 3 subdomains within the pVHI. The functional score is determined by adding the scores from the first 7 questions and the physical score by adding the final 7 questions. The questions and point values for responses are given in Figure 9–4.

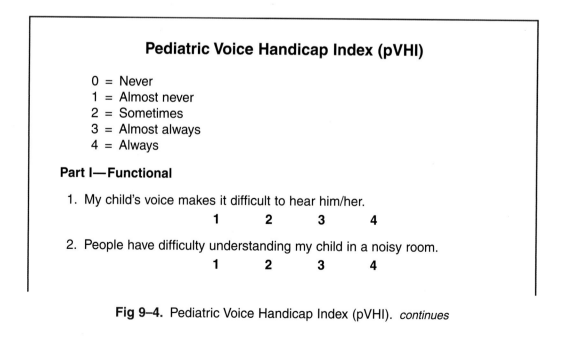

Fig 9–4. Pediatric Voice Handicap Index (pVHI). *continues*

3. At home, we have difficulty hearing my child when he/she calls through the house.

          1   2   3   4

4. My child tends to avoid communicating because of his/her voice.

          1   2   3   4

5. My child speaks with friends, neighbors, or relatives less often because of his/her voice.

          1   2   3   4

6. People ask my child to repeat him/herself when speaking face-to-face.

          1   2   3   4

7. My child's voice difficulties restrict personal, educational and social activities.

          1   2   3   4

Part II—Physical

8. My child runs out of air when talking.

          1   2   3   4

9. The sound of my child's voice changes throughout the day.

          1   2   3   4

10. People ask, "What's wrong with your child's voice?"

          1   2   3   4

11. My child's voice sounds dry, rasp, and/or hoarse.

          1   2   3   4

12. The quality of my child's voice is unpredictable.

          1   2   3   4

13. My child uses a great deal of effort to speak (eg, straining).

          1   2   3   4

14. My child's voice is worse in the evening.

          1   2   3   4

15. My child's voice "gives out" while speaking.

          1   2   3   4

16. My child has to yell in order for others to hear him/her.

          1   2   3   4

Fig 9–4. *continues*

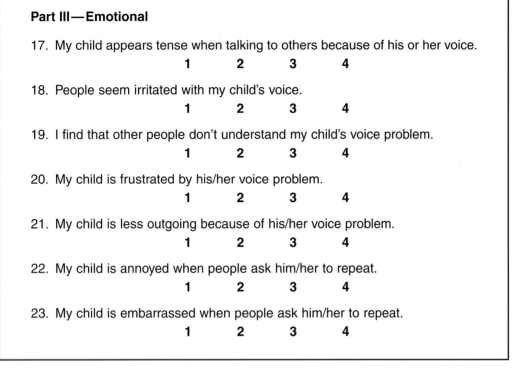

Part III—Emotional

17. My child appears tense when talking to others because of his or her voice.

    1   2   3   4

18. People seem irritated with my child's voice.

    1   2   3   4

19. I find that other people don't understand my child's voice problem.

    1   2   3   4

20. My child is frustrated by his/her voice problem.

    1   2   3   4

21. My child is less outgoing because of his/her voice problem.

    1   2   3   4

22. My child is annoyed when people ask him/her to repeat.

    1   2   3   4

23. My child is embarrassed when people ask him/her to repeat.

    1   2   3   4

Fig 9–4. *continued*

FUTURE DIRECTIONS

Quantitative analysis of voice outcomes following medical or surgical intervention is imperative if we are to advance the field of pediatric laryngology. Although we are gradually gathering normative data for both acoustic and quality of life instruments, widespread acceptance of their use has been slow to develop. Pediatric voice quality of life instruments are now available, but seem not to be utilized as often as they might be. There are now three such devices to choose from. It will be important, as we go forward, to adopt a standard instrument so that we can both track the voice results in our patients and compare results across institutions.

REFERENCES

1. Hartnick CJ. Validation of a pediatric voice quality-of-life instrument. *Arch Otolaryngol.* 2002;128:919–922.
2. Gliklich RE, Glovsky RM, Montgomery WW. Validation of a voice outcome survey for unilateral vocal cord paralysis. *Otolaryngol Head Neck Surg.* 1999;120:153–158.
3. Hartnick CJ, Volk M, Cunningham M. Establishing normative voice-related quality of life scores within the pediatric otolaryngology population. *Arch Otolaryngol Head Neck Surg.* 2003;129:1090–1093.
4. Boseley ME, Hartnick CJ. Assessing the outcome of surgery to correct velopharyngeal insufficiency with the pediatric voice outcomes survey. *Int J Pediatr Otorhinolaryngol.* 2004;68:1429–1433.

5. Hogikyan ND, Sethuraman G. Validation of an instrument to measure Voice-Related Quality of Life (V-RQOL). *J Voice.* 1999;13:557–567.

6. Boseley ME, Cunningham MJ, Volk MS, Hartnick CJ. Validation of the pediatric voice-related quality-of-life survey. *Arch Otolaryngol Head Neck Surg.* 2006;132:717–720.

7. Jacobson B, Johnson A, Grywalsky C. The Voice Handicap Index (VHI): development and validation. *Am J Speech Lang Path.* 1997;6:66–70.

8. Rosen CA, Lee AS, Osborne J, Zullo T, Murry T. Development and validation of the voice handicap index-10. *Laryngoscope.* 2004; 114:1549–1556.

9. Zur KB, Cotton S, Kelcher L, Baker S, Weinrich B, Lee L. Pediatric Voice Handicap Index (pVHI): a new tool for evaluating pediatric dysphonia. *Int J Pediatr Otorhinolaryngol.* 2007;71:77–82.

Laryngopharyngeal Reflux and the Voice

Steven C. Hardy

INTRODUCTION

Gastroesophageal reflux disease (GERD) is a relatively common problem encountered by otolaryngologists. Symptoms in the adult population include throat clearing, chronic throat irritation, chronic hoarseness, and chronic cough.[1] Infants, on the other hand, often present initially with complaints of frequent "spitting up" during feeds. Others have a more worrisome history to include failure to thrive, hematemesis, anemia, or recurrent pneumonia.[2] It is these patients that often require a multidisciplinary approach to management. Pediatric otolaryngologists, working alongside our pediatric pulmonology and gastroenterology colleagues, play an important role in this regard. This chapter addresses the timing of evaluating children suspected to have GERD, the diagnostic tests currently available, and the treatment options that should be considered. This chapter aims to elucidate our role as otolaryngologists in treating GERD.

The true incidence of GERD in children is difficult to ascertain as many infants can spit up without any untoward complications. Premature infants, however, seem to have a higher likelihood of having reflux than other children. Marino found that in a group of 75 such patients, 63% were found to have GERD.[3] The good news is that the majority of these patients improve as they grow. It appears that 55% have resolution of their symptoms by 10 months of age and an additional 16% improve by 18 months.[4]

The reason for the apparent higher incidence of reflux in infants than in adults is likely multifactorial. There are several anatomic differences that have been noted. The angle between the esophagus and the axis of the stomach (angle of His) is more obtuse in the infant. Children with hiatal hernias are also more subject to GERD as the lower esophageal sphincter (LES) is exposed to negative intrathoracic pressure, rendering it less effective as a barrier to gastric acid. Although these anatomic factors play a role, currently it is believed that transient LES relaxation (TLESR) is the major factor causing clinically significant reflux in infants.[2]

In addition to these anatomic factors, physiologic considerations must also be considered. Infants are usually fed large fluid boluses in order to lengthen the duration of time between feeds. Children are also usually placed in a supine position following feeding. Food allergy can also masquerade as GERD. Some have proposed that allergy might be the cause in up to 42% of cases.[5] Increasing the frequency and decreasing the volume of feeds may be helpful in decreasing symptoms. Placing the infant in a prone, head-elevated position should decrease the incidence of reflux. Thickening feeds may also be beneficial. Finally, a trial of hypoallergenic protein hydrolysate infant formula can be considered before initiating a formal workup for GERD.[6]

Sutphen has advocated that children under the age of 12 months must have failure to thrive, weight loss, pulmonary disease, and/or an apparent life-threatening episode (ALTE) before a workup should be undertaken. Beyond the age of 12 months, persistent spitting up is adequate to pursue further testing.[6]

DIAGNOSTIC TESTS

Once the decision is made to evaluate for GERD, there are several tests that are in our armamentarium. These include an upper gastrointestinal series (upper GI series), pH-probe testing, impedance monitoring, and endoscopy. The upper GI series consists of having the child swallow barium during a fluoroscopic examination of the upper aerodigestive tract. We often involve our speech and swallowing therapist during this evaluation as they are often more adept at commenting on the oropharyngeal component of swallowing. This study can be helpful in determining whether there is any evidence of laryngeal penetration. It is also useful to look for anatomic abnormalities such as a hiatal hernia, esophageal stricture, or tracheoesophageal fistula. However, when it comes to evaluating for GERD, some feel that this study is limited as the child is being tested under nonphysiologic conditions.

The 24-hour pH probe has become the procedure of choice for the diagnosis of GERD in infants and children. This probe has traditionally been placed through the nose and is attached to an external monitor. The recordings that have been commonly recorded are the number of reflux episodes (pH < 4), the percentage of time that the pH is less than 4 (reflux index), the number of reflux events of at least 5 minutes in duration, the average esophageal acid clearance time per reflux episode, the longest reflux episode, and the total time of pH less than 4.[6] It should be noted that there has not been a consensus on the values of these various variables as predictors to clinical disease.[6] However, one study in children with pulmonary disease showed a correlation between duration of reflux and evidence of esophagitis on esophageal biopsy specimens.[7] Another study looked specifically at reflux index and time with a pH less than 4 as predictors of esophagitis. The sensitivity for detecting GERD was 96% and 93%, respectively. However, the specificity was only 50% for the reflux index and 88% for time with a pH less than 4.[8]

The number of positions within the esophagus being tested has also varied over the years. One published report documented the sensitivity and specificity for detecting GERD at the levels of the lower esophageal sphincter and pharynx improved to nearly

100% when a double-probe was utilized.[9] Another study showed that 46% of children who had normal pH readings at the distal probe had abnormal pH values at the proximal probe, suggesting that the pharyngeal probe is necessary.[10] Finally, a report on the use of a four-probe device (pharynx, proximal, middle, and distal esophagus) showed a 87% sensitivity and 93% specificity in detecting GERD and LPR.[11]

Another option for esophageal pH monitoring is the Bravo pH-monitoring system. The Bravo involves a pH-capsule, about the size of a gel cap, that is temporarily attached to the wall of the esophagus, usually during an endoscopic exam (Figs 10–1 and 10–2). The Bravo pH capsule measures the pH of the surrounding esophagus and transmits the information continuously via radio telemetry to a receiver worn on the patient's belt, or kept nearby. As with a pH probe, the patient (or caregiver) records symptoms he or she experiences in a diary by pressing buttons on the receiver. The Bravo pH capsule collects pH measurements for up to 48 hours. After the study, data from the receiver is uploaded to a computer and diary information is entered for analysis to aid in the diagnosis and plan treatment. The capsule is released from the esophageal wall and passes through the alimentary tract until discarded with the patient's feces. The obvious advantage that this device has over standard pH monitoring is that there is no need for a probe to stay in the nose, and thus is better tolerated by children.

There are inherent problems with having so many different types of measurements and different types of probes when trying to define what makes up an abnormal study. Even if the results are consistent with GERD, this does not necessarily correlate with the child's symptoms. Finally, a pH

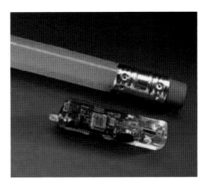

A

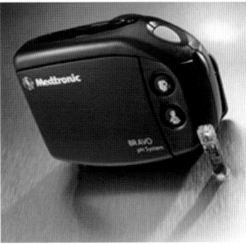

B

Fig 10–1. Bravo probe and receiver. **A.** The size is comparable to the size of a pencil eraser. **B.** The receiver is worn on the patient's belt.

probe study fails to address reflux of bile acids that have a pH greater than 5, but could still potentially be clinically significant.

One technique to better delineate a correlation of GERD with symptoms (particularly with pulmonary symptoms, such as apnea or ALTE) is to perform a Bernstein test. This test consists of placing a nasogastric tube into the esophagus and instilling alternating solutions of a low concentration of hydrochloric

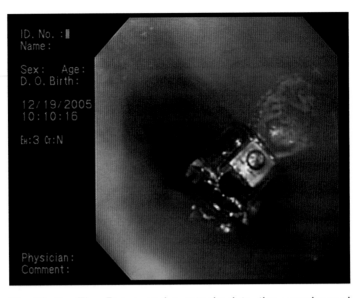

ID. No. :
Name:

Sex: Age:
D. O. Birth:

12/19/2005
10:10:16

EH:3 Gr:N

Physician:
Comment:

Fig 10–2. The Bravo probe attached to the esophageal mucosa.

acid and normal saline to see if the symptoms are reproduced. The second issue of nonacidic reflux is better addressed with multiple intraluminal impedance monitoring (MII). MII measures alterations in electrical impedance along multiple intraluminal electrodes during swallowing. This allows for detection of anterograde swallows and retrograde reflux, regardless of the acidity of the refluxate.[12] Perhaps the best evaluation for GERD would be a combination of a pH probe to measure acidity with MII to measure directional flow of fluid in the esophagus.

Endoscopy of the aerodigestive tract can be extremely useful when trying to make the diagnosis of GERD, particularly in those that have failed medical management. This group of children includes those with failure to thrive, chronic cough, and airway symptoms (including those with recurrent croup, pneumonias, and/or suspicion for aspiration). We have found it useful to include both our pediatric pulmonologist and gastroenterologist for this evaluation in the operating room.

The examination begins with a thorough inspection of the larynx with a 4.0-mm Hopkins rod telescope. Any signs of pharyngeal reflux are noted to include erythema and/or intra-arytenoid or true vocal fold edema. Also, care is taken to inspect for a laryngeal cleft as this could be the underlying cause for aspiration. A laryngeal mask airway is then placed to facilitate flexible bronchoscopy. A cobblestone appearance of the tracheal wall is a visual clue on endoscopy that the child may be aspirating (Fig 10–3). A bronchoalveolar lavage should be performed to confirm a suspicion of aspiration. Specifically, 100 macrophages are collected and stained with oil red O to test for lipid. Lipid-layden macrophages (LLM) become positive approximately 6 hours after a reflux episode and remain positive for up to 3 days.[13] The sensitivity for this test is believed to be near 85%.[14]

The child may be intubated prior to performing the esophagoscopy. A flexible grasping biopsy forceps is passed through the working port of the scope. Four sets of biopsies are taken from the duodenum, the stomach, and the distal and proximal esophagus. These specimens are examined for evidence of Barrett's esophagus or eosinophils which would suggest chronic reflux or allergic esophagitis. A endoscopic finding of "trachealization" or ringed appearance of the esophageal mucosal can be suggestive of esosinophilic esophagitis (Fig 10-4). Although uncommonly seen in the pediatric population, the clinician should also be aware of the distinct appearance of erosive esophagitis (Fig 10-5). This condition would obviously warrant more aggressive reflux therapy.

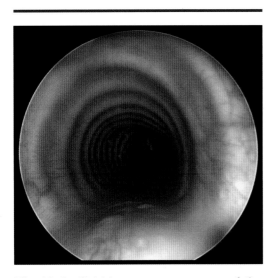

Fig 10–3. Cobblestone appearance of the tracheal mucosa is suggestive of aspiration.

Once the diagnosis of GERD is made by clinical suspicion, pH probe, or biopsy, the usual first step in treatment is through conservative management. Techniques such as formula changes (when allergy is suspected), thickening of feeds, smaller feeding size, suggestions for burping techniques,

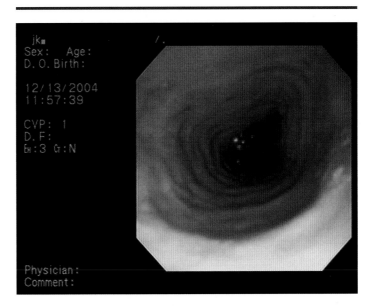

Fig 10–4. "Trachealization" of the esophagus suggesting the presence of eosinophilic esophagitis.

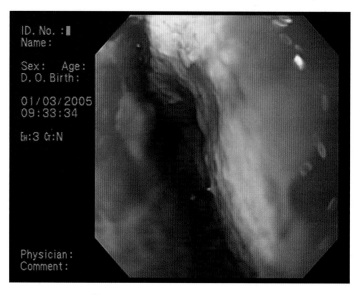

Fig 10–5. Erosive esophagitis.

and postcibal positioning therapy should all be entertained prior to beginning treatment with medications.[2,6,12] When necessary, medical treatment is successful in approximately 80% of cases.[15] Medications that have been used have included antacids, histamine receptor-2 (H_2) antagonists, proton-pump blockers, and prokinetic agents (Table 10–1).

MEDICAL MANAGEMENT

The use of antacids has been limited in the infant population due to the frequent feeding schedule and the potential risks from aluminum absorption. H_2 receptor anatagonists such as cimetidine and ranitidine, on the other hand, have been shown to be effective at treating both the clinical and histologic changes seen in children with GERD.[16-18] The prescribing physician should

be aware, however, that these drugs can rarely cause gynecomastia, diarrhea, and abnormalities in vitamin D or hepatic metabolism.[19] These risks seem to be less common with the use of ranitidine.[6] Treatment is usually carred on for 6 to 8 weeks for healing of mucosal irritation. Treatment can continue in order to prevent reinjury by reflux.

If more severe GERD is suspected, proton-pump blockers have become an important therapeutic option. These medications, which include omeprazole and lansoprazole, perform their action by inhibiting the proton-potassium ATPase enzyme system.[2] The common pediatric doses are listed in Table 10–1. Treatment with proton-pump inhibitors is generally 6 to 8 weeks minimum, as is the case for histamine receptor blockers. At one time there was a fear that long-term use of proton-pump blockers could lead to gastrinoma formation. This concern has not been proven to be true.[20]

Table 10–1. List of Commonly Prescribed Antireflux Medications and Doses

Medication	Dosage
Magnesium-aluminum hydroxide	0.5 ml/kg/dose PO before meals and qhs
Cimetidine	5-10 mg/kg/dose PO qid
Ranitidine	1-4 mg/kg/dose PO bid or tid
Metoclopramide	0.1 mg/kg/dose PO before meals and qhs
Omeprazole	1.0 mg/kg/dose, or 20 mg PO qd

Prokinetic agents are the last class of drugs to consider when treating clinically significant GERD. Otolaryngologists typically are hesitant to prescribe these drugs as the safety of both metoclopramide and cisapride has been questioned. The former has been associated with diarrhea, extrapyramidal symptoms, and dystonias. Cisapride, on the other hand, has been associated with serious cardiac arrhythmias, such as torsades de pointes and prolonged QT interval, and is no longer available in the United States.[6] It should be mentioned, however, that cisapride has been shown in a placebo-controlled, double-blind, 8-week trial to improve both pH scores and histologic changes in the esophagus.[21]

SURGICAL MANAGEMENT

Surgery is reserved for those children with diagnosed GERD who have failed medical management. The two most common operations are the Thal and Nissen fundoplications. The Thal is a 270-degree anterior wrap of the fundus of the stomach around the distal esophagus, whereas the Nissen is a 360-degree wrap. Indications for a wrap include failure to thrive, reflux-induced aspiration, peptic stricture, Barrett's esophagus, and ALTE. Failure rates for the Nissen fundoplication vary from 3 to 40% after 4 to 9 years.[22]

CONCLUSION

Gastroesphageal reflux is very common during infancy. Often, this is not clinically significant and requires no further diagnostic studies or medical treatment. Most of these children can be managed by educating the parents on how to feed and by general reassurance. Occasionally changes to the type of formula the child is being given can be beneficial as well. However, children with a more worrisome history (failure to thrive, hematemesis, anemia, or recurrent pneumonia) require a more thorough evaluation.[2] The tests for GERD that are currently available to us all have advantages and disadvantages. A 24-hour pH probe with the addition of esophageal biopsies should be considered for the most severe cases. Bravo probes can be done if the child is an appropriate candidate. Addition of impedance testing may be beneficial in cases where nonacidic reflux is believed to be the causative agent. Once the diagnosis is made, 85% of children can be managed with medical therapy alone.

REFERENCES

1. Koufman JA. The otolaryngologic manifestations of gastroesophageal reflux disease (GERD): a clinical investigation of 225 patients using ambulatory 24-hour pH monitoring and an experimental investigation of the role of acid and pepsin in the development of laryngeal injury. *Laryngoscope.* 1991;101:1-78.

2. Tsou MV, Bishop PR. Gastroesophageal reflux in children. *Otolaryngol Clin North Am.* 1998;31:419-434.

3. Marino M, Assing E, Carbone M, et al. The incidence of gastroesophageal reflux in preterm infants. *J Perinatol.* 1995;15: 369-371.

4. Khalaf MN, Porat R, Brodsky NL, Bhandari V. Clinical correlations in infants in the neonatal intensive care unit with varying severity of gastroesophageal reflux. *J Gastroenerol Nutr.* 2001;32:45-49.

5. Iacono G, Carroccio A, Cavataio F, et al. Gastroesopageal reflux and cow's milk allergy in infants: a prospective study. *J Allergy Clin Immunol.* 1996;97:822.

6. Sutphen JL. Pediatric gastroesophageal reflux disease. *Gastroenterol Clin North Am.* 1990;19:617-629.

7. Baer M, Maki M, Nurminen J, et al. Esophagitis and findings of long-term esophageal pH recording in children with repeated lower respiratory tract symptoms. *J Pediatr Gastroenterol Nutr.* 1986;5:187-190.

8. Vandenplas Y, Franckx-Goossens A, Pipeleers-Marichal M, et al. Area under pH 4: advantages of a new parameter in the interpretation of esophageal pH monitoring data in infants. *J Pediatr Gastroenterol Nutr.* 1989; 9:34-39.

9. Contencin P, Narcy P. Gastropharyngeal reflux in infants and children. *Arch Otolaryngol Head Neck Surg.* 1992;118:1028-1030.

10. Little JP, Matthews BL, Glock MS, et al. Esophageal pediatric reflux: 24-hour double-probe pH monitoring of 222 children. *Ann Otol Rhinol Laryngol.* 1997;169:1-16.

11. Haase GM, Meagher DP, Goldson E, et al. A unique teletransmission system for extended four-channel esophageal pH monitoring in infants and children. *J Pediatr Surg.* 1987;22:68-74.

12. Malloy EJ, Fiore JM, Martin RJ. Does gastroesophageal reflux cause apnea in preterm infants? *Biol Neonate.* 2005;87:254-261.

13. Zalzal GH, Tran LP. Pediatric gastroesophageal reflux and laryngopharyngeal reflux. *Otolaryngol Clin North Am.* 2000;33:151-161.

14. Nussbaum E, Maggi JC, Mathis R, et al. Association of lipid-laden alveolar macrophages and gastroesophageal reflux in children. *J Pediatr.* 1987;110:190-194.

15. Andze GO, Brandt ML, Vil DS, et al. Diagnosis and treatment of gastroesophageal reflux in 500 children with respiratory symptoms: the value of pH monitoring. *J Pediatr Surg.* 1991;26:295-300.

16. Cucchiara S, Staiano A, Romaniello G, et al. Antacids and cimetidine treatment for gastroesophageal reflux and peptic oesophagitis. *Arch Dis Child.* 1984;59:842-847.

17. Cucchiara S, Gobio-Casali L, Balli F, et al. Cimetidine treatment of relux esophagitis in children: an Italian multicentric study. *J Pediatr Gastroenterol Nutr.* 1989;8:150-156.

18. Shepherd RW, Wren J, Evans S, et al. Gastroesophageal reflux in children. *Clin Pediatr.* 1987;26:55-60.

19. Hebra A, Hoffman MA. Gastroesophageal reflux in children. *Pediatr Clin North Am.* 1993;40:1233-1251.

20. Berlin R. Omeprazole: gastrin and gastric endocrine cell data from clinical studies. *Dig Dis Sci.* 1991;36:129.

21. Cucchiara S, Staiano A, Capozi C, et al. Cisapride for gastro-oesophageal reflux and peptic oesophagitis. *Arch Dis Child.* 1987; 62:454-457.

22. Cilley R. Management of gastroesophageal reflux in children. *Curr Opin Pediatr.* 1991; 27:260.

The Role of the Pediatric Pulmonologist

Kenan E. Haver

INTRODUCTION

Voice is generated by the modulation of airflow through the vocal folds. The production and maintenance of airflow requires the coordinated function of both the muscles of respiration and those muscles and structures involved in maintaining the caliber of both the large and small airways. Conditions that impair the function of the respiratory muscles, decrease the caliber by constricting the smooth muscle in the small airways, or affect the normal movements of the vocal folds can each affect the voice. This chapter discusses how pulmonary function studies may be useful in assessing respiratory muscle strength, detecting bronchoconstriction, and identifying inspiratory flow limitation[7] (Table 11–1).

ANATOMY AND PHYSIOLOGY OF THE UPPER AND LOWER AIRWAY

The vocal folds make complete contact with each other during phonation with each vibration transiently closing the gap between them which cuts off the escaping air.[1] When the air pressure in the trachea rises as a result of this closure, the folds are blown apart, while the vocal processes of the arytenoid cartilages remain in apposition. This creates an oval-shaped gap between the folds and some air escapes, lowering the pressure inside the trachea. Rhythmic repetition of this movement creates a pitched note. The pitch, volume, and timbre of the sound produced can be altered by the shape of chest and neck,

Table 11–1. Maximal Respiratory Pressures.[10]

	Maximal Inspiratory Pressure	Maximal Expiratory Pressure
Poor effort	Decreased	Decreased
Fatigue	Decreased	Decreased
Neuromuscular disease	Decreased	Decreased
Increased lung volume	Decreased	Normal
Decreased lung volume	Normal	Decreased

Conditions to consider in patients with decreased maximal respiratory pressures. Used with permission from Medical Algorithms Project, *Maximal Inspiratory and Maximal Expiratory Pressures*, Chapter 8, Pulmonary and Acid-Base, Copyright (©) 2006–2007, Institute for Algorithmic Medicine, Houston, Texas.

and the position of the lips, tongue, jaw, palate, and airway. The vocal folds themselves can loosen or tighten and change their thickness.

Airflow in the respiratory system begins with the active process of inhalation, which is principally dependent on the function of the diaphragm. With each contraction, the diaphragm flattens which enlarges the thoracic cavity. The diaphragm also elevates and stabilizes the lower rib cage.[2] During normal breathing, most of the accessory muscles are silent. However, these muscles may be recruited to stabilize the chest or abdominal wall to improve the efficiency of the diaphragm under certain conditions.

Airflow is increased during inspiration by negative pressure generated at the margins of the air column, a phenomenon referred to as the Bernoulli effect. The acceleration of flow as the air enters a narrowed passage, known as the Venturi effect, tends to reduce the diameter of the airways. These forces are resisted by the structural elements of the airway and the tone of the airway muscles. The upper airway must also be kept patent during inspiration and therefore the function of the alae nasi, phayngeal wall muscles, genioglossus, and arytenoid muscles also play an important role.[2]

Exhalation is generally a passive process. The lungs have a natural elasticity; as they recoil from the stretch of inhalation, air flows back out until the pressures in the chest and the atmosphere reach equilibrium. However, with active or forced exhalation, as when singing, the abdominal and internal intercostal muscles are used to generate abdominal and thoracic pressure which forces air out of the lungs.[3]

MEASURING RESPIRATORY MUSCLE STRENGTH

Muscle weakness needs to be considered in the evaluation of patients with voice-related problems. Muscle weakness, either congenital or acquired, can impair respiratory muscle function, decrease airflow, and subsequently affect the voice. Voice changes have been associated with a variety of diseases that affect the muscles of respiration, including Guillain-Barré syndrome, myasthenia gravis, muscular dystrophies, and poliomyelitis.[4] Spinal injuries can also directly impact the muscles of respiration. Finally, respiratory muscle strength can be affected by deconditioning, which can be caused by debilitating diseases, mechanical ventilation, malnutrition, or immobilization.

Establishing the cause for the weakness is important to select appropriate therapy. Even when specific therapy is not available to treat the disorder, inspiratory muscle training (IMT) may help patients strengthen and improve their voice. Additional benefits from IMT include decreased perception of exertional dyspnea, enhanced cough, and improved airway clearance.[5]

Measuring respiratory muscle strength is straightforward. Both the maximum inspiratory pressure (MIP—the highest pressure developed during inspiration) and maximum expiratory pressure (MEP—highest pressure developed during expiration) can be measured and compared to controls. Patients with disorders that affect respiratory muscle strength may have impaired MIPs and MEPs. These can be measured quite easily at the mouth using a pressure meter. Normal values have been published for both adults and children. Caution is needed in the interpretation of the studies as values in the lower quarter of the normal range are compatible both with normal strength and with mild to moderate weakness. A normal MEP with a low MIP suggests isolated diaphragmatic weakness. These tests are volitional and require full cooperation. Accordingly, an abnormal result may be due to lack of motivation and does not necessarily indicate reduced inspiratory or expiratory muscle strength.[6]

Clinical Case

Jennifer is an 18-year-old young woman who is an aspiring singer with a history that included an interrupted aortic arch and ventricular septal defect who presented with a hoarse voice and chronic aspiration. She was found to have a paralyzed left vocal fold and underwent a left ansa cervicalis to recurrent laryngeal nerve anastomosis procedure with a fat graft injection laryngoplasty. Over the next year, she regained the ability to eat orally without evidence of aspiration and her conversational voice had markedly improved. However, as she was an avid singer, she still noted difficulty with sustaining notes. She asked if another procedure would help. Videostroboscopy suggested that she has good glottal closure with no significant glottal gap and no apparent mucosal wave abnormalities.

Her surgical options were reviewed which included a revision thyroplasty. Physical examination revealed her chest was clear to auscultation, but her breath sounds were diminished bilaterally. Her diaphragm moved appropriately by palpation. We measured her maximal inspiratory (MIP) and expiratory pressures (MEP) to evaluate the strength of her respiratory muscles. Her MIP was very low at 24 cm H_2O and her MEP was at the low end of the normal range at 85 cm H_2O. Her reduced respiratory muscle strength may have been due, at least in part, to deconditioning. She was referred to a respiratory muscle strength-training program, where she would breathe in and out against progressively increasing resistance. Her respiratory muscle strength increased significantly following her participation in the program. Her maximal respiratory pressures increased to a MIP of 32 (improved but still below the range of normal) and her MEP increased to 107. Along with the changes seen in her maximal respiratory pressures, she reported improvement in her ability to sing and no longer desires further surgical intervention. This case illustrates how pulmonary function studies helped establish the cause for her weak voice. With this information we were able to direct her to nonoperative therapy. We can continue to monitor her progress by regular reevaluation of her respiratory muscle strength.

Measuring Respiratory Muscle Strength Using the Sniff Test

Another test of muscle strength is the sniff test. This is a short, sharp voluntary inspiratory maneuver performed through one or both unoccluded nostrils. It involves contraction of the diaphragm and other inspiratory muscles. The sniffs need to be a maximal effort to be a useful test of respiratory muscle strength. This is relatively easy for most willing subjects, but may require some practice. Subjects should be instructed to sit or stand comfortably, and to make sniffs using maximal effort starting from relaxed end expiration. Detailed instruction on how to perform the maneuver are generally not necessary, and may, in fact, be counterproductive. However, subjects should be encouraged to make maximal efforts, with a rest between sniffs. Most subjects achieve a plateau of pressure values within 5 to 10 attempts. When done properly, the maneuver achieves rapid, fully coordinated recruitment of the inspiratory muscles.[6]

MEASURING SMALL AIRWAY OBSTRUCTION

The lower respiratory tract plays a key role in voice production by delivering airflow to the vocal folds. Airflow can be impaired by intrinsic or extrinsic compression of the airways. Asthma, which is characterized by chronic inflammation and smooth muscle dysfunction in the small airways, can present with both breathlessness and dyspnea. Asthma is the most common obstructive pulmonary disease in children and is characterized by reversible airway obstruction. Patients with asthma often present with dyspnea, but during a severe exacerbation may appear breathless and unable to complete sentences. Small airway obstruction can be detected by pulmonary function tests, even when the patient appears well and the chest is clear to auscultation.

Changes in pulmonary function that are insignificant with normal speech have been shown to lead to performance impairment for both amateur and professional singers. In a study of singers with voice problems (including vocal fatigue) who did not have causal laryngeal pathology, the investigators found that they had bronchodilator responsive airway obstruction. The singers, when treated for asthma, were shown to have improvement in their performance-related difficulties. The authors concluded that singers who present with complaints of impaired vocalization, such as vocal fatigue, decreased control, and excessive muscular tension, should be evaluated for increased airway reactivity as a possible cause of their complaints.[7]

Restrictive lung disease, which can be differentiated from obstructive lung diseases with spirometry and other tests of pulmonary function, can arise from interstitial lung disease or limitations to chest wall movement such as chest wall deformities. These deformities can include scoliosis, space-occupying intrathoracic processes (large bullae or congenital cysts), and alveolar filling defects (lobar pneumonia or pleural effusions).

Spirometry is the best method for documenting airflow obstruction. Spirometry measures the volume of air inspired and expired as a function of time, and is by far the most frequently performed test of pulmonary function in children. Pulmonary function tests enable clinicians to establish mechanical dysfunction in children with respiratory symptoms, quantify the degree of dysfunction, and define the nature of the dysfunction (Table 11-2).[8] Table 11-3 illustrates how spirometry can differentiate an obstructive from a restrictive process.

Figure 11-1 illustrates a normal flow-volume loop obtained during a respiratory maneuver that includes both inspiration and forced exhalation, whereas Figure 11-2 is a flow-volume loop of a patient with asthma for comparison. A reliable study requires patient effort and cooperation, accurate testing equipment, as well as a skilled and knowledgeable staff. Although the maneuvers needed to obtain measurements appear straightforward, studies are only valid if they reflect maximal effort and are reproducible. Children over the age of 6 can often perform adequately, although children as young as age 3 years have been shown to be able to perform spirometry with coaching. Each test needs to be repeated twice, and two studies need to have results within 5% of each other before the study can be reported as accurate.[9]

Table 11–2. Uses of Pulmonary Function Studies in Children

- To establish pulmonary mechanical abnormality in children with respiratory symptoms
- To quantify the degree of dysfunction
- To define the nature of pulmonary dysfunction (obstructive, restrictive, or mixed obstructive and restrictive)
- To aid in defining the site of airway obstruction as central or peripheral
- To differentiate fixed from variable and intrathoracic from extrathoracic central airway obstruction
- To follow the course of pulmonary disease process
- To assess the effect of therapeutic interventions and guide changes in therapy
- To detect increased airway reactivity
- To evaluate the risk of diagnostic and therapeutic procedures
- To monitor for pulmonary side effects of chemotherapy or radiation therapy
- To aid in prediction of the prognosis and quantitate pulmonary disability
- To investigate the effect of acute and chronic disease processes on lung growth

Modified with permission from Castile R, Pulmonary Function Testing in Children. In *Kendig's Disorders of the Respiratory Tract in Children*, 7th edition. Edited by Chernick V, Boat TF, Wilmott RW, and Bush A. Philadelphia, Pa: Saunders; 2006:168.8

Table 11–3. Characteristics of Obstructive and Restrictive Patterns of Lung Disease (FVC = forced vital capacity, FEV_1 = forced expiratory volume over 1 second)

Measurement	Obstructive	Restrictive
FVC	Normal/Decreased	Decreased
FEV_1	Decreased	Decreased
FEV_1/FVC	Decreased	Normal

Obstructive and restrictive lung diseases can be distinguished by expiratory flow measurements. FVC = forced vital capacity; FEV_1 = forced expiratory volume in the first second.

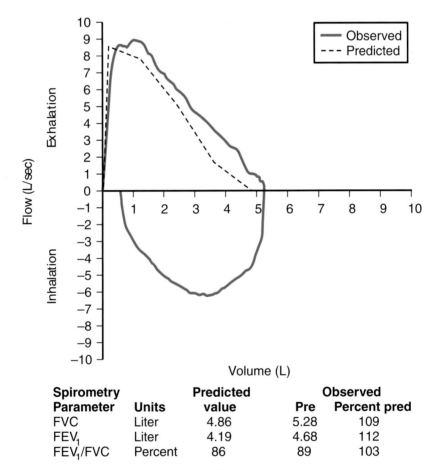

Spirometry Parameter	Units	Predicted value	Observed Pre	Observed Percent pred
FVC	Liter	4.86	5.28	109
FEV_1	Liter	4.19	4.68	112
FEV_1/FVC	Percent	86	89	103

Fig 11–1. Normal pulmonary function test. The normal flow-volume curve obtained during forced expiration rapidly ascends to the peak expiratory flow. Shortly after reaching the peak expiratory flow, the curve descends with decreasing volume following a reproducible shape that is independent of effort. In this normal flow-volume curve, the FEV_1/FVC, FEV_1, and FVC are all within the normal range for this patient's age group. The shapes of both the inspiratory and expiratory limbs are normal as well.

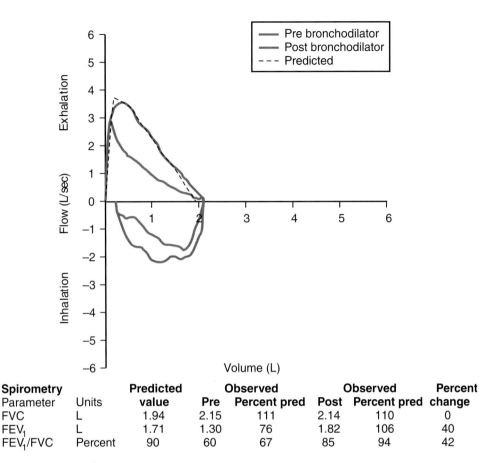

Spirometry Parameter	Units	Predicted value	Observed Pre	Observed Percent pred	Observed Post	Observed Percent pred	Percent change
FVC	L	1.94	2.15	111	2.14	110	0
FEV_1	L	1.71	1.30	76	1.82	106	40
FEV_1/FVC	Percent	90	60	67	85	94	42

Fig 11–2. Pulmonary function test demonstrating a reversible obstructive defect. The forced expiratory volume over one second (FEV_1) as a percentage of forced vital capacity (FVC) is decreased in patients with airway obstruction. The prebronchodilator curve shape (blue) is scooped. Following administration of a short-acting bronchodilator, the curve shape (brown) appears normal and there is an increase in both the FEV_1/FVC and FEV_1. This child has asthma and demonstrates a marked increase in FEV_1 after treatment with a short-acting bronchodilator. Reversible airflow obstruction is one of the hallmarks of asthma.

With a forced maneuver, the volume exhaled from full inhalation in the first second is referred to as the forced expiratory volume in the first second (FEV_1). The maneuver is completed when the subject has completed exhaling as fast as possible after a maximal inhalation. The maximal exhalation is referred to as the forced vital capacity (FVC). Normally, a child should be able to exhale more than 80% of the total lung volume in the first second of exhalation. Children with obstructive lung disease have a decreased ability to exhale. If the volume exhaled in the first second divided by the volume of full exhalation (FEV_1/FVC) is less than 80%, then airway obstruction is present (see Figure 11–2). The FEV_1 needs to be interpreted in the context of FVC as a low FEV_1 itself is not sufficient to make the diagnosis of airflow obstruction.

Spirometry cannot, however, provide data about absolute lung volumes because it measures the amount of air entering or leaving the lung, rather than the amount of air in the lung. Thus information about functional residual capacity (FRC) and lung volumes calculated from FRC (total lung capacity and residual volume) must be computed via different means. These tests include gas dilution and body plethysmography. Gas dilution is based on measuring the dilution of nitrogen or helium in a closed circuit connection to the lungs, whereas body plethysmography calculates lung gas volumes based on changes in thoracic pressures.

In addition to diagnostic uses, spirometry is used to assess the indication and efficacy of treatment. For example, the obstruction in those with asthma is usually reversible, either gradually without intervention or much more rapidly after treatment with a bronchodilator. An improvement in FEV_1 of 12% and 200 mL is considered a positive response.[9] In addition to confirming the diagnosis of asthma, the degree of airflow obstruction, as indicated by the FEV_1, is one indication of asthma control. A low FEV_1 or an acute decrease from baseline may reflect a child whose asthma is not under good control and therefore potentially at greater risk for an exacerbation.

Many children with a history strongly suggestive of asthma, even with a corroborating family history, may have a normal physical examination and normal spirometry when seen between exacerbations. Provocative testing can be used to induce bronchoconstriction in these patients. Cold air, exercise, and methacholine are commonly used to induce bronchoconstriction after a baseline study has been performed.[9] This can be reversed with the administration of a bronchodilator once the study has been completed.

CENTRAL AIRWAY OBSTRUCTION

One of the most common causes of central airway obstruction in children is due to paradoxical vocal fold motion (PVFM). PVFM involves excessive muscle tension that causes the vocal folds to involuntarily adduct during inhalation which restricts the airway opening. Often without a specific organic etiology, PVFM can masquerade as asthma, gastroesophageal reflux, vocal fold paralysis, or a functional voice disorder. PVFM may also be seen as a comorbid condition in these same patients. In some cases, PVFM may precipitate an apparent upper airway obstructive emergency, resulting in unnecessary endotracheal intubation, cardiopulmonary resuscitation, or tracheostomy. Other common presentations include laryngitis, hoarseness, choking, or stridor. Triggers include singing, shouting, exercise, and stress or anxiety. Exposure to cigarette smoke or viral infections may also trigger episodes of PVFM in the susceptible host.

The diagnosis of PVFM can be challenging. In addition to helping differentiate fixed from variable airway obstruction, spirometry may help to identify children with PVFM. This suggestive information can be gleaned from distinctive changes in the configuration of the graphic representation of inspiratory and expiratory flow volumes plotted against time or flow-volume loops. The flow-volume loop of a child with paradoxical vocal fold motion may appear normal between episodes, only taking on the characteristic shape on the flow-volume curve when the vocal cords are adducted. The observation that the obstruction is evident only intermittently helps establish the diagnosis and direct appropriate therapy.

A fixed central airway obstruction, such as tracheal stenosis, may obstruct both inspiration and expiration, flattening the flow-volume curve for each (Fig 11–3). Variable obstruction will tend to affect one part of the ventilatory cycle. When inhaling, the chest expands and draws the airways open. The chest and intrathoracic airways collapse during exhalation. Variable extrathoracic lesions tend to obstruct on inhalation more than exhalation, whereas intrathoracic lesions, such as tracheomalacia, will typically have a more pronounced effect on exhalation. Tracheomalacia will often produce both expiratory stridor, which may worsen with exercise and respiratory infections, and a characteristic truncation of the expiratory limb of the flow-volume curve.

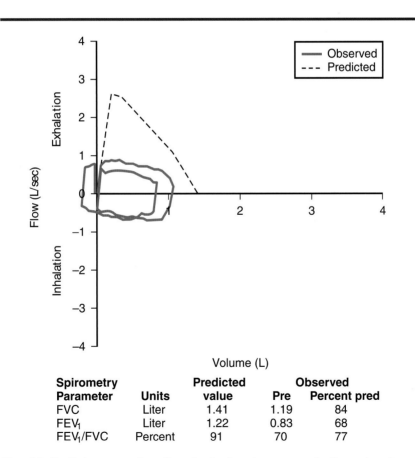

Spirometry Parameter	Units	Predicted value	Observed	
			Pre	Percent pred
FVC	Liter	1.41	1.19	84
FEV_1	Liter	1.22	0.83	68
FEV_1/FVC	Percent	91	70	77

Fig 11–3. Pulmonary function test showing an extrathoracic airway obstruction. The FEV_1/FVC, FEV_1 and FVC are all within the normal range. However, both the inspiratory and expiratory limbs of the flow volume loop are flattened. This child has severe subglottic stenosis, which developed at the site of her tracheotomy 2 years after the tube had been removed.

CONCLUSION

Pulmonary function studies, including measurement of respiratory muscle strength and flow-volume curves, can be very useful for establishing the diagnosis in a variety of disorders that affect speech. In disorders where there is a question of muscle weakness, or where monitoring muscle strength is important, inspiratory and expiratory muscle strength can be easily measured. Spirometry not only can help establish the diagnosis of airflow obstruction, but also can help determine reversibility. Reversible airflow obstruction is characteristic of asthma, allowing the differentiation from other obstructive disorders. Careful review of the flow-volume loops can provide evidence of airflow obstruction that may not otherwise be appreciated.

REFERENCES

1. *The New Grove Dictionary of Music and Musicians.* In: Sadie S, Tyrrell J, eds. *Vol 6. Edmund to Fryklund.* Oxford: Oxford University Press;1980.

2. Chernick V, West JB. The functional basis of respiratory disease. In: Chernick V, Boat TF, Wilmott RW, Bush A, eds. *Kendig's Disorders of the Respiratory Tract in Children.* 7th ed. Philadelphia, Pa: Saunders Elsevier; 2006.

3. Forster RE, DuBois AB, Briscoe, WA, Fisher, AB. *The Lung, Physiologic Basis of Pulmonary Function Tests.* 3rd ed. Chicago, Ill: Year Book Medical Publishers, Inc; 1986.

4. Laghi F, Tobin MJ. Disorders of the respiratory muscles. *Am J Respir Crit Care Med.* 2003;168,10–48.

5. Koessler W, Wanke T, Winkler G, et al. Two years' experience with inspiratory muscle training in patients with neuromuscular disorders. *Chest.* 2001;120:765–769.

6. ATS/ERS Statement on Respiratory Muscle Testing. *Am J Resp Crit Care Med.* 2002; 166:518–624.

7. Cohn JR, Sataloff RT, Spiegel JR, Cohn JB. Airway reactivity induced reversible voice dysfunction in singers. *Allergy Asthma Proc.* 1997;18(1)1–5.

8. Castile R: Pulmonary function testing in children In: Chernick V, Boat TF, Wilmott RW, Bush A, eds. *Kendig's Disorders of the Respiratory Tract in Children.* 7th ed. Philadelphia, Pa: Saunders Elsevier; 2006.

9. National Asthma Education and Prevention Program. *Full Report of the Expert Panel: Guidelines for the Diagnosis and Management of Asthma* (EPR-3). 1st ed. Pending, National Heart, Lung, and Blood Institute, National Institutes of Health; 2007:1–6064.

10. Medical Algorithms Project. (Chapter 8), Pulmonary and acid-base. *Maximal Inspiratory and Maximal Expiratory Pressures.* Institute for Algorithmic Medicine: Houston, Tex: Copyright (©) 2006-2007.

Voice Therapy for the Child with a Vocal Disorder

Jennifer Allegro

INTRODUCTION

Voice intervention for the child with a voice disorder can take on many different forms. The speech-language pathologist working within the pediatric population should be receptive to the use of varied and nontraditional approaches to improve voice quality. Information obtained from a comprehensive perceptual, acoustic, and stroboscopic assessment of vocal functioning is critical in establishing an appropriate therapy program for the child. A detailed discussion of the comprehensive voice assessment conducted by the speech-language pathologist and otolaryngologist specialized in the evaluation and treatment of pediatric voice disorders can be found in Chapter 5. In addition to incorporating findings from the comprehensive voice assessment, a successful voice therapy program must take into account underlying medical factors, behavior and psychosocial factors, functional communication needs of the child,

and most importantly, the role and involvement of the caregivers in the child's daily voice activities.

THE ROLE OF THE SPEECH-LANGUAGE PATHOLOGIST

A speech-language pathologist works individually or as part of a multidisciplinary team to help adults and children communicate effectively and efficiently.[1] Speech-language pathologists evaluate and treat adults and children with voice, language, speech, fluency, and other related communication or swallowing disorders. Voice therapy is a type of treatment provided by the speech-language pathologist to address dysphonia —deviations in vocal quality, pitch, and/or volume. A speech-language pathologist working within pediatric voice disorders will have a strong interest in vocal pathology and will have likely pursued additional training throughout their career in the identification and treatment of voice disorders.

Speech-language pathologists provide voice therapy to children in a variety of settings including specialized pediatric voice clinics, hospital outpatient/inpatient clinics, children's treatment centers, private clinics, public health units, and school boards. There are several types of service delivery models for the provision of voice therapy. Indirect service delivery models may include patient education, parent workshops, and classroom consultation, whereas direct service delivery models include individual and group voice training sessions. Individual or group therapy sessions may range from half an hour to 1 hour, with the frequency of therapy dependent on a number of factors such as the severity of the child's voice disorder, the child's progress in therapy, and the availability of speech-language pathology services within a given geographical region.

THERAPY CONSIDERATIONS FOR THE PEDIATRIC POPULATION

There are many existing voice therapy programs designed for adults with voice disorders. Therapy techniques from adult therapy programs are routinely adapted to accommodate the child and his or her presenting voice dysfunction. However, there are inherent differences in voice intervention approaches between children and adults. Adults with voice disorders typically recognize the presence of a voice problem, are motivated for change, and understand the causal relationship between voice use and symptoms. On the contrary, children with voice disorders are frequently unaware of the existence of a voice problem and have a limited understanding of the cause-and-effect relationship of voice behaviors and their symptoms.[2,3] Subsequently, children will typically require a greater amount of time spent in therapy focusing on awareness and explanation of the voice disorder. In addition, when adapting adult therapy approaches for children the underlying motivation level, developmental and cognitive status, and expressive/receptive language level must be taken into consideration.

One of the primary challenges in voice therapy with children is motivation for voice change. Voice therapy techniques are taught to children with carryover and reinforcement into the child's life by caregivers, family, and school personnel. However, for voice therapy to be successful it is important that a main motivation for improvement stem from the child. Determining the child's maturational level and "readiness" for direct voice therapy is necessary prior to commencing direct therapy.

The cognitive and development levels of the child will have direct implications on voice behaviors, as well as other general behaviors that indirectly impact therapy. For children who have never had a "normal" voice quality, explanations and activities targeted to improve voice may be more difficult not only because of developmental age but also because the child may not have an internal representation or memory of a "normal" voice.[4] The use of motivating and engaging materials can be introduced early in therapy to facilitate the child's general awareness of the voice disorder. In addition to existing therapy programs which provide strategies for different phases of therapy[2] there have also been recent developments in computer programs and interactive software packages that target the pediatric population.

The clinician's awareness of the child's expressive and receptive language levels is necessary to ensure appropriate therapy goals and to facilitate progress with therapy. The language used during therapy for the pediatric patient must be meaningful, with concrete and modified terminology to explain voice production and therapy techniques. The use of age-appropriate language and concrete examples facilitates understanding of the target vocal technique and increases the likelihood of compliance with practice exercises. A multimodality approach incorporates the use of verbal, written, audio, and visual cues to teach concepts and voice exercises to the young child. For example, when working with a preschool-age child, the description "motor sound" (of a boat, airplane, etc.) for bilabial trill may be more appropriate to describe the target vocal exercise. Also, clinician feedback on the child's voice use and vocal exercise techniques during the session should be tangible and frequent.

Therapy for the young child will typically be play-based with structured activities to engage the child and caregiver.[4] Therapy outcomes will be maximized if caregivers are actively engaged in carryover therapy of goals, implement vocal hygiene patterns and voice techniques, and provide frequent models of healthy voice production during daily activities.[2,5-8] For the school-age, preteen, and older teenager, more direct treatment activities can be introduced (eg, vocal drills) as well as more direct discussions of potentially harmful vocal behaviors common during the teen years (eg, cheerleading, shouting during sports, smoking). Depending on cognitive and developmental levels, older teenagers may participate in voice therapy programs very similar to those existing for adults.

The concept of early identification and intervention is paramount when working with children with voice disorders. Clinicians have long known—albeit anecdotally—that if left untreated voice disorders will typically not improve spontaneously. There are limited longitudinal studies investigat-ing the long-term prevalence patterns of voice disorders in children. For example, Powell et al's longitudinal study revealed that school-age children who were identified with a voice disorder and who did not receive any therapy continued to present with dysphonia for up to 5 years after the initial screening.[9] This highlights the importance of early intervention and therapy target-ed to meet the needs of the child and family.

USE OF OUTCOME MEASURES IN VOICE THERAPY FOR CHILDREN

The overall goal for the child with a voice disorder is optimal voice quality and laryngeal function. Pre- and post-treatment perceptual, objective, stroboscopic, and QOL measurements are essential in determining the overall effectiveness of any therapy program. At the Centre for Paediatric Voice and Laryngeal Function at The Hospital for Sick Children in Toronto, Canada, multidimensional voice evaluations are performed initially to obtain baseline data and at completion of therapy to obtain outcome data. Perceptual and objective evaluations assist in the decision-making process for therapy goals and activities, facilitate monitoring of progress with therapy, and document changes in voice. As such, therapy goals should be measurable and incorporate the use of multidimensional voice parameters.[10]

Direct voice therapy is an important part of the overall treatment plan of a child with a voice disorder. Early identification and intervention is advocated; however, voice therapy is also highly effective in patients with a long-standing history of dysphonia.[10]

The efficacy of voice therapy has been investigated and substantiated for a wide range of voice disorders in both adults and children.[10-15] A comprehensive outline of clinical trials and efficacy studies can be found in Ramig and Verdolini's[16] review of the literature up to 1998 and in the more recent technical report from the American Speech-Language-Hearing Association in 2005.[17]

INDIRECT AND DIRECT THERAPY TECHNIQUES

Voice therapy aims to minimize inappropriate voice use and to restore normal phonatory function within the context of an underlying organic and/or nonorganic laryngeal pathology. To address the multifactorial nature of voice disorders in children and to maximize therapy outcomes, therapy programs should be comprehensive and combine both indirect and direct treatment techniques.[11,14] Therapy programs for children typically evolve through several important phases: an initial period of general awareness of voice production and vocal behavior; a period of more specific awareness of the vocal behaviors requiring change; a period of direct voice therapy or vocal exercise activities; and finally, generalization or carryover activities.[2,5]

INDIRECT THERAPY TECHNIQUES

Indirect therapy techniques include (1) education on normal and disordered voice production and disorders, and (2) vocal hygiene (Table 12-1). The educational component of any therapy program includes an overview of normal and healthy voice production, with a discussion of laryngeal structure and function suitable to the child's age and developmental/cognitive level. Various activities, interactive models, and computer software programs can be incorporated into the educational sessions to facilitate understanding and increase motivation levels. Andrews and Summers[2] outline in detail numerous activities and strategies for the education and awareness phases of voice therapy. For young children in particular, it is advisable that the child's caregiver(s) be involved in the educational sessions to ensure consistency of terminology and to ensure the entire family has a

Table 12–1. Indirect and Direct Therapy Techniques

Indirect Therapy	Direct Therapy
Patient and Family Education	Resonant Voice Techniques
Vocal fold anatomy and physiology	Vocal Function Exercises
Normal and disordered voice production	Voice Facilitating Techniques
Patient awareness to voice disorder	Confidential Voice
Vocal Hygiene	Biofeedback Programs
Voice misuse/overuse	Manual Circumlaryngeal Therapy
Hygiene strategies	Relaxation Techniques
Daily voice behavior checklists/charts	

similar understanding of voice production during the child's daily activities. During this phase, it is also important to differentiate the child's voice disorder from any other speech or fluency disorders that may be present. Supplemental written information of the topics discussed is recommended, as families may be receiving a great deal of information within a relatively short time frame.

The second component of indirect therapy is vocal hygiene. Vocal hygiene attempts to address vocal behaviors that may be impacting the child's voice production. Vocal hygiene aims to eliminate potentially harmful voice patterns and promote healthy voice by advocating: hydration for the laryngeal mechanism; reduction of exposure to irritants such as cigarette smoke; elimination of habitual and frequent throat clearing/coughing; and reduction or elimination of misuse/overuse voice patterns (e.g., "funny" voices, shouting, etc.). The use of voice checklists and logs of voice behaviors are typically introduced during this stage of therapy. An important component of vocal hygiene for the pediatric voice patient is providing feasible alternatives to the child and family. For example, alternatives to throat clearing may include the dry swallow or forced yawn techniques. Or, to address excessive vocal strain and shouting, voice-facilitating techniques to improve projection of the child's voice may be considered. For older school-age and teenage patients, the clinician may want to discreetly track the frequency of vocal misuse patterns (e.g., throat clear, cough) during the session and later share this with the patient. Patients and families will often express they are unaware of the frequency of habitual vocal misuse patterns. At the Hospital for Sick Children, Toronto, Canada, a summary of vocal hygiene and voice use patterns is also provided to families in a brochure format.

DIRECT THERAPY TECHNIQUES

The following sections are intended to provide an overview of the more common direct voice therapy techniques which have traditionally been used with adults and are often adapted for the pediatric population. Table 12-1 summarizes the direct therapy techniques discussed in the upcoming section.

Direct voice therapy for children consists of vocal exercises aimed to: optimize the balance of voice production and the laryngeal mechanism; facilitate improved breathing during voice production; and achieve appropriate quality, pitch, and loudness with minimal laryngeal effort. The specific techniques and vocal exercises chosen by the clinician will vary with the specific area(s) of deficit and the underlying etiology of the child's voice disorders. Many techniques can be used successfully with children if the clinician adopts a creative and flexible approach to the voice task hierarchies and cuing strategies. For example, it is difficult to isolate and target clavicular versus diaphragmatic breathing with young children. However, with the use of small-group therapy sessions, peer interaction, and multimodality cues, posture, shoulder, and neck tension can be addressed.[18] Alternatively, rather than targeting breathing in isolation, it may be more appropriate to use more concrete speech tasks to facilitate coordination of breath and voicing (eg, having the child move from a voiceless sound to a voiced sound across the phonemes /f/ and /v/).[18]

Resonant Voice Therapy

Resonant voice is a common therapy approach in the fields of both adult and pediatric voice disorders. The aim of resonant voice therapy programs is to achieve the strongest possible voice with the least amount of effort and least impact on the vocal folds.[7-8] Resonant voice techniques are based on motor learning principles and attempt to establish a new motor pattern which optimizes phonation efficiency and minimizes the likelihood of vibratory impact stress and/or vocal fold injury.[19,20] During resonant voicing the vocal folds are in a "barely adducted" position. Verdolini et al established that this laryngeal posture was reliably distinguished from hyperadduction (during "pressed" voice quality) and hypoadduction (during "breathy" voice quality) adults with nodules and with normal larynges.[19] The technique incorporates a "forward focus" and oral vibratory sensations within the context of "easy phonation." The approach emphasizes the role of processing sensory and kinesthetic information to monitor the "feel" of voicing and to concentrate on the auditory feedback. There are several variations of the resonant therapy approach with different procedural differences.[7-8,19-21] However, among the varied approaches there is general consensus that resonant techniques require: the mastery of a basic voice training gesture; daily and frequent practice to facilitate a new motor pattern; and a gradual progression to increasingly complex tasks within a voice-task hierarchy.[21] The basic training gesture varies across authors and includes the vowel /i/, the semivowel "y" (ybuzz), and humming (/m/). The basic training gesture is first established in isolation, with a gradual move into syllables, words, phrases, and conversation. Studies investigating the efficacy of resonant voice techniques have been limited to the adult voice patient.[12,14,15,19] Resonant voice techniques have been proven to be effective in treating adult teachers with voice disorders, as measured by multidimensional outcome parameters including acoustic, perceptual, stroboscopic, and functional measurements.[14-15]

Vocal Function Exercises

A second common therapy approach in the field of adult voice disorders and often adapted for children is vocal function exercises. The underlying premise of vocal function exercises is that the laryngeal mechanism is a muscular system that may become strained and imbalanced.[7-8] The laryngeal mechanism is compared to other muscular systems in the body that may become strained and imbalanced. Similar to resonant techniques, vocal function exercises are a neuromuscular training approach. The goal of this approach is to balance the subsystems of voice (airflow, laryngeal musculature, tone) and to restore balance, strength, and ease of phonation. The program consists of four specific exercises that are practiced at home for a period of 6 to 8 weeks. The exercises consist of maximum vowel prolongations and pitch glides using specific pitch and phonetic (sound) contexts.[21] The exercises are produced as softly as possible and are combined with a forward placement of the tone. It is speculated that by improving the "strength, endurance and coordination" of the systems involved in voice production, the exercises eventually help to rehabilitate the voice and prevent negative vocal effects from extended voice use.[7]

The efficacy of vocal function exercises as a technique to improve voice production was initially substantiated in adult females with normal voice qualities.[13] In their study, Stemple et al identified that vocal function exercises had positive physiologic effects, particularly with improved airflow rates, frequency ranges, and maximum phonation times.[13] Roy et al also evaluated the effectiveness of vocal function exercises in teachers with voice disorders.[21] In their randomized trial consisting of a vocal function exercises group, a vocal hygiene group, and a nontreatment control group, Roy et al identified that the only group that reported functional improvements in voice as measured on the VHI was the group that adhered to the vocal function exercises therapy program.[21]

Therapy programs such as Resonant Voice and Vocal Function Exercises are built on the frequent use of nasal consonants. These programs utilize humming, nasal consonants, and nasalized vowels in the initial stages and then gradually shift to non-nasal consonants with varied pitch and loudness levels. Titze[22-23] describes the theoretical underpinnings of these voice exercises within the context of vocal tract shaping, vocal tract compliance, and occlusions within the vocal tract. Voice activities that create semiocclusions of the vocal tract—such as lip trills, bilabial fricatives, raspberries, tongue trills, humming, sighing, or phonation into tubes/straws—result in heightened interaction between the glottis and the supraglottal tract and facilitate more efficient phonation.[22-24] In addition, heightened kinesthetic and sensory feedback is created by the conversion of aerodynamic energy to acoustic energy within the vocal tract and behind the location of the semi-occlusion.[22-24] These exercises are effective in optimizing vocal fold vibratory functioning secondary to a vocal fold mass or compensatory muscle tension.[25]

Case Study: Muscle Tension Dysphonia

Resonant voice techniques and vocal function exercises have proven beneficial in determining stimulability for improvement in children with voice disorders. The use of bilabial trills, humming (eg, nasals consonant), and sighing ("uh hm") are very useful techniques for a variety of voice disorders in children.

Background: J.D. is a 9-year-old male who presented with a 6-week history of aphonia following an URTI. He was seen in clinic approximately 2 months following the URTI and after multiple community ENT and ER visits. Numerous external stressors were identified during the initial patient-family interview. Also noteworthy is a previous 1½-year history of inconsistent voice loss.

Assessment Findings: Perceptually J.D. presented with severe dysphonia, fluctuating from a whisper to significantly strained voice quality. Laryngostroboscopy revealed severe supraglottic compression, with lateral compression and ventricular fold vibration. The true vocal folds could not be visualized. The initial stroboscopic findings were used to explain voice production and the patient's current muscle tension dysphonia.

Diagnostic Therapy: Within the initial diagnostic therapy session, a combination of indirect and direct techniques were introduced, including: vocal function exercises, resonant voice, visual/audio biofeedback, and voice production education/counseling. Resonant voice techniques and vocal function exercises were used to determine stimulability and to establish ease of voicing. Bilabial trills were initially introduced followed by voice tasks using humming and "m" prolongation, with gradual shaping to consonant-vowel phonetic contexts. Intermittent periods of voicing were noted during stimulability tasks. The brief periods of voicing were gradually lengthened and shaped into words, phrases, and eventually conversational speech levels. Significant improvement in voicing was noted and J.D. was able to achieve near-normal voicing quality within the first session. Ongoing voice therapy and monitoring was recommended to maintain initial therapy gains and to further improve J.D.'s voice quality.

Relaxation Techniques

The goal of many relaxation approaches to voice therapy is to eliminate compensatory muscle tension and extraneous muscular effort during voice production.[25-26] Many children with voice disorders will present with some degree of inappropriate muscle tension, typically within the jaw, neck, or shoulder region. Children often benefit from visual cues (mirror, pictorial images, adult models) to explain and differentiate between inappropriate and appropriate muscle tension within these regions. Various stretching and relaxation programs are available that aim to address excessive muscle tension by direct stretching of the affected muscles in the head and neck region (eg, jaw, tongue, shoulder stretches).

Circumlaryngeal Massage/ Laryngeal Reposturing Techniques

Circumlaryngeal massage and laryngeal reposturing techniques have been successful in addressing voice disorders in adults.[27,28]

The technique involves direct palpation of the laryngeal mechanism and is often used to reduce musculoskeletal tension in hyperfunctional voice disorders. Direct palpation of the hyoid bone and thyroid cartilage is conducted while the patient is instructed to voice (hum, prolonged vowel), with gradual removal of tactile cues during voicing.[27,28] Laryngeal reposturing and circumlaryngeal massage is often difficult to implement in young children, due to the invasive nature of the technique compared to other traditional approaches, and also because of the underlying anatomy/physiology of the young larynx. Older school-age and teenage children may be more receptive to the use of direct palpation and may demonstrate benefit from use of laryngeal massage. Studies have validated the use of manual circumlaryngeal therapy, particularly for adult patients with functional voice disorders.[27,28] The studies suggest that vocal gains with manual laryngeal musculoskeletal tension are often made quickly in therapy and maintained in the long-term.

Facilitating Techniques

There are a number of techniques that are used to target specific voice symptoms. These techniques attempt to eliminate or reduce functional voice misuse and facilitate the patient to produce improved phonation by directly modifying the voice symptom. Examples of the voice facilitating techniques initially described by Boone include respiration training, digital manipulation, altering tongue position, pitch inflections, chewing exercises, and ear/auditory training.[6-8] The facilitating techniques commonly used with children include altering tongue position, eliminating hard glottal attacks, the yawn-sigh approach, open-mouth exercises, change of loudness and pitch, and voice rest. Lee et al[29] illustrated the efficacy of direct voice therapy using three types of facilitating techniques—easy voice onsets, manual circumlaryngeal, and humming phonation—in children aged 4 to 12 years of age with muscle tension dysphonia and/or vocal fold nodules. The study confirmed the efficacy of therapy using a combination of voice facilitating techniques.[29]

Elimination of hard glottal attacks and promotion of easy voice-onset is a well-known technique in pediatric voice therapy. This is a particularly useful technique to teach easy coordination of airflow and phonation and to reduce laryngeal tension.[6] Elimination of hard glottal onsets can be introduced by using a "sigh" or "h"-phonation. With this technique the child is initially taught to insert the phoneme "h" in front of an initial vowel or voiced consonant (eg, "hhhhegg" for "egg"). The "h-insertion allows the child to 'feel' the easy-onset of air intra-orally while producing the following vowel without abrupt adduction and release of the vocal folds.[29]

The yawn-sigh facilitating voice technique is also a child-friendly and engaging technique for children. In this technique the child is instructed to pretend to yawn and end with a sigh, gradually shaping this posture into real sounds and words. The ultimate goal is to lower the larynx in order to reduce laryngeal tension and foster easy airflow and phonation.[6-7]

Confidential Voice Therapy

Confidential voice is a technique used less frequently in therapy with very young children. Confidential voice therapy is also referred to as "breathy phonation" and is essentially a voiced whisper. In this approach, patients are instructed to use a soft "breathy" voice with reduced volume. Con-

fidential voice techniques may be beneficial in children with appropriate cognitive levels to distinguish between voiced and voiceless whispering. The clinician must be vigilant to discourage productions that are simply reduced in intensity, or with increased "pushing" of air, or with reduced mouth opening and increased laryngeal tension.[6] Confidential voice production is intended to be used as an interim therapy approach to foster mucosal repair following traumatic laryngeal pathology, hyperfunctional voice use, or surgery.[6]

CONCLUSION

Voice therapy techniques developed for adults are routinely adapted and applied to the pediatric voice patient. Voice therapy involves indirect methods of education and vocal hygiene, coupled with direct vocal exercises and behavioral changes to obtain optimal phonation. A multifaceted therapy approach is essential in the management of pediatric voice disorders. The lack of efficacy studies for voice therapy in children highlights the importance of future clinical trials comparing the effectiveness of different therapy techniques in children.

REFERENCES

1. Canadian Association of Speech-Language Pathologists and Audiologists. *Speech-Language Pathology*. Retrieved November 2007 from http:// www.caslpa.ca .
2. Andrews ML, Summers AC. *Voice Treatment for Children and Adolescents.* San Diego, Calif: Singular Thomson Learning; 2002.
3. Trani M, Ghidini A, Bergamini G, Presutti L. Voice therapy in pediatric functional dys-

phonia: a prospective study. *Int J Pediatr Otolaryngol.* 2007;1:379–384.

4. Hooper CR. Treatment of voice disorders in children. *Lang Speech Hearing Serv Schools.* 2004; 35:320–326.

5. Andrews ML. *Manual of Voice Treatment: Pediatrics Through Geriatrics.* 2nd ed. San Diego, Calif: Singular Publishing Group; 1999.

6. Colton RH, Casper JK. *Understanding Voice Problems: A Physiological Perspective for Diagnosis and Treatment.* 2nd ed. Baltimore, Md: Williams & Wilkins; 1996.

7. Stemple JC, Glaze LE, Klaben BG. *Clinical Voice Pathology: Theory and Management.* 3rd Ed. San Diego, Calif. Singular Publishing Group;2000.

8. Stemple JC. *Voice Therapy Clinical Studies.* 2nd ed. San Diego, Calif. Singular Publishing Group;2000.

9. Powell M, Filter MD, Williams B. A longitudinal study of the prevalence of voice disorders in children from a rural school division. *J Commun Disord.* 1989;22:375–382.

10. Speyer R, Wieneke GH, Dejonckere PH. Documentation of progress in voice therapy: perceptual, acoustic, and laryngostroboscopic findings pretherapy and posttherapy. *J Voice.* 2004;18:325–340.

11. Carding PN, Horsley IA, Docherty GJ. A study of the effectiveness of voice therapy in the treatment of 45 patients with nonorganic dysphonia. *J Voice.* 1999;13:72–104.

12. Simberg S, Sala E, Tuomainen J, Sellman J, Ronnemaa A. The effectiveness of group therapy for students with mild voice disorders: a controlled clinical trial. *J Voice.* 2006;20 (1):91–109.

13. Stemple JC, Lee L, D'Amico B, Pickup B. Efficacy of vocal function exercises as a method of improving voice production. *J Voice.* 1994;8:271–278.

14. Roy N, Weinrich B, Gray SD, Tanner K, Stemple JC, Sapienza CM. Three treatments for teachers with voice disorders: a randomized clinical trial. *J Speech Lang Hear Res.* 2003; 46(3):670–688.

15. Chen SH, Hsiao TY, Hsiao LC, Chung YM, Chiang SC. Outcome of resonant voice therapy for female teachers with voice disorders: perceptual, physiological, acoustic, aerodynamic, and functional measurements. *J Voice.* In press.

16. Ramig LO, Verdolini K. Treatment efficacy: voice disorders. *J Speech Lang Hear Res.* 1998;21:S101–S116.

17. American Speech-Language-Hearing Association. *The Use of Voice Therapy in the Treatment of Dysphonia* [Technical Report]. Retrieved March 2007 from: http:// www.asha.org/policy .

18. Hunt J, Slater A. *Working with Children's Voice Disorders.* Oxon, UK: Speechmark Publishing Limited; 2003.

19. Verdolini-Marston K, Burke M, Lessac A, Glaze L, Caldwell E. Preliminary study of two methods of treatment for laryngeal nodules. *J Voice.* 1995;9:74–85.

20. Verdolini K, Druker DG, Palmer PM, Samawi H. Laryngeal adduction in resonant voice. *J Voice.* 1998;12:315–327.

21. Roy N, Gray SD, Simon M, Dove H, Corbin-Lewis K, Stemple JC. An evaluation of the effects of two treatment approaches for teachers with voice disorders: A prospective randomized clinical trial. *J Speech Lang Hear Res.* 2001;44:286–296.

22. Titze IR. Acoustic interpretation of resonant voice. *J Voice.* 2001;15:519–528.

23. Titze IR. Voice training and therapy with a semi-occluded vocal tract: rationale and scientific underpinnings. *J Speech Lang Hear Res.* 2006;49:448–459.

24. Smith CG, Finnegan EM, Karnell MP. Resonant voice: spectral and nasendoscopic analysis. *J Voice.* 2005;19:607–622.

25. Emerich KA. Nontraditional tools helpful in the treatment of certain types of voice disturbances. *Curr Opin Otolaryngol Head Neck Surg.* 2003;11:149–153.

26. Rammage L, Morrison M, Nichol H. *Management of the Voice and Its Disorders.* 2nd ed. San Diego, Calif: Singular Thomson Learning; 2001.

27. Roy N, Bless DM, Heisey D, Ford CN. Manual circumlaryngeal therapy for functional dysphonia: an evaluation of short- and long-term treatment outcomes. *J Voice.* 1997;11: 321–331.

28. Roy N, Leeper HA. Effects of the manual laryngeal musculoskeletal tension reduction technique as a treatment for functional voice disorders: perceptual and acoustic measures. *J Voice.* 1993;7:242-249.

29. Lee E-K, Son Y-I. Muscle tension dysphonia in children: voice characteristics and outcome of voice therapy. *Int J Pediar Otorhino-laryngol.* 2004;69:911-917.

Working with the Pediatric Singer: A Holistic Approach

Robert Edwin

INTRODUCTION

Children sing. Whether it be nursery rhymes at home, songs in school choruses, show tunes on Broadway, or arias in opera, children sing. In my large private voice studio, over two-thirds of my students are under the age of 18. They represent but the tip of a very substantial "iceberg" of pediatric singers who want to study the art of singing. Add to that the many children who wish to sing better for amateur performance or for purely personal reasons, and the iceberg swells significantly. Yet, despite this large population so eager to be taught, the opinion still exists among many voice care providers and pedagogues that children should not study singing until after puberty.

This opinion, however, flouts the fact that no scientific, pedagogic, physiologic, or psychologic evidence exists indicating teaching children to sing is inherently harmful to their bodies, minds, or spirits. That is not to say children or others cannot do harmful things to the voice. Most voice care professionals are well aware of the damage improper, ill-advised, or excessive voice use can inflict, but it will be argued here that properly trained young singers with age-appropriate vocal technique and repertoire are less likely than untrained singers to hurt themselves or allow themselves to be hurt by other people. For more support on this pedagogic point of view, please reference the American Academy of Teachers of Singing 2002 statement, "Teaching Children to Sing," at the end of this chapter (Appendix 13).

BEGINNING SINGERS

When do children start to sing? We know from numerous clinical studies that respiration and phonation begin at birth. Intonation (cooing, squealing, laughing) normally develops within the first 4 months of life. Articulation begins at around 4 months, with consonant-vowel alternations called babble following at 7 to 10 months. The first words with intentional accent and variation of pitch appear at 10 to 13 months. Before a child is 2 years old, two-word combinations are being used. It is important to note that after 7 or 8 months of age a child will stop using the sounds he does not hear on a regular basis and will use only those he hears most frequently.

An analysis of these data reveals that the necessary elements for singing—respiration, phonation, resonation, and articulation—are in place at a very early age. It follows then that the opportunity to teach children to sing can also occur at a very early age.

In this teacher's studio, such opportunities occur frequently. Like many of my colleagues in dance and instrumental music, I take great delight in introducing young children to a wonderful art form through the use of age-appropriate and voice-appropriate technique and repertoire that challenges but does not overly tax their minds and bodies.

A HOLISTIC PEDAGOGIC APPROACH

The voice does not exist in a vacuum. It is not like any other musical instrument. It issues forth from the very fiber of every human being, the result of the activity of flesh and blood, mind and body, psyche and soma. The voice is as individual as the individual who creates it.

A singing teacher's initial session with the pediatric singer can yield much information about that young person's uniqueness. As the singer sings a song or does a vocal exercise, we watch and listen and assess his or her voice technique including posture (slouched, rigid, or balanced), breathing (high or low in the body), phonation (breathy, pressed, or flow), resonation (nasal, covered, or balanced), and articulation (sloppy, overpronounced, or clear). We evaluate acting skills and emotive qualities (passive, phony, or evocative), repertoire preferences (Bach to rock, and places in between), and personality traits (shy to brazen, defensive to vulnerable, nervous to confident, and more places in between).

As singing is both an intuitive, talent-based activity as well as a learned behavior capable of being taught, we evaluate what the singer has given us to work with and immediately begin to formulate strategies that may help the singer achieve a higher level of efficiency and expressiveness. In the initial session and in subsequent sessions, effective teachers of singing will establish rapport and maximize their effectiveness by acquainting themselves with the aspects of their young students' lives that affect their singing. That would include understanding and respecting the uniqueness and individuality of their pediatric singers: their hopes and dreams, their likes and dislikes, how they access information, what their learning modes are, and their medical history. The singing instructor might also want to learn more about their singers' friends and family, their personal habits such as diet, sleep patterns, and hygiene, as well as their musical heritage.

ROLE-PLAY AS VOCAL TECHNIQUE

It is not an oxymoron to say that instructing the pediatric singer should take the form of "serious play," as functional activities and creativity join forces to provide a comfortable, dynamic, and playful learning environment.

By making role-play or "characterization" a part of vocal technique, the mind and body are disciplined simultaneously.

Actor and singer are always working together in partnership. Student singers learn how to create appropriate mental environments and increase attention span so they can respond confidently and positively to technical and artistic demands. Furthermore, role-play or "storytelling" encourages the singer to create a character and scene and establish a context for singing each individual vocal exercise or song. Thus, the singer as storyteller can execute any task while retaining control of his environment even as outside influences such as voice teachers, conductors, choral directors, managers, agents, and parents are directing him.

BODY ALIGNMENT

Vocal instruction should begin with body alignment. In our very casual society, some of us have come to associate good posture with superiority or even arrogance. Children do not want to feel out of place, so they often stand as many of their peers stand—in a slouch. If students can understand good posture as both a storytelling issue as well as a primary component of vocal efficiency, they may be more willing to move from the reality of the peer pressure slouch to the created reality of the storyteller whose role requires them to have a more efficient and dynamic physical presence.

Exercises for Body Alignment

The simplest exercise to establish good individual body alignment is to have the singer fully extend her arms over her head while easily flexing the knees. That action lifts the rib cage (the primary player in posture), elevates the sternum, and lines up the rest of the body. Singers with poor posture

may experience discomfort when their bodies are placed in an unfamiliar position. They need to be reassured that, in time, their muscles will adjust to this new and more efficient position.

For the singer to better understand balanced posture, have her explore the extremes of posture in a role-play. Ask her to portray a girl who is shy or lacking in self- confidence. Most likely she will slouch over with a collapsed rib cage and rounded shoulders to model that hypoposture. Then, ask her to portray a girl who is over confident or "stuck up." Most likely she will exaggerate a lifted rib cage, pull back on the shoulders, and lock the knees to model hyper posture. Now repeat the initial exercise with the arms comfortably over the head and the knees slightly flexed to re-establish balanced posture and a sense of a confident individual. More intense and specific work on body alignment can be done through disciplines such as the Alexander technique and Feldenkrais method.

BREATH MANAGEMENT

The development of an "I'm-in-charge-and-having-fun" storyteller can also aid in breath management training. The singer need not be a shy, rib cage-dropping, shallow-breathing person; or a tense, rib cage-stretching, shoulder-raising person, but rather a confident, ribcage-elevated, lower torso-expanding, deeper breathing individual.

Exercises for Breath Management

First, have the singer take very shallow, small breaths as the shy boy with his upper torso collapsed. Then, have him take very high, big breaths raising his shoulders as if he were the "Big, Bad Wolf" in "The Three Little Pigs." Next, have the singer put his hands in a V shape on the lower part of his rib cage as Superman or Peter Pan would. Without taking a breath, have him pull in and tense his abdominal muscles ("tummy" to the younger students), then release them. Repeat this exercise a few times. Next, have him exhale while contracting his abs. Then, have him relax his abs as he inhales the next breath. Patience and numerous repetitions will eventually allow for a more spontaneous release of the abs that triggers the efficient intake of air.

Exhalation, the "support" part of the breath, can be easily demonstrated by hissing like a snake. The "hisssssss" will provide resistance so the singer feels the abs contracting and managing the airflow under pressure. The singer should eventually feel his hands on his sides move out as the rib cage, abs, and back all expand on inhalation. He then needs to learn to keep that expansion throughout the exhalation phase of the breath cycle so the air is used most efficiently.

PHONATION

Phonation, too, can be strongly influenced by the storytelling process. The extremes of singing span the traditional English Choir School use of exclusively upper register or "head voice" singing, to the so-called "Annie" school of singing where lower register or "chest voice" dominant belting is used exclusively.

It is, of course, necessary for the entire voice to be developed, strengthened, and coordinated to create a functionally healthy and efficient voice. The thyroarytenoid muscles (TA) and the cricothyroid muscles (CT) share responsibility for creating vocal fold thickening and stretching, respectively, and one isolated from the other is simply bad vocal pedagogy for any age group and any style of singing. The goal in phonation is to avoid the extremes of pressed and breathy, and create that balanced vocal fold posture called flow phonation.

Exercises for Phonation

The pediatric vocalist will usually have a preferred style of singing and, hence, a register preference. Once again, through storytelling techniques and characterization, the less preferred register can be engaged. For example, an Annie-type belter can be asked to imagine herself as a very young opera singer. As the child shifts from her dominant identity to that of the opera singer, her cricothyroid muscles ("head voice") will have a greater chance to participate more actively in phonation. Be aware that for her to achieve a CT-dominant vocal fold posture, it may be necessary to choose vocal exercises or songs that are above her normal belt range. C above middle C (C5) is a good starting point for triads (1-3-5-3-1 or, do-mi-sol-mi-do) and scales (1-2-3-4-5-4-3-2-1) with the "oo" [u] vowel, as in the word, "you," usually being the easiest vowel for a strong belter/weak soprano to produce.

For the boy or girl with a weak or non-existent TA-dominant sound, a strongly, stubbornly, rudely, and loudly sung "no!" on middle C (C4) pitch or below will often trigger the dormant lower register or "chest voice."

As a warm-up or cool-down exercise, humming and chewing simultaneously on moderate pitches is one of the most beneficial. It is especially helpful for voices that have sung too long, too high, or too loud.

RESONATION

Yet another component of singing, resonation, can be addressed via storytelling. The three primary resonating cavities—the throat, the mouth, and the nose—provide almost inexhaustible combinations of sound textures as they amplify and reinforce frequencies created by the vocal folds. As the pediatric singer, to his or her detriment, often copies adult singers and adds too much thickness in vocal fold configuration and too much weight in resonance-coupling, finding the right balance or timbre for each child's voice should be a major goal of the voice instructor.

Exercises for Resonation

The full spectrum of resonance can be explored through characterization. For example, using triads, scales, or arpeggios, the pediatric singer can create a *Wizard of Oz* "Wicked Witch" storyteller to sing bright, treble-dominant, or even nasal sounds. Conversely, the "cowardly lion" character can create the dark, bass-dominant, covered sounds. Those two characters can then be given singing instruction to create a more balanced chiaroscuro, bright/dark sound, appropriate to the age and individual vocal instrument of the student.

Have the singer sing a triad (1-3-5-3-1) starting in a comfortable, medium to low pitch range (middle C) first as the "Wicked Witch" using the evil laugh, "heh, heh, heh, heh, heh." Ask the singer to sing it through her nose while scrunching up her face. (Pointing a crooked finger while singing is optional.) Move the triad up and down in half-steps to hear if such resonance can be kept consistent throughout the usable voice range. Make sure the sound is not pushed or pressed.

Next, have the singer create the "Cowardly Lion" character to sing the opposite extreme: a hollow, woofy sound with little or no treble or bright resonance. The same triad can be used, this time with the phrase, "Oh dear, Do-ro-thy." Once again, be on the alert for pushed or pressed phonation. The next step is to ask the singer to resing both phrases with a prettier sound, one that has a little of the Wicked Witch, a little of the Cowardly Lion, but mostly Dorothy. Experiment with the textures so the singer can hear the entire spectrum of her resonant voice.

ARTICULATION

Articulation also falls under the storytelling banner as sloppy, mumbled word formation, or crisp, clean pronunciation is assigned to specific characters. Actively and efficiently engaging the articulators—the lips, the teeth, the tongue, and the soft palate—will help the pediatric singer release excessive tensions as well as improve the intelligibility of both speech and song. Note that role-play may at times hit a bit too close to home so, initially, care must be taken to make the storyteller characters unthreatening to the student's core personality and behavior. For example, a child with a severe speech defect may react negatively to an exercise and character role-play that highlights her problem.

Exercises for Articulation

On a five-note diatonic scale (1-2-3-4-5-4-3-2-1), have the singer sing the alphabet with each letter being repeated on each note of the scale (a-a-a-a-a-a-a-a-a, b-b-b-b-b-b-b-b-b, etc). Listen and look for problems caused by malfunctioning articulators (lisps, tongue thrusts, retracted tongue, palatal rigidity). Do not take this exercise too high because the singer will begin to lose intelligibility as the notes go above the musical staff (G5). Next, ask the singer to repeat the exercise with two different characters, "Crisp," who overpronounces each letter, and "Sloppy," who underpronounces each letter. Once again, the extremes will help to define the middle or balanced position for each pediatric singer. This same exercise can be done with names, numbers, and food groups, and can serve a variety of pedagogic goals, such as phonation and resonation objectives. The exercises can also be interactive with the student providing input on the content such as names of friends or favorite foods.

MUTATION: THE "CHANGE OF VOICE"

One of the most rewarding pedagogic opportunities comes during the adolescent voice change as both the student's voice and psyche are guided through the turbulent waters of laryngeal growth. The instructor can use constantly changing storyteller modes and continual reinforcement of technique, especially the use of the upper register (falsetto or head voice) which acts as a counterbalance as the lower register (chest voice) heads "southward." One can play man's/woman's voice, boy's/girl's voice, and child's voice games exploring old and new timbres and vocal fold postures. Let the larynx dictate what it wants to do and in what range it wants to do it. Accept the narrowing of vocal range as a natural and temporary part of the transition process. Because of their ongoing singing through

mutation, male singers, especially, rarely experience the embarrassing register shifts and yodels of their untrained counterparts. For that alone, they seem forever grateful for singing lessons.

REPERTOIRE

Not all children aspire to be the next famous operatic or classical singer. Pavarotti, Hampson, Horne, or Battle may not be on any of their music listening devices, so the child voice pedagogue should be prepared to address and affirm, if they are willing and able, Contemporary Commercial Music (nonclassical) singing techniques and styles such as pop, rock, rhythm and blues, gospel, Tejano, jazz, and folk. Regardless of the style of singing, classical to CCM, teachers need to continually remind their young charges not to copy the adult voices they hear either live or on recordings. Student singers should be encouraged to develop voice techniques, styles, and repertoire that suit their age, their instrument, and their personality. For example, low-voiced, pediatric belters should avoid the temptation to try for a role in *Annie*. That show has been blamed for many a voice disorder, yet it is a very doable and vocally safe show for child singers with very high belt voices. Conversely, high-voiced singers should avoid repertoire whose pitch range stays in the low extreme of their vocal compass.

It is important to note here that no one voice technique can serve all the diverse styles of singing. Voice techniques are implemented to support the style and repertoire being sung. Just as a classically trained young soprano is not prepared to do the aforementioned *Annie* unless she is also simultaneously working on her belting and mixing voice technique, neither is an *Annie*-type belter prepared to sing in the opera, *The Magic Flute,* unless she, too, has developed a classical voice technique.

CONCLUDING THOUGHTS

Whether teaching the "Annie" and "Oliver" on Broadway, or the "Annie" and "Oliver" in the local synagogue show, a singing instructor needs to understand how to teach children and what to teach children. A basic knowledge of both child and adult psychology as well as vocal anatomy and physiology is essential. Critical is the recognition that children are not "miniature adults" to be trained with the same techniques and expectations.

The voice teacher needs to establish a child-friendly learning environment. The standard components of singing—posture, breath management, phonation, resonation, articulation, and interpretation—need to be addressed in a patient, creative, and playful manner. Also, the standard assortment of vocalises, lip and tongue trills, triads and scales need to be reshaped so that the exercises are perceived as games rather than dull, repetitive drills. Important, too, is the teacher's sensitivity to the ever changing bodies and minds of his or her student singers. As vocal and emotional limits expand and contract, the teacher must be able to adjust the lessons to keep the singer within these continually evolving boundaries.

On that same note, teachers should find out if the children will receive at home the kind of encouragement that will allow them to develop their own vocal identities. Even if parents or guardians are living out their own performing fantasies through the child, it is still possible for that child to grow independently as long as the child is allowed strong personal input in the learning process. The process tends to break down if an adult tries to dominate the child's musical will, or if the child is singing only to please the family.

The role of the pediatric voice pedagogue will not be a comfortable one for all teachers of singing. Teaching children to sing requires an even greater commitment beyond technique and repertoire. The child's constantly changing body and evolving mind challenge continuity with regard to predictability of either vocal or emotional stability. Every lesson should begin with, "where are you and your voice today?" The answer strongly influences the direction of the session. It is a wise and skillful teacher who looks, listens, and then begins the day's lesson.

On a personal note, my hope is that more singing teachers will join me in this fascinating and rewarding endeavor. Unfortunately, at this writing, there are simply too few of us willing and able to serve the needs of pediatric singers.

APPENDIX 13

AMERICAN ACADEMY OF TEACHERS OF SINGING

www.voiceteachersacademy.org

Member
National Music Council

Chair
Robert C. White, Jr.
600 West 116th Street
New York, NY 10027-7042

Vice Chair
Jean Westerman Gregg
11 Old Quarry Road
Woodbridge, CT 06525-1005

Secretary
Jeannette L. LoVetri
317 West 93rd Street, #3B
New York, NY 10025-7236

Treaurer
Jan Eric Douglas
777 West End Avenue
New York, NY 10025-5551

Publications Officer
Robert Gartside
20 Loring Road
Lexington, MA 02421-6945

Adele Addison
Elaine Bonazzi
Claudia Catania
Lindsey Christiansen
Jan Eric Douglas
Robert Edwin
Shirlee Emmons
Robert Gartside
Jean Westerman Gregg
Katherine Hansel
Hilda Harris
Helen Hodam
Barbara Honn
Marvin Keenze
Paul Kiesgen
Antonia Lavanne
Jeannette LoVetri
Elizabeth Mannion
John McCollum
Joyce McLean
Klara Meyers
Richard Miller
Dale Moore
Gordon Myers
Louis Nicholas
Russell Oberlin
Chloe Owen
Julian Patrick
John B. Powell
George Shirley
Richard Sjoerdsma
Craig Timberlake
Robert C. White, Jr.
Beverly Wolff
Edward Zambara

TEACHING CHILDREN TO SING
A Statement by the American Academy of Teachers of Singing
November 2002

From their first cry at birth to their last sigh at death, human beings are sound-producing creatures. We know from numerous clinical studies that respiration and phonation occur at birth. Intonation (humming, cooing, squealing, laughing) normally develops in the first four months of life. Articulation and the first words occur at about one year of age. Before a child is two years old, two-word combinations are being used.

Analysis of such data reveals that the necessary elements for singing – respiration, phonation, resonation, and articulation – are in place at a very early age. It follows then that the opportunity to teach children to sing more efficiently and expressively can also occur at a very early age. There continues to this day, however, a controversy as to when, and even if, the training of young singers should begin. The **American Academy of Teachers of Singing** addresses the topic of teaching children to sing.

Acutely aware of the physical damage improper, excessive, or ill-advised singing can cause, the Academy in the past has recommended that children not engage in formal voice studies. However, upon further investigation, no scientific, pedagogical, or physiological evidence indicates that child voice pedagogy is inherently harmful to children's bodies, minds, or spirits.

The Academy now recognizes that there are benefits to teaching children to sing. In fact, well-trained singers of any age are less likely than untrained singers to hurt their vocal instruments or to allow their instruments to be hurt by others. Observing our fellow pedagogues in dance and instrumental music, we find they have identified and successfully acted on the potential to instruct interested and motivated young children in their respective disciplines. Clearly, these teachers have developed age-appropriate technical exercises and repertoire that challenge but do not overly tax the young body and mind. They are astutely aware that children are not "miniature adults," and should not be taught as such.

The Academy believes that teachers of singing should take their cue from the aforementioned colleagues to develop and utilize age-appropriate vocal exercises and repertoire that support the natural inclination of children to express themselves in singing and song. The quantity and quality of musical talent as well as the interest of each child, however, will vary greatly. Therefore, the Academy suggests three general categories of child singer:

Category one includes children for whom singing is but one activity to which they are exposed along with other disciplines such as mathematics, science, history, language, physical education, art, dance, and spirituality. For them, gaining an appreciation of and experience in the recreational joy of singing may be sufficient. Venues where this exposure occurs include home, school, and places of worship.

Category two includes children for whom singing is a recreational activity they wish to pursue more intensely. These children may express an interest in private voice lessons to improve basic vocal technique and develop repertoire. Venues include select choirs and choruses, and solo opportunities at school, clubs, sporting events, and places of worship.

2

Category three includes children for whom singing is a professional or pre-professional activity that subjects their vocal technique, performance skills, and repertoire to highly critical evaluation and scrutiny. For these children to deal successfully with the added physical and emotional demands a singing career requires, formal voice training should be considered a necessity. Venues include opera, music theater, recording, pageants, film, radio, and television.

Regardless of the categories of the singers, training should be in the hands of qualified teachers who understand both **how** to teach children and **what** to teach children. A basic knowledge of child vocal anatomy and physiology, age appropriate vocal technique and repertoire, and child psychology is essential for successful instruction. Teachers must know, for example, that a child's vocal instrument cannot sustain the larger and fuller tonal spectra adult vocal instruments are capable of producing. Teachers must also avoid repertoire that exceeds the physical, intellectual, and emotional understanding of the young student singer.

Critical to the pedagogical process is the establishment of a child-friendly learning environment. Elements such as posture, breath management, phonation, resonation, articulation, and interpretive skills need to be addressed in a patient, creative, and playful manner. Using standard pedagogical tools such as lip and tongue trills, scales, triads, and arpeggios, the singing teacher must endeavor to create exercises that resemble games rather than repetitive drills. For example, abdominal breathing activity can be explored by having the child "pant like a dog." Scales and other vocalises can be done using numbers, colors, names, or even items found in the studio. Role play and storytelling suggestions ("be a happy singer," or "pretend you are saying something very important") can help to focus the exercises by providing a context for their use. As lessons continue, the instructor must be sensitive to the growing and changing bodies and minds of the child singers, closely monitoring them to see if the students are singing within or beyond their vocal and emotional limitations. This is especially true during male puberty since rapid physical growth can radically alter and even temporarily destabilize the vocal instrument.

Important, too, is a willingness to work with the child's preference in music. Not all children wish or need to sing classical repertoire. Therefore, the teacher may need to address nonclassical singing styles such as music theater, pop, rock, jazz, gospel, Latino, country, rhythm and blues, and folk music, and provide vocal techniques to authentically support these and other vocal music categories. No matter what the vocal style, however, teachers need to remind their young students not to imitate the fuller, more mature adult voices they hear, but to develop a vocal sound that suits their own age, voice, and personality.

Since children are not independent beings, teachers must be able to effectively communicate with parents and guardians regarding their child's training, choice of repertoire, and potential for growth. Adults pushing unwilling young singers into training and performance environments need to be tactfully confronted and encouraged to let the children participate in the decision-making process.

In summary, singing is a natural and spontaneous activity for a majority of children. The **American Academy of Teachers of Singing** supports and encourages the teaching of children to sing. As in other activities in which youngsters are involved, singing can be accomplished on many levels from recreational to professional. At all levels, however, there should be qualified instructors willing and able to help young singers on their musical journeys.

Benign Lesions of the Pediatric Vocal Folds: Nodules, Webs, and Cysts

J. Scott McMurray

INTRODUCTION

The evaluation and management of hoarseness in children remains a highly controversial but also often speculative problem. Hoarseness in children is often neglected or overlooked as a transient and self-limiting problem. Many assume a stance of "benign" neglect to avoid potential iatrogenic aggravation of the laryngeal pathology. This attitude is often justified as a means to avoid potential life-lasting injury to the vocal folds. Common goals, however, for those who actively treat or use benign neglect for dysphonic children are their protection from harm and their improved quality of life. With advances in diagnostic tools, a better understanding of the developing layers of the vocal folds, better measures of the impact on quality of life, and refinements in surgical techniques and their indications, the treatment of hoarseness in children will dramatically change and the stance of

benign neglect will be determined as less than benign (Fig 14-1).

If we consider each dysphonic child as our own, we should worry about the worst, see what is there and treat what we find. Our experiences reinforce the need to visualize the larynx and accurately diagnose the cause of the dysphonia in the child. Too often, dysphonic children will be ignored as simply having something they will outgrow until they are found to have obstructing papillomata in severe respiratory distress (Fig 14-2). The psychological, social, and academic impact of dysphonia on a child is often underplayed as well. It has been shown that dysphonic children are often perceived as dirty, cruel, ugly, unfair, small, weak, slow, clumsy, or sick based solely on their vocal quality and no visual cues.[1] The assessment of the impact on perceptions of quality of life is also in its infancy. New tools are being designed to help determine the impact of dysphonia on children.[2] I believe that we will find that the dysphonic and

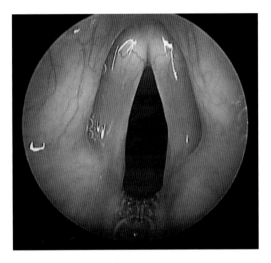

Fig 14–1. Endoscopic view of a normal 6-year-old larynx during direct micro-laryngoscopy. Note the relatively small membranous vocal fold to vocal process ratio when compared to an adult. This may concentrate vibratory trauma to a small area in the child than the adult.

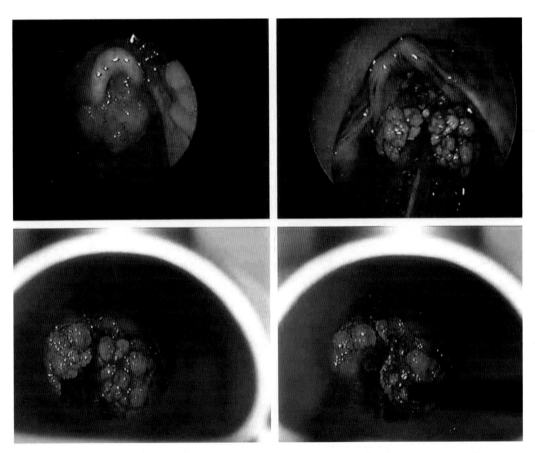

Fig 14–2. Young boy with severe papilloma. For 5 months he had been assumed to have a functional voice disorder until he began having breathing dificulties as well.

pressed voiced child perceives significant impairments to quality of life compared to the child with a normal voice. As better tools to measure perceived quality of life in children of all ages are developed, the true impact will be determined.

Recent review of the outcomes of children with nodules moving on to adolescence revealed that 29% of the nodules persisted and only 44% of children with nodules achieved a normal voice in adolescence.[3] All children were given vocal hygiene or voice therapy and only a few had surgery. This review suggests that a significant number of children do not improve simply with puberty and laryngeal maturation. The means for visualizing the vibrating pedi-

atric vocal fold are improving dramatically (Fig 14-3). Distal-chip cameras of smaller size, greater resolution, and brighter lighting will give the pediatric laryngologist the same capabilities of the adult laryngologists. It should be emphasized that if the diagnosis is uncertain or if what seems to be appropriate management is not demonstrating progress, direct microlaryngoscopy should be considered for a reassessment and perhaps more accurate diagnosis of the underlying pathology. As with any disease process, appropriate management relies on an accurate diagnosis.

This chapter addresses general overviews of benign glottic pathology. General approaches to each pathologic condition are

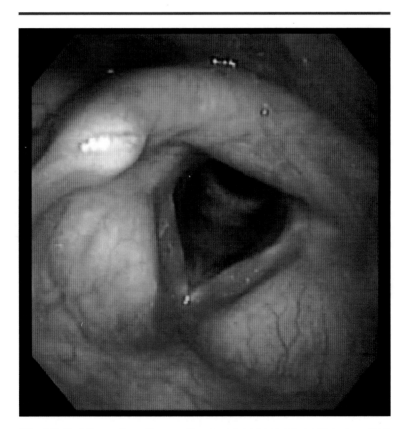

Fig 14–3. View of an 8-year larynx at nasopharyngoscopy using a distal-chip digital nasopharyngoscope.

outlined. Voice therapy, the main treatment paradigm for laryngeal disorders of adults and children is not specifically addressed in this chapter.

In the evaluation of the dysphonic child, many historical points need clarification. The duration and timing of the hoarseness is important. When did it start and who noticed it first. Was the hoarseness present since birth or did it come later? The severity and impact on the child's life must be assessed. Does the hoarseness wax and wane centered on a constant baseline of vocal quality or is the general baseline of the hoarseness progressively worsening? Are there associated breathing issues or swallowing concerns? Associated medical conditions such as asthma, environmental allergy,[3,4] chronic rhinosinusitis and cough, laryngopharyngeal reflux,[5-7] and snoring must be evaluated (Fig 14-4). A thorough voice use or abuse history should also be taken. Each of these historical points may lead us to a general idea of where inflammation or trauma to the vocal folds may be coming from. The appropriate management of concomitant medical conditions may be a prerequisite to successful management of the dysphonia.

VOCAL FOLD NODULES

Vocal nodules (Fig 14-5) are the most common cause of dysphonia in children. Although the incidence in the general pediatric population has not been extensively studied, one group from Turkey demonstrated that 36% of all school-aged children have some benign pathology of the vocal folds.[8] Dysphonia was found in the general population in 21.6% of boys and 11.7% of girls of school age.

Nodules are intense fibronectin deposits in the superficial layers of the vocal fold

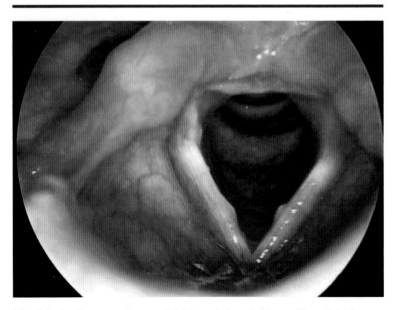

Fig 14–4. Symmetric vocal fold nodules during office rigid laryngoscopy with signs of laryngopharyngeal reflux.

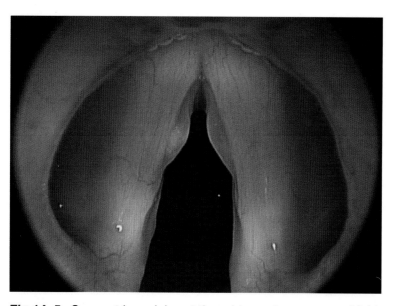

Fig 14–5. Symmetric nodules at the mid-membranous vocal fold.

often coupled with basement membrane zone injury as indicated by thick collagen type IV bands.[9] They are often centered in the mid-portion of the vibrating vocal fold and are generally symmetric to quasisymmetric (Fig 14–6). Although thought to come from vocal trauma or voice abuse, the exact inciting event leading to cyclic injury is not truly understood. Children with nodules often have a hard glottal attack and louder more pressed voices. The increased mass of the vocal folds caused by the nodules may incite a louder more strained voice. This may perpetuate the nodules but does not necessarily answer the question of their origin. Is the hard-pressed voice causing the nodules or are the nodules causing the hard pressed voice?

Further study will be required into the underlying ultrastructure and development of the layers of the vocal fold before a definitive cause will be determined. There is some controversy regarding the age when the layers of the superficial lamina propria

begin and complete their differentiation. The latest studies by Boseley and Hartnick indicate that the lamina propria may have the same ultrastructure of an adult by the age of 7 years.[10] This may be important for surgical considerations. It is not known if surgery prior to complete development of the layers of the superficial lamina propria will cause abnormal maturation and scarring or if the active differentiation and development of these layers will be protective and aid in healing. Furthermore, molecular and genetic differences in the vocal folds of hoarse and normal voicing children may play a more important role than presently understood.[11-14]

Vocal nodules generally affect boys more often than girls.[7] There is a bimodal presentation in age around 3 to 5 years and then again at 8 to 10 years. After the age of 13, dysphonia from vocal nodules becomes primarily a problem of young women. In a longitudinal study, 21% of children with prepubescent vocal nodules continued to have

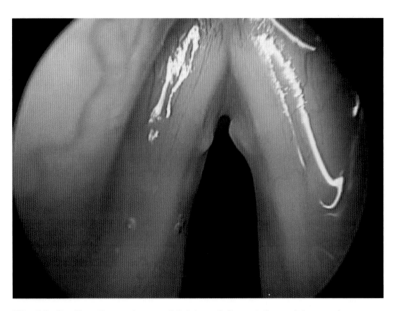

Fig 14–6. Small rough vocal fold nodules at the mid-membranous portion of the vocal fold.

dysphonia into adolescents despite voice therapy.[3] It is important, then, to discover if treating nodules at an earlier age may decrease the dysphonia seen after puberty. There is currently no widely accepted rating scale for vocal nodules in children. It is difficult to compare treatment strategies without a consistent grading scale. Shah and Nuss have recently reviewed their experience and have proposed a grading scale.[15] Their scale uses a three-point system determined by the configuration of the larynx, which is modified as "d" or "s," depending on whether the nodules are discrete or sessile. The grade 1 to 3 defines the laryngeal configuration, with 1 having a normal contour, 2 having an anterior glottic chink, and 3 having an hourglass appearance and glottic gap. Further study is required to determine the utility of their scale.

Shah and Nuss in another paper found that 75% of the children they evaluated with vocal nodules exhibited significant muscle tension disorder. This hyperfunction or muscular tension disorder correlated with nodules size.[7] It is unclear if the hyperfunction was a result of the nodule size or if the nodule size caused the increased vocal tension. They also found that 25% of the children with nodules had signs of laryngopharyngeal reflux. The presence of reflux did not correlate with nodule size, however. Their series of over 600 children illustrates the notion that not all nodules are the same (Figs 14-7 through 14-15). There may be several interrelated causes for the dense fibronectin and collagen deposition at the basement membrane and therefore treatment paradigms may need to vary depending on the cause and distribution of the nodule.

The typical history of a child with nodules consists of intermittent hoarseness that worsens with voice use and improves with voice rest. The baseline of vocal clarity generally does not worsen with time; however, the frequency of hoarseness and the duration

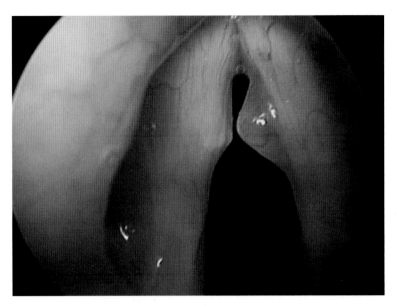

Fig 14–7. Right vocal fold polyp with left vocal fold nodule.

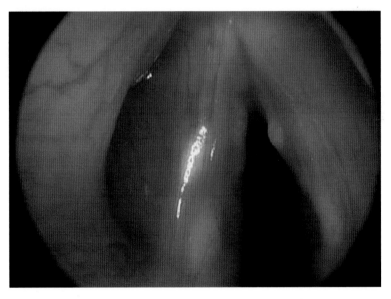

Fig 14–8. Small quasisymmetric nodules in the mid-membranous vocal fold.

with hoarseness may increase. It would be considered very unusual to have associated dysphagia. Aphonia may be experienced, symptoms of associated larygopharyngeal reflux, allergy, and chronic cough should also be noted.

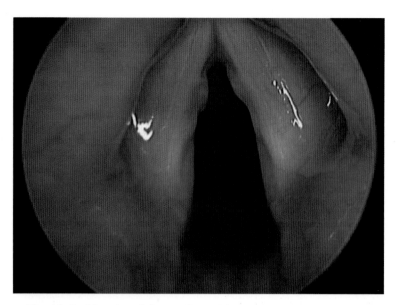

Fig 14–9. Vocal nodules at the mid-membranous vocal fold.

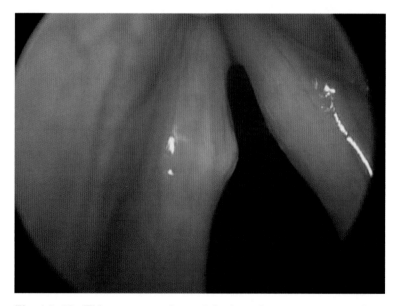

Fig 14–10. This asymmetric nodule has the appearance of an intracordal cyst.

The diagnosis is confirmed with indirect laryngoscopy. Either fiberoptic or rigid laryngoscopy should be performed to visualize the larynx. Stroboscopy may be helpful to distinguish subtle pathologies of the vocal folds such as the differentiation of

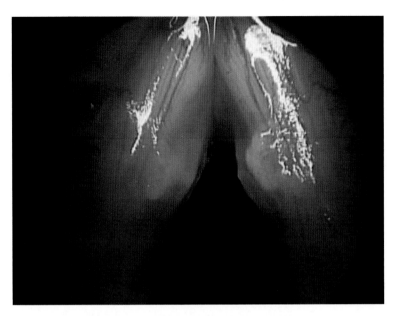

Fig 14–11. Rough appearing nodules.

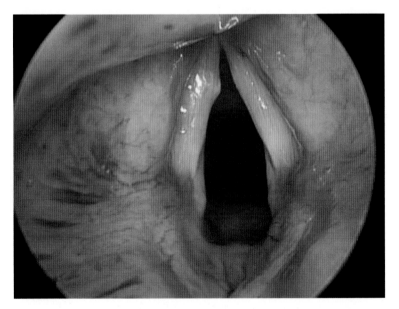

Fig 14–12. Asymmetric vocal nodule on the left vocal fold.

vocal nodules from intracordal cysts. If this cannot be determined, a trial of voice therapy and adjuvant medical therapy may be indicated with a follow-up examination. Nodules generally improve with voice therapy. In the case of a unilateral intracordal

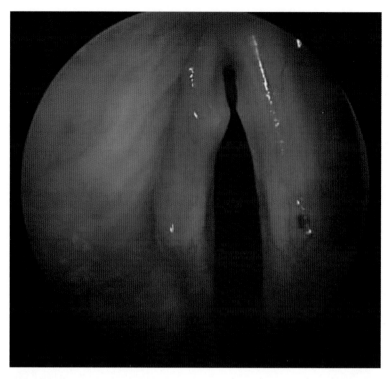

Fig 14–13. Vocal nodules at the mid-membranous vocal fold. The left nodule is slighter larger than the right nodule.

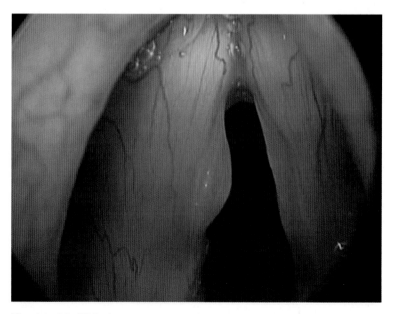

Fig 14–14. This is an asymmetric vocal nodule on the left vocal fold.

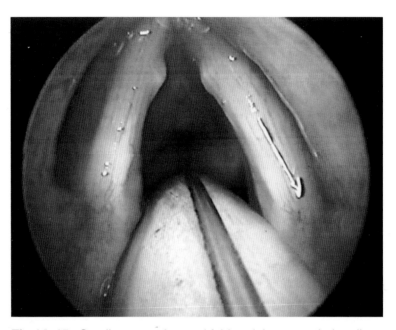

Fig 14–15. Small symmetric vocal fold nodules seen during direct microlaryngoscopy.

cyst with a contralateral nodule, the nodule and the surrounding edema of the vocal fold may improve with conservative management allowing the intracordal cyst to become more defined and easier to diagnose. If the diagnosis is still in question, direct microlaryngoscopy should be considered with palpation of the vocal folds. Proper management always relies on an accurate diagnosis (Fig 14–16).

Typically, treatment of vocal fold nodules consists of vocal hygiene, voice therapy, and behavioral management for possible reflux. Occasionally if signs and symptoms are significant for laryngopharyngeal reflux, proton-pump inhibitors are used over 3 to 4 months as an empiric antireflux therapy trial. There are currently no hard data regarding the efficacy of reflux management in the treatment of vocal nodules in children.

Other sources for potential laryngeal irritation or causes for laryngeal injury such as chronic throat clearing should be sought and treated if present. Postnasal drip from chronic adenoidal hypertrophy, chronic sinusitis, or environmental allergy may be another source for sticky mucus on the vocal folds. Environmental allergy treatment, nasal saline lavage, or surgical treatment for adenoidal or adenotonsillar hypertrophy for chronic sinusitis may be beneficial to the child with vocal nodules. The association has been made with these disease entities contributing to hoarseness but the efficacy of their treatment has not been studied.

Surgery has nearly been abandoned for the treatment of vocal nodules. This, in part, has come from the adage that the nodules will disappear with the onset of puberty. Previous surgical techniques may also have resulted in vocal fold scarring which may be lifelong. Overzealous removal of vocal fold mucosa or deep thermal injury from lasers may have contributed to these poor

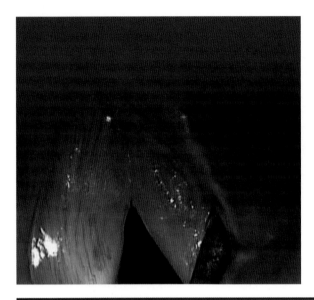

Fig 14–16. This boy had dysphonia from what looked like vocal nodules. When he failed voice therapy and medical management, direct microlaryngoscopy was performed. A sulcus vocalis was identified. This required surgical excision due to the severity of his dyphonia.

outcomes. Finally, many surgeons who have removed vocal nodules have been frustrated when some return. Successful surgical management requires proper patient selection and the development of proper surgical techniques. There are currently no reliable data on which to base the decision of when or how to remove nodules in children. It is not always an easy task to determine if a child has mastered proper voice use techniques. As with adults, good voice use may deteriorate into poor voice use depending on the circumstances. Surgical techniques for the management of vocal fold nodules will need to be developed to remove the fibrous scarring at the basement membrane zone while saving the overlaying epithelium and not disturbing the developing layers of the lamina propria. The latest techniques for removal of nodules include a superficial mucosal incision adjacent to the lesion with a dissection toward the nodule in the most superficial layers of the lamina propria. The underlying fibrous tissue is then dissected off the overlaying mucosa either with microsurgical techniques or powered microresection. Care is taken to preserve the mucosa. Voice rest followed by proper voice use is prescribed in the postoperative period.

Proper patient selection is the key to successful surgical outcomes. Adequate mastery and adherence to voice therapy and a desire for vocal improvement are required from the patient at a minimum. There are a number of children who are motivated and are experts at proper voice use, who continue to have significant hoarseness due to the mass effect and stiffening of their vocal folds by their vocal nodules. These children are prime candidates for surgical intervention.

As for treatment modalities, Kazunori Mori followed 259 children with hoarseness.[16] Presented as retrospective case reports, his patients received four different modalities; (1) vocal hygiene, (2) voice therapy, (3) surgery and voice therapy, and (4) no treatment except reassurance. As a retrospective review, the severity of the voice disorder in each group was not controlled and may have been stratified unevenly into the different treatment groups. Sixteen percent in the vocal hygiene group improved, 52% percent in the voice therapy group improved, 56% percent in the reassurance group improved, and 89% in the surgery group improved. Regardless of the treatment modality, there was a dramatic improvement in voice after puberty that did not differ among the groups. He reiterated, however, that 12% of his patients continued to have dysphonia after puberty. He concluded that surgery was helpful in motivated patients who needed immediate help from their voice disorder. If immediate help was not required, voice therapy could be attempted, but the outcome was generally based on motivation. Although much of the dysphonia will resolve after puberty, dysphonic patients deserve close follow-up and individually tailored management.

Many treating physicians are concerned about the age at which interventions are appropriate. We give each child the benefit of the doubt regarding their ability to follow and adhere to voice therapy. The sessions are tailored to the child's age. Rest periods between groups of therapy sessions are given so that the child does not become bored or overburdened with the therapy. If a child is too young or immature and does not grasp the concepts or is incapable of performing the task, it is revisited after a break to reinforce what has been learned and assess the readiness of the child to proceed. Overall, the treatment of the dysphonic child is tremendously rewarding.

VOCAL FOLD CYSTS

Vocal fold cysts may also cause hoarseness in children. Cysts seen on the vocal folds are either congenital or acquired. Congenital cysts are either mucus-retention cysts filled with thick mucus such as that seen in a mucocele (Fig 14–17) or epidermal cyst filled with keratinous material (Fig 14–18).

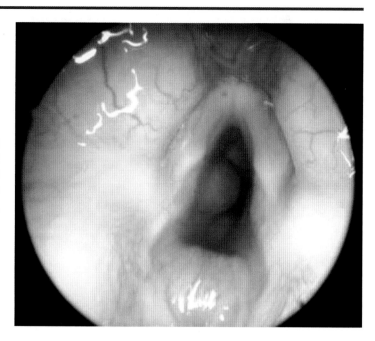

Fig 14–17. Large submucosal cyst in the immediate subglottis causing airway and voice disturbance.

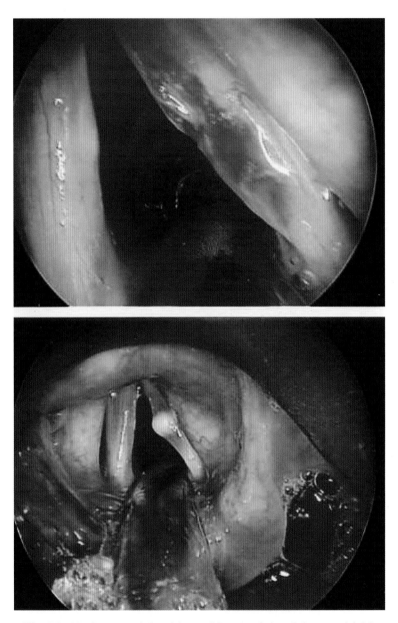

Fig 14–18. Intracordal epidermoid cyst of the right vocal fold.

Surgical excision is generally required for intracordal cysts. Careful dissection is required using microlaryngeal surgical techniques. Care is taken to completely remove the intracordal cyst as residual cyst wall will cause a recurrence. Rupture of the cyst during removal does not portend failure but careful inspection and complete removal of the cyst wall is still required.

As stated in the section on nodules, sometimes the diagnosis of an intracordal cyst is difficult to make, especially with mucus-retention cysts as they may mimic vocal nodules in appearance. Intracordal vocal fold cysts generally are unilateral, however. Epidermal cysts have a whitish appearance as they are filled with keratinous debris. If the diagnosis is in question, initial voice therapy may decrease the edema surrounding the intracordal cyst as well as decrease the contralateral nodule caused by the trauma of the cyst on the opposite vocal fold. This may make the diagnosis more clear and surgical management may proceed. If an accurate diagnosis is not possible with indirect laryngeal visualization, direct microlarygoscopy with palpation and possible vocal fold exploration should be considered.

Occasionally, acquired mucus-retention cysts of the subglottis may cause hoarseness or airway embarrassment. When recognized, these cysts are generally amenable to marsupialization with sharp instruments, electrocautery, or laser.

ANTERIOR GLOTTIC WEBS

Anterior glottic webs may be congenital or acquired. They cause dysphonia by changing the portion of the vocal fold allowed to vibrate and generate sound. As a band spanning from leading edge to leading edge of the true vocal fold they do not allow airflow across the membranous vocal fold and prevent the mucosal wave from propagating (Fig 14–19). Acquired glottic webs are generally iatrogenic (Fig 14–20). Repeated microsurgical resection of recurrent respiratory papillomata may result in the formation of an anterior glottic web (Fig 14–21). These webs are still difficult to treat but are generally thinner than congenital webs and are contained to the glottis without extension into the subglottis.

Congenital glottic webs, however, are causes by a problem of recannulization of the glottis during fetal development. They

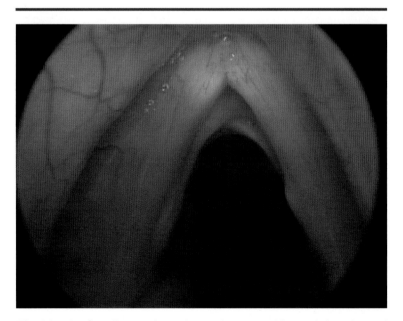

Fig 14–19. Small complex microweb seen with associated vocal fold nodule

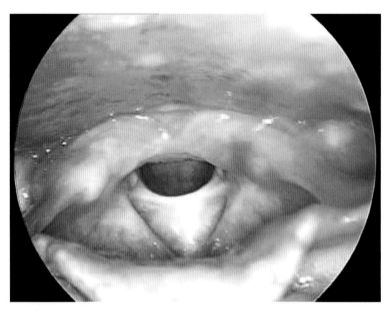

Fig 14–20. Severe glottic web caused by carbon dioxide laser treatments of recurrent respiratory papilloma.

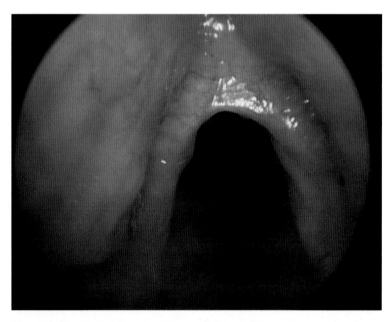

Fig 14–21. This is a small iatrogenic glottic web resulting from the treatment of recurrent respiratory papilloma.

may present with variable severity but often include thickening of the anterior cricoid cartilage (Fig 14-22). This may be seen as a "sail" sign in the subglottis on lateral neck radiographs. Treatment of congenital glottic webs generally requires treatment of the narrowed cricoid as well (Fig 14-23). An association with velocardiofacial syndrome (deletion of 22q) has been reported and children with congenital webs of the glottis should also have a genetic workup.[17]

The goal of surgical correction of an anterior glottic web is restoration of the vibrating vocal folds. A sharp anterior commissure is difficult to obtain without the placement of a keel to keep the edges of the anterior vocal fold from healing together. Keels may be placed externally with a laryn-gofissure or internally via an endoscopic approach. As surgical techniques advance, the endoscopic placement of a laryngeal keel has become more commonplace.

Treatment of the narrowed cricoid relies on the same principles of laryngotracheal reconstruction with augmentation of the cartilage framework with an autologous cartilage graft. In severe cases with cricoid involvement, the subglottic component is addressed initially with expansion laryngotracheoplasty and a keel is placed secondarily to resolve any residual webbing of the glottis. There are anecdotal reports of endoscopic repair of glottic webs with cricoid narrowing via endoscopic approach with an endoscopic anterior cricoid split using a sickle knife and primary endoscopic

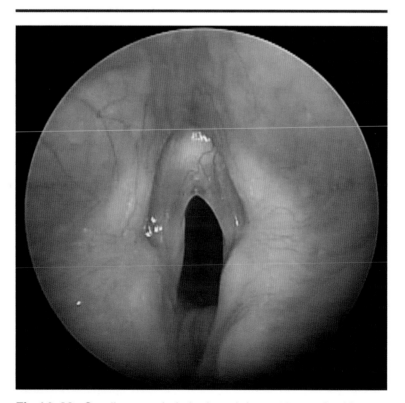

Fig 14–22. Small congenital glottic web in an 18-month-old causing mild stridor and dysphonia.

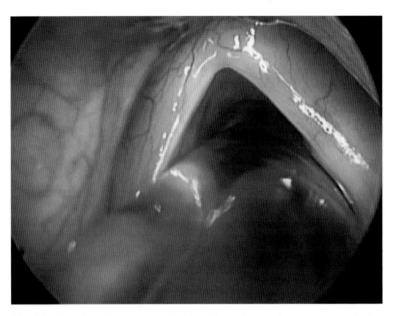

Fig 14–23. Result of congenital glottic web repair using an anterior costal cartilage laryngotracheoplasty.

placement of a keel. This technique sounds promising but larger case series will be needed to determine the indications and limitations of the technique.

CONCLUSION

Common laryngeal pathology in children fortunately is often benign. The appropriate treatment of some of these pediatric vocal fold lesions remains to be determined as the subspecialty of pediatric voice is still in its infancy. Above all, no lifelong irreparable harm should come to the developing vocal folds of the child. It should be pointed out, however, that significant prejudice is imparted on the child with dysphonia and so these children should not be ignored. As tools to measure perception of quality of life are developed, I believe significance impair- ments will be discerned in the dysphonic child. Continued study of the differentiating layers of the vocal fold will help direct us as to when surgical interventions are possible to achieve positive benefits. Overall, evaluating and managing dysphonic children is a rewarding and gratifying part of the pediatric otolaryngology practice.

REFERENCES

1. Ruscello DM, Lass NJ, Podbesek J. Listeners' perceptions of normal and voice-disordered children. *Folia Phoniatr (Basel)*. 1988; 40(6):290–296.
2. Boseley ME, Cunningham MJ, Volk MS, Hartnick CJ. Validation of the Pediatric Voice-Related Quality-of-Life survey. *Arch Otolaryngol Head Neck Surg.* 2006;132(7): 717–720.

3. De Bodt MS, Ketelslagers K, Peeters T, et al. Evolution of vocal fold nodules from childhood to adolescence. *J Voice.* 2007;21(2): 151-156.

4. Hocevar-Boltezar I, Radsel Z, Zargi M. The role of allergy in the etiopathogenesis of laryngeal mucosal lesions. *Acta Otolaryngol Suppl.* 1997;527:134-137.

5. Halstead LA. Role of gastroesophageal reflux in pediatric upper airway disorders. *Otolaryngol Head Neck Surg.* 1999;120(2):208-214.

6. Mandell DL, Kay DJ, Dohar JE, Yellon RF. Lack of association between esophageal biopsy, bronchoalveolar lavage, and endoscopy findings in hoarse children. *Arch Otolaryngol Head Neck Surg.* 2004;130(11): 1293-1297.

7. Shah RK, Woodnorth GH, Glynn A, Nuss RC. Pediatric vocal nodules: correlation with perceptual voice analysis. *Int J Pediatr Otorhinolaryngol.* 2005;69(7):903-909.

8. Akif Kilic M, Okur E, Yildirim I, Guzelsoy S. The prevalence of vocal fold nodules in school age children. *Int J Pediatr Otorhinolaryngol.* 2004;68(4):409-412.

9. Gray SD, Hammond E, Hanson DF. Benign pathologic responses of the larynx. *Ann Otol Rhinol Laryngol.* 1995;104(1):13-18.

10. Boseley ME, Hartnick CJ. Development of the human true vocal fold: depth of cell layers and quantifying cell types within the lamina propria. *Ann Otol Rhinol Laryngol.* 2006;115(10):784-788.

11. Gray SD. Cellular physiology of the vocal folds. *Otolaryngol Clin North Am.* 2000; 33(4):679-698.

12. Gray SD, Chan KJ, Turner B. Dissection plane of the human vocal fold lamina propria and elastin fibre concentration. *Acta Otolaryngol.* 2000;120(1):87-91.

13. Gray SD, Titze IR, Alipour F, Hammond TH. Biomechanical and histologic observations of vocal fold fibrous proteins. *Ann Otol Rhinol Laryngol.* 2000;109(1):77-85.

14. Hammond TH, Gray SD, Butler JE. Age- and gender-related collagen distribution in human vocal folds. *Ann Otol Rhinol Laryngol.* 2000;109(10 pt 1):913-920.

15. Shah RK, Feldman HA, Nuss RC. A grading scale for pediatric vocal fold nodules. *Otolaryngol Head Neck Surg.* 2007;136(2): 193-197.

16. Mori K. Vocal fold nodules in children: preferable therapy. *Int J Pediatr Otorhinolaryngol.* 1999;49(suppl 1):S303-S306.

17. Miyamoto RC, Cotton RT, Rope AF, et al. Association of anterior glottic webs with velocardiofacial syndrome (chromosome 22q11.2 deletion). *Otolaryngol Head Neck Surg.* 2004;130(4):415-417.

Managing Juvenile Recurrent Respiratory Papillomatosis and Care of the Voice

Matthew B. Patterson
Seth M. Pransky

INTRODUCTION

Juvenile recurrent respiratory papillomatosis (JRRP) is a rare disease characterized by wartlike growths (Fig 15-1) in the aerodigestive tract with potentially devastating consequences despite its benign histopathology. As the larynx is the most common site of disease involvement, the implications for vocal function and voice abnormalities are readily apparent. In addition, repetitive surgical management to remove JRRP can predispose to well-intentioned but overzealous management with potential long-term impact on vocal fold function. Even with advances in the tools used to manage this disease there is great risk of chronic and irreversible change to the voice. Fortunately, greater understanding of the pathophysiology, natural history, and evolving treatments of

JRRP now affords the luxury of prioritizing voice in the management of this recalcitrant disease.

Epidemiology

JRRP is defined as disease onset prior to age 12 and is the most common benign neoplasm of the larynx in the pediatric population. The incidence is estimated at 4.3 per 100,000 children,[1] with 75% being diagnosed by their fifth birthday[2] and boys and girls affected essentially equally.[3] However, our experience is that JRRP is not uncommonly diagnosed in the first year of life and there can be a delay as long as one year from onset of the predominant symptom of hoarseness to ultimate diagnosis. In one study, 75% of affected children were the firstborn, vaginally delivered infants of primigravid, teenage women of low socioeconomic

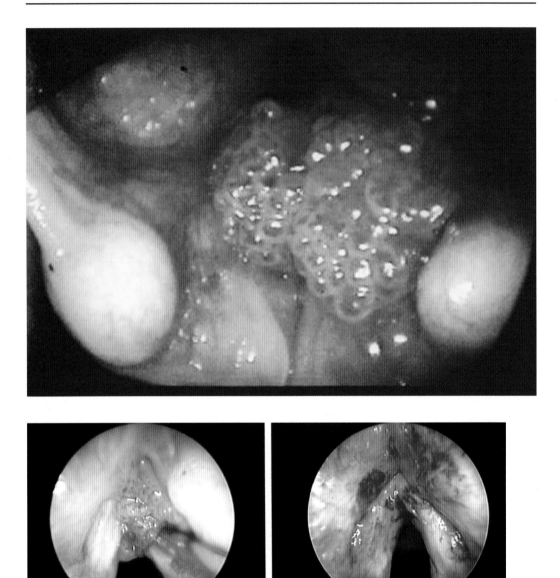

Fig 15–1. The classic appearance of pedunculated, exophytic, "cauliflowerlike" papillomas with diffuse laryngeal involvement.

status.[4] Diagnosis at a younger age corresponds to greater severity of disease, more frequent surgical intervention, and greater risk of progressive disease.[5,6]

The disease is caused by human papillomavirus (HPV), and vertical transmission from mothers with genital condylomata to newborns is generally accepted. In one series, 7 of every 1000 births to women with genital warts resulted in newborns with JRRP, corresponding to an odds ratio of 231 compared to vaginal deliveries from unaffected women.[7] However, the incidence of JRRP in offspring of women with genital condylomata is still surprisingly small, estimated at 1 in 400 delivered vaginally from a mother with a history of disease in the genital tract.[8] In addition, cesarean section is not necessarily protective and not currently recommended by the American College of Obstetrics and Gynecology as an elective option to prevent disease.

The recurrent nature of the disease subjects the patient to repetitive surgeries with a high cumulative cost. In a review of a national registry of children with RRP, patients underwent more than 19 lifetime procedures, averaging more than 4 per year.[9] More than 15,000 procedures are performed annually in the United States on children with JRRP at an estimated cost of over $150 million.[1] The estimated lifetime cost to treat one case ranges from $60,000 to $470,000.[10]

Pathophysiology

Nearly all cases of JRRP are caused by HPV types 6 and 11, the same types found in genital condylomata. Isolation of other HPV types within JRRP is extremely rare, and the rare involvement with types 16 and 18 is associated with a risk of malignant transformation. HPV type 11 is associated with a more aggressive disease course and greater likelihood of distal airway spread compared with type 6.[11] The presence of viral particles or DNA within the aerodigestive tract is not sufficient for infection or subsequent development of papillomas. HPV can lie dormant within otherwise healthy mucosa, and is replicated along with host cells. The exact mechanism which results in active infection and papilloma growth is still unknown, although key viral coded proteins are known to bind to and inhibit the tumor

suppressing gene products p53 and pRB within the host cell.[12] Local immune dysfunction has been considered as a component to the development of disease in JRRP.

Papillomas typically occur in regions where ciliated and squamous epithelium are juxtaposed, and readily form in similar interfaces from iatrogenic causes such as a tracheostomy.[13] The most common regions affected by RRP are the upper and lower ventricle margins, the undersurface of the vocal folds, the laryngeal surface of the epiglottis, the carina, and bronchial spurs, the nasal limen vestibule, and the nasopharyngeal surface of the soft palate.[4] Injury to adjacent normal tissue from surgical intervention or extraesophageal reflux can lead to proliferation of disease. Tracheotomy patients tend to have earlier presentation and more widespread disease, and the procedure itself may hasten spread distally into the trachea and pulmonary parenchyma.[14]

Clinical Presentation and Evaluation

Symptoms of varying degrees of respiratory obstruction are the most common presentation of JRRP. Hoarseness is most often the chief complaint, and, as noted above, delay in diagnosis from the onset of symptoms of greater than a year is not atypical. For this reason, children can also present with stridor or respiratory distress at the time of initial diagnosis. Patients are often treated for croup, asthma, allergies, or vocal nodules in the interim. At times the definitive diagnosis is made because of the development of significant stridor. Rarely, a patient will present with failure to thrive, recurrent pneumonias, or an acute life-threatening airway event.

A thorough history of a child with hoarseness is critical to establish the diagnosis of JRRP from other causes. The nature and timing of the symptoms, prior airway trauma or intubation, congenital anomalies, significant comorbidities, and associated symptoms must be addressed. Maternal history of vaginal or cervical condylomata should be assessed and follow-up recommended. A slowly progressive inspiratory or biphasic stridor is suggestive of a glottic or subglottic lesion that requires visualization.

A complete physical examination with visualization of the pharynx and larynx is typically sufficient to make a definitive diagnosis. In the stable patient without acute airway compromise, flexible nasolaryngoscopy is performed on the awake patient to assess anatomy, presence of lesions, and laryngeal function. Patients presenting with tachypnea, cervical hyperextension, air hunger, hypoxia, or other signs of acute respiratory compromise may require evaluation in the operating room by direct laryngoscopy with endotracheal intubation if necessary.

Prior to or at the time of initial surgical treatment, direct laryngoscopy is performed in the operating room under general anesthesia. Photo or video documentation of disease extent is very helpful if not essential to monitor effectively the subsequent response to therapy and to communicate findings with parents. A staging system developed by Derkay and Coltrera is in common use to allow reliable communication of findings between providers.[15]

TREATMENT OF RECURRENT RESPIRATORY PAPILLOMATOSIS

No predictive medical or surgical cure exists for JRRP, and surgical debulking of disease is the mainstay of treatment to control symptoms ranging from hoarseness to life-threatening airway compromise. The goals of any particular intervention will vary with the disease status of the patient, although there are common themes. Securing a safe airway by decreasing critical tumor burden is always of paramount importance. However, improving voice quality likely prompts the most visits to the operating room overall and is used as a guide to intervene before significant airway obstruction occurs. Accomplishing these two goals is ideally done in a manner that preserves underlying normal structures, increases the time between interventions, avoids the need for tracheotomy, and reduces the likelihood of morbidity and complications. A biopsy for HPV typing should be performed at the initial surgery for prognostic purposes, and typically it is not necessary to repeat this at subsequent excisions unless clinical indicated or to look for changes brought about by therapeutic intervention.

It is critical to recognize that surgical treatment itself becomes an integral part of the disease process. This is currently unavoidable for several reasons. First, it is not possible to determine an effective margin of disease because healthy cells can still contain latent virus that will become active in the future. Second, trauma to adjacent healthy tissue at the time of surgery can lead to spread of disease. Third, the disease is recurrent and typically requires multiple procedures over the lifetime of the patient. Finally, overly aggressive excision of papilloma can result in scar and web formation with significant consequences for voice. Therefore, with repetitive interventions as the mainstay of management, there is likely to be some negative impact on the laryngeal structures. Although essentially unavoidable, it is still necessary to maintain constant awareness of this unique interaction to improve outcomes, particularly in regard to voice.

Adjuvant treatments to surgery are expanding and show promise in lengthening the interval between surgical interventions and possibly decreasing the time to disease remission. Given the risks of general anesthesia and the potential complications of repetitive surgery, these agents can result in substantial improvements in quality of life for patients. Voice is now a critically recognized entity in the overall management of patients with JRRP. Medicines and techniques that help preserve normal laryngeal anatomy and physiology represent major advances in treatment.

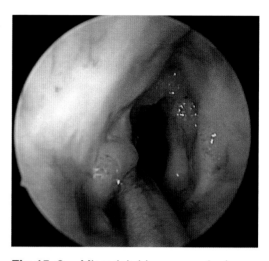

Fig 15–2. Microdebrider removal of exophytic, pedunculated papilloma.

Surgical Treatment

Surgical tools for excision of recurrent respiratory papillomas are microlaryngoscopic cold steel instruments, the microdebrider, or various lasers. Cold steel excision, once the only option, is still utilized for removal of disease, predominantly in the adult form of RRP, which tends to be less aggressive and recurrent compared to JRRP.[16] Until recently, the CO_2 laser was the favored method of treatment in the pediatric population.[12] Currently, the microdebrider is the preferred instrument for the surgical management of JRRP, especially when the disease is pedunculated and exophytic (Fig 15–2).[17] Ultimately, the disease status and anatomy of the patient determine the most effective intervention at the time of surgery.

Effective communication and cooperation with the anesthesiologist prior to and during surgery on RRP is critical. The bulk and location of disease along with the desired treatment modality will determine the appropriate method of ventilation. Pediatric anesthesiologists have become increasingly familiar with and comfortable with maintaining the airway using spontaneous ventilation and adjuvant anesthetic agents.

This provides the best view of the larynx and extent of disease and the best access for removal. Endotracheal intubation may be required initially for excessive disease and at times jet ventilation or apneic techniques are employed.

Microdebrider

The microdebrider is a powered instrument with oscillating blades and suction that is compatible with most of the goals of surgical treatment of JRRP. The device allows very precise removal of tumor with fine control of depth of excision and no surrounding thermal damage. It eliminates the other inherent risks and costs of laser use including fire, longer surgical times, release of HPV DNA into the air, distal airway damage, and scar formation. A randomized prospective trial comparing the CO_2 laser and microdebrider found the use of the latter was associated with more rapid voice improvement, decreased cost, and shorter operative time.[18] Others have found similar benefits for reduced time, cost, and surrounding tissue damage.[19,20] The microdebrider is still limited in very fine or sessile disease and papilloma that involve the anterior commissure or ventricles and maintains the potential for surrounding tissue mechanical trauma. Knowledge of the blade sizes and cutting surfaces as well as the recommended speed of the oscillating debrider blade are essential in reducing iatrogenic damage from the microdebrider.

CO₂ Laser

The CO_2 laser was the mainstay for treatment of JRRP for decades. Its effective wavelength is absorbed by water in tissues, and combined with the operative microscope results in precise vaporization of papilloma. The technique is bloodless, and advances in the technology reduced surrounding tissue damage. However, CO_2 laser treatment is limited to line of sight disease, is costly, and carries significant risks. (At present the line of sight difficulty may be obviated by the newly developed flexible CO_2 laser.) The risk of airway fire requires a laser safe endotracheal tube. HPV DNA may be released in the plume, placing operating room personnel at risk.[21] In addition, the development of anterior and posterior glottic scars and webs was reported in several series, with rates as high as 36%.[19] Part of this may be due to surrounding thermal injury from the laser. Therefore, this technique may place voice preservation at risk.

Angiolytic Lasers: Pulsed Dye Laser, Pulsed KTP Laser

The 585-nm pulsed dye laser and 532-nm pulsed KTP laser overcome many of the limitations of the CO_2 laser. These wavelengths are absorbed by oxyhemoglobin, resulting in subepithelial microvascular damage and involution with relative sparing of the epithelium. Therefore, bilateral glottic lesions can be treated in the anterior commissure without subsequent web formation as has been demonstrated in practice (Fig 15–3).[22] The fibers can be passed through a flexible scope, suction device, rigid bronchoscope side port, or adaptor and can be used in adults in a clinic setting under local anesthesia. With a 2-mm depth of penetration, it is well suited for smaller, sessile lesions, but it is not effective for large exophytic papillomas. From a voice preservation perspective, this laser treatment holds promise in the treatment of lesions in the anterior commissure and ventricle as well as the free edge of the vocal folds and infraglottic region and has already demonstrated improved voice satisfaction in patients after treatment.[23,24] However, as compared to the microdebrider, there is a longer period of voice recovery with hoarseness persisting for 5 to 7 days after treatment.

Adjuvant Therapies

In a query of American Society of Pediatric Otolaryngology members, adjuvant treatments were required in 20% of JRRP patients.[17] Typical criteria include greater than 4 surgeries per year, rapid return of aggressive disease, and distal airway spread.[14] The rarity of the disease is a significant challenge to well-controlled, randomized, prospective trials on the effectiveness of these treatments. The majority of evidence available consists of case series using various antiviral therapies. Due to the lack of adequate controls, it is difficult to judge if these therapies are altering a disease process that inherently demonstrates wide variability both within and between patients in terms of natural history. However, in those

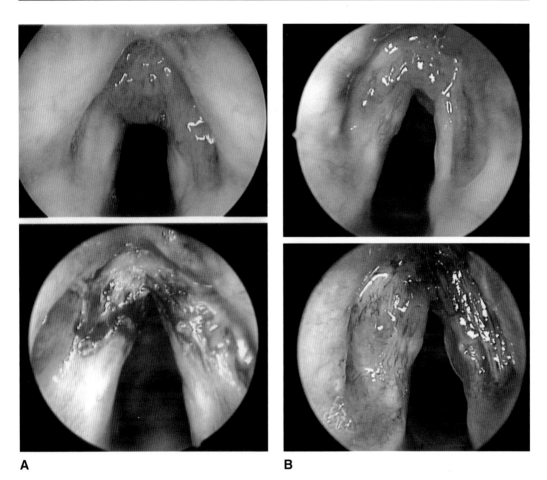

A   **B**

Fig 15–3. A. Anterior commissure involvement of RRP with significant impact on voice. Removal using the pulsed dye laser. **B.** Pulsed dye laser removing anterior commissure disease extending onto right true vocal fold.

patients with aggressive disease requiring surgery as often as every 6 weeks, adjuvant therapy that reduces tumor burden will likely reduce frequency of intervention and likely reduce long-term voice changes.

Interferon α-2a

Interferon α is produced naturally by infected leukocytes and exerts antiviral activity via activation of proteins that interfere with various stages of the virus life cycle.

Systemic administration to JRRP patients demonstrated significant effectiveness in multi-institutional, randomized trials.[25] However, it is associated with significant side effects including an influenzalike illness, neuropsychiatric complications, neutropenia, and thrombocytopenia. In addition, prolonged therapy lasting up to several years is necessary and a rebound phenomenon is observed in up to one-third of patients with initial clinical response following cessation of therapy.[25]

Cidofovir

Intralesional injection of cidofovir has received a great deal of attention over the past decade as an adjuvant treatment for JRRP. It is approved by the Food and Drug Administration for the systemic treatment of cytomegalovirus retinitis in HIV patients, and the mechanism for activity against HPV is not clearly established. Several uncontrolled case series have demonstrated effectiveness of cidofovir in concentrations of 5 to 10 mg/mL,[25] including a series of severely affected children with a mean follow-up of 51.6 months.[26] Systemic administration is associated with potential nephrotoxicity, hepatotoxicity, and neutropenia. Concern also exists about both vocal fold thickening from the injection and possible carcinogenic effects of local administration. However, local injection is not associated with significant systemic concentrations and animal studies failed to demonstrate significant scarring or tumorigenicity at concentrations used in humans.[27]

Despite numerous anecdotal reports of cidofovir effectiveness, the overall risks and benefits are difficult to establish given the lack of large, well-controlled studies. The mechanism of action, definitive toxicity profile, and optimum treatment dose and timing are undefined. Despite these limitations, the cumulative evidence does suggest that cidofovir is a relatively safe and useful adjunct in the treatment of aggressive or poorly controlled JRRP refractory to standard therapy. Benefits include increasing surgical interval, improving quality of life, decreasing the chance for iatrogenic damage to the larynx, and potentially hastening remission.

Indole-3-Carbinol

Indole-3-carbinol is a nutrient naturally found in cruciferous vegetables and is a nutri-

tional supplement approved by the Food and Drug Administration. It affects estrogen metabolism to favor the production of 2-hydroxyestrone over 16α-hydroxyestrone, with a proposed effect of decreasing the risk of hormone-dependent tumors, including RRP.[28] It is a systemic therapy without significant side effects, although long-term use has been associated with bone density concerns. It has been reported to be effective in treating adult onset RRP in various case series.[25] It does not appear to be as useful in children and no large, prospective, well-controlled study has been published to date to verify the benefits of indole-3-carbinol.

Immune Modulation

The most beneficial form of therapy is, of course, prevention. At present there is now an FDA-approved quadrivant vaccine (Gardasil-Merck) indicated for the prevention of disease caused by human papillomavirus (HPV) types 6, 11, 16, and 18. A second, bivalent vaccine (Cervarix-GSK) is on the horizon. From the point of view of management of JRRP the quadrivalent vaccine, which includes types 6, and 11 would be preferred over a vaccine that did not cover these HPV types.

Results of the phase 3 study on the highly effective quadrivalent vaccine against human papillomavirus types 6, 11, 16, and 18 were recently published.[29] The trial was targeted at women for the prevention of anogenital disease. Given the high prevalence of genital HPV in the population at large and the risk of JRRP from vertical transmission, it seems reasonable that widespread vaccination could significantly impact the incidence of JRRP. This will likely take many years to become apparent. Gardasil has been approved for use in girls and women 9 to 26 years of age; it is currently recommended in the vaccine schedule published by the American Academy of Pediatrics and consists of three injections spaced over 6 months.

A targeted vaccine for treatment of HPV-related disease is under development. Heat-shock protein E7 (HspE7) is a recombinant fusion protein consisting of heat-shock protein Hsp65 of *Mycobacterium bovis* BCG and the E7 protein from HPV type 16. An open-label trial on children with JRRP was conducted using three subcutaneous injections over 8 weeks that demonstrated significant increases in intersurgical interval with only mild to moderate injection-site reactions.[31] Further studies are pending.

Management of Extraesophageal Reflux Disease

Extraesophageal reflux has been suggested to exacerbate RRP. In a retrospective review of children undergoing multiple surgical procedures, those treated with antireflux regimens developed laryngeal webs significantly less often compared with those not treated.[32] The authors recommended prophylactic antireflux regimens for patients undergoing procedures that disrupt the laryngeal mucosa to prevent soft-tissue complications.

JUVENILE RECURRENT RESPIRATORY PAPILLOMATOSIS AND THE VOICE

The recurrent nature of this disease and its propensity for laryngeal involvement make voice complaints a universal feature and concern both during and after treatment. It is remarkable that many patients who have undergone upward of 60 to 80 procedures maintain as good a voice as they do.

Papillomas of the anterior commissure and inferior aspect of the vocal folds can be extremely difficult to access and safely manage surgically. Even when these lesions are accessible, overly aggressive excision can lead to soft tissue complications such as scars and webs leading to voice deficits. Regardless of the particular surgical technique used, the underlying disease process remains the same. Until a cure is discovered or vaccination becomes universal, surgery will remain a necessary tool to manage symptoms until disease remission. Although slow regression tends to occur at the onset of puberty,[33] the cumulative result of the disease and treatment over time can lead to lifelong poor voice quality.

The Rady Children's Hospital Experience

Our experience with JRRP is extensive with more than 20 active patients in varying stages of disease and management at any time. At the initial procedure, suspension microlaryngoscopy using spontaneous ventilation (Parsons or Benjamin laryngoscope, Karl Storz Endoscopy-America Inc, Culver City, Calif) and bronchoscopy is performed, extent of disease documented with photographs before and after surgical manipulation (photographs are taken at each procedure permitting rapid comparison of disease state throughout the treatment period), biopsy with HPV typing is sent, and debulking of gross, bulky disease carried out using a powered laryngeal microdebrider (Xomed, Jacksonville, Fla). Disease in the anterior commissure region is not manipulated at all. Disease is staged according to the system established by Derkay and Coltrera.[15] No perioperative steroids are administered and patients are discharged home on the same day.

Follow-up endoscopy is scheduled 4 to 6 weeks later in an effort to assess rapidity and location of regrowth. At this junction multiple modalities of treatment are readied, including the microdebrider and the 585-nm pulsed dye laser (PDL). Preoperative discussion with the family reviews the issues of airway management and voice management and use of the PDL for sensitive areas, such as the anterior commissure, difficult to reach areas such as the ventricles and infraglottic regions, and for finer, sessile lesions. Bulky disease is removed with the microdebrider. If the PDL is used the family is told to expect some degree of increased hoarseness for approximately 5 to 7 days, after which they can anticipate overall improvement in the voice. Follow-up endoscopies are scheduled based on the age of the patient, the extent of papilloma regrowth, concerns for airway obstruction, and the status of the voice.

A comprehensive discussion of all available adjuvant therapies is held with the parents of those patients with severe disease. In our institution, severe disease is defined as patients requiring surgery every 8 weeks or less to maintain a patent airway. First-line adjuvant therapy is intralesional cidofovir at a concentration of 5 mg/mL. The family is made aware that there will be 4 or 5 injections carried out at two 3-week intervals and then the need for continued injections is reassessed (Fig 15–4). Injec-

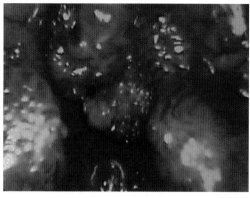

A

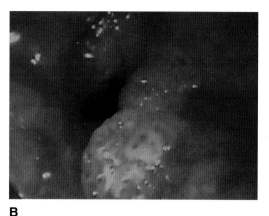

B

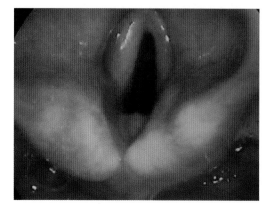

C

Fig 15–4. A. Severe diffuse RRP. **B.** Same patient 1 year later after monthly debulking procedures to preserve airway. **C.** Same patient 2 weeks later after initial injection with cidofovir. (This patient required 4 injections and ultimately has had durable remission with >6 years follow-up).

tions are performed with either a straight laryngeal needle (Leurlock, Straight 8598B, Karl Storz Endoscopy-America Inc, Culver City, Calif) or with a gastrointestinal sclerosing needle (Bard, Billerica, Mass) passed through the side port of a pediatric bronchoscope in the setting of difficult to reach lesions. For laryngeal disease usually 1 to 1.5 mL is injected into the various sites of involvement, including the anterior commissure region. The injection is done at the base of the lesion after debridement or laser of the overt disease. A small wheal is raised at the sites of injection with great care taken not to compromise the airway. Patients are monitored with monthly complete blood counts, chemistry panels, and liver function tests for potential toxicities and repeat biopsies are sent every other treatment session. We have now injected approximately 20 children with cidofovir and have seen complete and durable remission in almost 60% of cases and significant improvement in disease in another 20%. Ultimate voice results have been very good, although there is often some degree of mild persistent raspiness. There are patients who do not seem to respond to cidofovir, especially when they present with extensive prior surgical manipulation and scarring of the laryngeal tissues. We have not encountered any significant adverse effects from the cidofovir. Although there may be some thickening of the laryngeal mucosa with the cidofovir, this is difficult to distinguish from the thickening that occurs with other surgical manipulation of the larynx.

As mentioned above, there is some evidence that extraesophageal reflux disease can exacerbate RRP. Consequently, whenever there is extensive disease in the larynx, spread of disease beyond the larynx, or if the child is receiving cidofovir injections, GERD management is instituted with either an H2 blocker or a proton-pump inhibitor, along with dietary and positional manipulation. At times an esophagogastroduodenoscopy with biopsy is carried out by our pediatric GI colleagues to look for spread of disease into the esophagus, overt evidence of GERD, and for evidence of coexistent disease such as *H. pylori* or eosinophilic esophagitis.

The patient with scar or web formation in the setting of active JRRP presents a challenge. Whenever possible, treatment of these soft-tissue complications is delayed until a clinically significant level of remission of papillomas is achieved. At that time, they are treated the same as in a patient without JRRP. However, an important consideration is that a web may hide papilloma that does not resolve until it is uncovered and treated directly.

Layers of Expertise

In addition to the pathophysiology and treatment modalities used, there are many factors that likely contribute to voice outcomes in JRRP. Although these potential pitfalls are unavoidable in some circumstances, and certainly not ameliorated by the rarity of the disease, they must still be taken into account when considering voice outcomes. The treatment setting provides the foundation for multiple layers of expertise necessary to successfully manage this disease. A dedicated children's hospital with subspecialty departments covering a wide referral base is most likely to encounter enough patients with JRRP to gain facility in treating it. Outcomes in such a setting reflect the cumulative experience of the surgeon and anesthesiologist whose effective cooperation is so critical. Understanding the need for a "shared airway" and having expertise in spontaneous ventilation is typically required for optimal management. In addition, awareness of "cutting edge" therapies, and access to, and experience with different surgical tools and adjuvant therapies that increase surgical intervals and limit soft-tissue complications may be more readily available at an institution that treats a high volume of JRRP patients. As pediatricians become more aware of JRRP and refer voice abnormalities earlier, younger patients with smaller airways will be referred making all of the above issues even more important. In addition, continuing research into the various modalities often used in adult laryngeal disease, such as the ongoing studies by the editor (C.J.H.) and the author (M.B.P.) on angiolytic laser treatment, are critical.

Speech Therapy

At what point does speech therapy play a therapeutic role in the child with JRRP? Now that greater attention is given to functional outcomes of treatment, this question becomes increasingly important. A series of 4 prepubescent children with at least 12 months of remission from JRRP reported normal voice satisfaction on the voice-related quality of life questionnaire that was not significantly different from controls.[34] However, objective analysis of these patients in the same study showed more hoarseness, lower average fundamental frequency, and a higher relative average perturbation. Although a very small study, the results reflect what seems obvious to those who care for these patients. Voice quality is clearly affected during active disease and beyond remission even if it is not considered significant by the young patient. The appropriate timing and effectiveness of speech therapy for these children remains to be determined. We have begun to involve our speech therapists in management of the chronic hoarseness issues with these patients once the need for aggressive and repetitive surgical intervention has diminished. However, our results with speech therapy are too preliminary to make any recommendations for when these patients should be referred and for how long therapy should be continued.

REFERENCES

1. Derkay CS. Task force on recurrent respiratory papillomas. A preliminary report. *Arch Otolaryngol Head Neck Surg*. 1995;121:1386–1391.
2. Cohn AM, Kos JT II, Taber LH, Adam E. Recurring laryngeal papilloma. *Am J Otolaryngology*. 1981;2:129–132.
3. Armstrong LR, Derkay CS, Reeves WC. Initial results from the National Registry for Juvenile-Onset Recurrent Respiratory Papillomatosis. RRPTask Force. *Arch Otolaryngol Head Neck Surg*. 1999;125:743–748.
4. Kashima HK, Shah F, Lyles A, et al. A comparison of risk factors in juvenile-onset and adult-onset recurrent respiratory papillomatosis. *Laryngoscope*. 1992;102:9–13.
5. Reeves WC, Ruparelia SS, Swanson KI, et al. National registry for juvenile-onset recurrent respiratory papillomatosis. *Arch Otolaryngol Head Neck Surg*. 2003;129:976–982.
6. Ruparelia S, Unger ER, Nisenbaum R, et al. Predictors of remission in juvenile-onset recurrent respiratory papillomatosis. *Arch Otolaryngol Head Neck Surg*. 2003;129:1275–1278.
7. Silverberg MJ, Thorsen P, Lindeberg H, Grant LA, Shah KV. Condyloma in pregnancy is strongly predictive of juvenile-onset recurrent respiratory papillomatosis. *Obstet Gynecol*. 2003;101:645–652.
8. Shah K, Kashima H, Polk BF, Shah F, Abbey H, Abramson A. Rarity of cesarean delivery in cases of juvenile-onset respiratory papillomatosis. *Obstet Gynecol*. 1986;68:795–799.

9. Armstrong LR, Derkay CS, Reeves WC. Initial results from the national registry for juvenile-onset recurrent respiratory papillomatosis. RRP Task Force. *Arch Otolaryngol Head Neck Surg.* 1999;125:3-8.

10. Bishai D, Kashima H, Shah K. The cost of juvenile-onset recurrent respiratory papillomatosis. *Arch Otolaryngol Head Neck Surg.* 2000;126:935-939.

11. Rabah R, Lancaster WD, Thomas R, Gregoire L. Human papillomavirus-11-associated recurrent respiratory papillomatosis is more aggressive than human papillomavirus-6-associated disease. *Pediatr Dev Pathol.* 2001;4:68-72.

12. Stamataki S, Nikolopoulos TP, Korres S, Felekis D, Tzangaroulakis A, Ferekidis E. Juvenile recurrent respiratory papillomatosis: still a mystery disease with difficult management. *Head Neck.* 2007;29:155-162.

13. Kashima H, Mounts P, Leventhal B, Hruban RH. Sites of predilection in recurrent respiratory papillomatosis. *Ann Otol Rhinol Laryngol.* 1993;102:580-583.

14. Derkay CS. Darrow DH. Recurrent respiratory papillomatosis. *Ann Otol Rhinol Laryngol.* 2006;115:1-11.

15. Derkay CS, Malis DJ, Zalzal G, Wiatrak BJ, Kashima HK, Coltrera MD. A staging system for assessing severity of disease and response to therapy in recurrent respiratory papillomatosis. *Laryngoscope.* 1998;108:935-937.

16. Zeitels SM, Casiano RR, Gardner GM, Hogikyan ND, Koufman JA, Rosen CA. Voice and Swallowing Committee, American Academy of Otolaryngology Head and Neck Surgery. Management of common voice problems: Committee report. *Otolaryngol Head Neck Surg.* 2002;126:333-348.

17. Schraff S, Derkay CS, Burke B, Lawson L. American Society of Pediatric Otolaryngology members' experience with recurrent respiratory papillomatosis and the use of adjuvant therapy. *Arch Otolaryngol Head Neck Surg.* 2004;130:1039-1042.

18. Pasquale K, Wiatrak B, Woolley A, Lewis L. Microdebrider versus CO_2 laser removal of recurrent respiratory papillomas: a prospective analysis. *Laryngoscope.* 2003;113:139-143.

19. El Bitar MA, Zalzal GH. Powered instrumentation in the treatment of recurrent respiratory papillomatosis: an alternative to the carbon dioxide laser. *Arch Otolaryngol Head Neck Surg.* 2002;128:425-428.

20. Patel N, Rowe M, Tunkel D. Treatment of recurrent respiratory papillomatosis in children with the microdebrider. *Ann Otol Rhinol Laryngol.* 2003;112:7-10.

21. Kashima HK, Kessis T, Mounts P, Shah K. Polymerase chain reaction identification of human papillomavirus DNA in CO_2 laser plume from recurrent respiratory papillomatosis. *Otolaryngol Head Neck Surg.* 1991;104:191-195.

22. Franco RA Jr, Zeitels SM, Farinelli WA, Anderson RR. 585-nm pulsed dye laser treatment of glottal papillomatosis. *Ann Otol Rhinol Laryngol.* 2002;111:486-492.

23. Valdez TA, McMillan K, Shapshay SM. A new laser treatment for vocal cord papilloma—585-nm pulsed dye. *Otolaryngol Head Neck Surg.* 2001;124:421-425.

24. Zeitels SM, Franco RA Jr, Dailey SH, et al. Office-based treatment of glottal dysplasia and papillomatosis with the 585-nm pulsed dye laser and local anesthesia. *Ann Otol Rhinol Laryngol.* 2004;113:265-276.

25. Kimberlin DW. Current status of antiviral therapy for juvenile-onset recurrent respiratory papillomatosis. *Antiviral Res.* 2004;63:141-151.

26. Pransky SM, Albright JT, Magit AE. Long-term follow-up of pediatric recurrent respiratory papillomatosis managed with intralesional cidofovir. *Laryngoscope.* 2003;113:1583-1587.

27. Silverman DA, Pitman MJ. Current diagnostic and management trends for recurrent respiratory papillomatosis. *Curr Opin Otolaryngol Head Neck Surg.* 2004;12:532-537.

28. Rosen CA, Bryson PC. Indole-3-carbinol for recurrent respiratory papillomatosis: long-term results. *J Voice.* 2004;18:248-253.

29. Garland SM, Hernandez-Avila M, Wheeler CM, et al. Quadrivalent vaccine against

human papillomavirus to prevent anogenital diseases. *N Engl J Med.* 2007;356:1928-1943.

30. Pashley NRT. Can mumps vaccine induce remission in recurrent respiratory papilloma? *Arch Otolaryngol Head Neck Surg.* 2002;128:783-786.

31. Derkay CS, Smith RJH, McClay J, et al. HspE7 treatment of pediatric recurrent respiratory papillomatosis: final results of an open-label trial. *Ann Otol Rhinol Laryngol.* 2005;114: 730-737.

32. Holland BW, Koufman JA, Postma GN, McGuirt WF Jr. Laryngopharyngeal reflux and laryngeal web formation in patients with pediatric recurrent respiratory papillomas. *Laryngoscope.* 2002;112:1926-1929.

33. Pransky SM, Kang DR. Tumors of the larynx, trachea and bronchi. In: Bluestone CD, Stool SE, Alper CM, et al, eds. *Pediatric Otolaryngology,* 4th ed. Philadelphia, Pa: Saunders; 2003:1558-1572.

34. Lindman JP, Gibbons MD, Morlier R, Wiatrak BJ. Voice quality of prepubescent children with quiescent recurrent respiratory papillomatosis. *Int J Pediatr Otorhinolaryngol.* 2004;68:529-536.

16

Pediatric Unilateral Vocal Fold Immobility

J. Andrew Sipp
Christopher J. Hartnick

INTRODUCTION

Although an individual's experience may vary, most pediatric otolaryngologists or laryngologists can expect to participate in the care of a patient under the age of 18 with unilateral vocal fold immobility (UVFI). Case series of tertiary care pediatric otolaryngology practices report 4 to 10 patients a year.[1-3] Unilateral vocal fold immobility in neonates is associated with stridor, poor feeding, or with symptoms associated with an incompetent larynx.[1,4] Generally, in this young age group the issues of airway and aspiration are more important than voice. Older children with UVFI, with or without aspiration, more commonly seek medical attention for severe dysphonia. Speech therapy is useful in UVFI and may be adequate in treating some cases; however, others require surgery for greater degrees of medialization.[3,5-6] Vocal fold medialization may be considered in pediatric patients with aspiration as well as in select pediatric patients with dysphonia secondary to UVFI. This chapter touches on the differential diagnosis and workup of pediatric UVFI, but then focuses on the surgical efforts to achieve an improved voice for children with UVFI.

PRESENTATION

Stridor is present in up to 70% young children with UVFI.[1,7] This is in contrast to adults. The smaller the larynx, the more likely stridor and airway compromise are present. Poor feeding, weak cry, cyanosis, and aspiration are common in neonates and young children.[1] Hoarseness and poor vocal projection are more often the chief complaints in older children and adolescents.

EVALUATION

History and physical examination should first determine the stability of airway. Once a stable airway is either assessed or established, the onset of symptoms in relation to birth, intubation, surgery, recent illness, or medical therapy can be explored. In addition to a detailed head and neck examination, the chest should not be overlooked. History and physical examination alone is successful in determining etiology of unilateral vocal fold paralysis in 2 out of 3 adults with UVFI.[8]

A complete evaluation of the airway should be considered even if the cause is evident. Synchronous airway lesions including laryngomalacia, tracheomalacia, subglottic stenosis, intubation granuloma, cricoarytenoid joint fixation, or laryngeal webs are present in up to 45% patients.[1] Upright, flexible laryngoscopy is helpful for evaluating supraglottic and glottic pathology and can be performed even in the neonate in the appropriate setting. We perform direct laryngoscopy and bronchoscopy under general anesthesia with a preoperative chest X-ray for most children with UVFI. Under direct laryngoscopy the arytenoids can be assessed for fixation. If the diagnosis remains elusive, imaging based on findings can be directed.[9]

Laryngeal EMG is an investigational tool that may provide helpful information in assessing prognosis of vocal fold recovery.[10] Recently, laryngeal EMG can be obtained using the NIM Response system (Medtronic ENT USA, Inc, Jacksonville, Fla) which is the same system used commonly for facial nerve monitoring. The electrodes can be inserted into the thyroarytenoid muscle under endoscopic guidance. The patient's level of anesthesia can be lightened in effort to witness a tracing consistent with a muscle unit action potential (MUAP). The LEMG tracings can be recorded to a disk drive and reviewed with a neurologist. The role of LEMG needs to be better clarified in the pediatric patient with vocal fold paralysis.

ETIOLOGY

Etiologies of UFVI are presented in Table 16–1.

Congenital UVFI

Neonates may present with a vocal fold palsy secondary to cervical trauma sustained during complicated or prolonged vaginal delivery.[2] Anatomic brain anomalies and additional cranial nerve palsies may also be seen in a child born with UVFI. "Cardiovocal syndrome" is a congenital left vocal fold paralysis with an associated thoracic vascular or cardiac abnormality.[2] No cause is identified in 30 to 50% of patients with UVFI at birth.[2,11]

Acquired UVFI

Surgical or Trauma UVFI

Iatragenic injuries account for the majority of cases of UVFI in children, most often after patent ductus arteriosus (PDA) ligation.[1,3,12] Rates of recurrent laryngeal nerve injury after PDA ligation between institutions vary widely (8–62%).[13-15] Extremely low birth weight (<1 kg) children undergoing PDA ligation appears to be at increased risk for UVFI.[14] UVFI is also associated with laryngeal trauma, prolonged intubation,

Table 16–1. Etiologies of UFVI

Congenital	Acquired
Birth Trauma	Idiopathic
Arnold-Chiari	Peripheral Neurologic Disease
Intrathoracic Cardiac or Vascular Abnormality	Charcot-Marie-Tooth
	Postviral Vagal Neuropathy
	Iatrogenic
	Prolonged intubation
	Neurosurgical procedures
	Thyroid surgery
	Drainage of neck abscess
	TEF repair
	Tracheal resection
	Congenital heart surgery
	PDA ligation
	Vascular malformation excision
	Laryngeal Trauma
	Neoplasia
	CNS neoplasm
	Hilar neoplasm
	Cervical neoplasm
	Medications
	Vincristine
	Infections
	Thryoiditis
	Lyme disease
	TB
	Polioencephalitis
	EBV
	Hydrocephalus

and cervical, neurologic, or cardiothoracic surgery.

UVFI Secondary to Infections

Numerous infectious agents can cause UVFI. Most are described in the adult literature, but the pediatric population is susceptible. Epstein-Barr virus,[16] polioencephalitis,[17] Lyme disease,[18] West Nile virus,[19] tuberculosis,[20] thyroiditis,[21] and post-URI[22] have all been reported.

UVFI Secondary to Neoplasms and Chemotherapy

Neoplasms of the central nervous system, neck, mediastinum, or hilum can cause vocal fold paralysis by invasion. UVFI in the setting of cancer may be related to recurrent laryngeal nerve neuropathy secondary to vinca alkaloid chemotherapy.[23] These agents (vinblastine, vincristine) are used to treat two common childhood malignancies—lymphoma and sarcoma.

PROGNOSIS

Data, albeit retrospective with nonstandardized follow-up, demonstrate that rates of vocal fold recovery vary with each etiology (Table 16–2). Knowledge of this data can help in guiding management decisions. However, the etiology of vocal fold paralysis does not predict the likelihood of recovery for each individual.

In one series, UVFI at birth carried a favorable prognosis. de Gaudemar described 62 children born with UVFI[2]; Seventy-three percent without a cardiac etiology recovered. Restoration of vocal fold movement happened early, with all 43 recoveries within the first 3 months of life and none recovering over the ensuing 5 years. However, this analysis classifies patients lost to follow-up as "not recovering." If patients lost to follow-up are excluded, the recovery rate for the noncardiac group was 42/44 (95%).[2] Children born with "cardiovocal syndrome" had only a 20% recovery rate.[2] Emery and Fearon reported only a 20% recovery for idiopathic, congenital vocal fold paralysis.[11]

Recurrent laryngeal nerve injury after PDA ligation does not have a high chance of recovering. A close look at two major articles reviewing this subject failed to report recovery in any of the 27 paralyses after PDA ligation followed out to 31 months.[13,14] The prognosis of recovery of vocal fold function after other cardiac procedures may be better. Koltai describes 11 children with acquired UVFI after surgery for congenital cardiac malformations (not including PDA); 9 (82%) had full motion within 3 to 8 months.[24]

Recovery rates for other types of iatrogenic surgical injury are fair. Daya reports 20 of 44 patients (46%) regaining function over 5 years following injury.[1] Emery and Fearon's report witnessed 15 of 25 patients (60%) with iatragenic peripheral nerve injury recovering between 2 and 22 months. There were no additional recoveries occurring during a 6-year observation.[11]

Most infectious causes are described in adult case reports, but with the exception

Table 16–2. Prognosis of Recovery of Vocal Fold Movement by Etiology. The numbers of patients studied and the number of patients who recovered functional movement are listed in fraction. Percent of patients who recovered are listed in parenthesis. The duration of follow-up for each patient in the study is listed in the third column.

Etiology	Recovered	Follow-up Period
Congenital		
Noncardiac	45/54 (83%)	1.5–13 years[1,11]
Cardiovascular Abnormality	1/5 (20%)	5 years[10]
Acquired		
PDA Ligation	0/27 (0%)	0–31 months[13,14]
Cardiac Surgery (non-PDA)	9/11 (83%)	3–8 months[25]
Peripheral nerve injury/Iatragenesis	27/45 (60%)	3 months to 6 years[1,11]
Idiopathic	5/5 (5%)	6 years[11]
Peripheral Neuropathy	0/2 (0%)	6 years[11]
Infectious	5/6 (83%)	7 months[16,18–21]

of polio, the prognosis for return of function is good. Vocal fold paresis secondary to invasive neoplasm can be expected not to recover. Acquired idiopathic UVFI in children is rare, but 4 of 4 children in a study by Emery and Fearon recovered.[11]

MANAGEMENT

The treatment of neonates, or children younger than school age, should focus on airway protection and alimentation. Tracheotomy can have a role, but is usually necessary only if synchronous airway lesions are present.[1] Speech therapy evaluation and modified barium swallow can clarify dietary recommendations. Enteral nutrition via gastric or nasogastric tubes may be needed, but simple thickening of feeds is often all that is necessary. If the airway is adequate and there are no feeding difficulties, no treatment is needed. As discussed earlier in this chapter, many children will recover movement of their vocal fold. Other patients learn to compensate. Pereira reported that although there were no recoveries of vocal fold function over 8 months, 5 of 7 neonates who acquired UVFI after PDA ligation did not require any dietary restrictions.[13] Two patients needed tube feeds, but they were removed within 3 months.

Speech therapy can strengthen compensatory methods of glottic closure while minimizing risk of hyperfunctional dysphonia. Administered twice weekly for an average of 12 sessions, speech therapy resulted in statistically significant improvements in jitter, shimmer, maximal phonation time, breathiness, and glottic closure for adults with UVFI.[5] Voice quality is less likely to be a chief complaint for children who are younger than school age. Compensation with speech therapy is sufficient for many children.[24] Some authors have described children with UVFI as having "a near normal voice (that) is the rule rather than the exception."[13]

VOCAL FOLD MEDIALIZATION

Most research concerning vocal fold medialization has been conducted in adult study populations. At the time of this writing, a Pubmed search of English language articles since 1966 using the phrase "vocal fold medialization" identifies 174 papers, whereas "pediatric vocal fold medialization" yields 3. Most published work investigating surgical intervention and UVFI in children describes treatment specifically for aspiration or does not distinguish which patients were treated primarily for voice.[3-4]

There is a degree of trepidation toward intervening surgically in the pediatric larynx. Spontaneous recovery of UVFI has been reported at 18 months in an adult[25] and as late as 4 years in a child.[1] Congenital bilateral vocal cord paralysis has recovered as late as 11 years.[1,11] The appropriate timing of surgical intervention for dysphonia, in the absence of aspiration, is a subject of debate. There are other concerns relating to the procedures themselves and how they are accomplished. Many children are not able to undergo phonosurgery under local anesthesia. Although thyroplasty can be performed under general anesthesia, this is not optimal for surgical correction of dysphonia as it precludes the opportunity for intraoperative vocal "tuning" to optimize results. Moreover, the anatomic alterations that result from most phonosurgical interventions are static, whereas the size, thickness, and composition of the larynx changes as a person progresses from childhood to adulthood.[26] Good results obtained at a young age may be lost in maturation. Because a poor voice is not life threatening, it may be prudent in some cases to wait for spontaneous recovery or to abstain from surgical intervention until after a child has gone through puberty in order to get the best result.

Although these concerns are valid, a child's voice quality affects interactions with peers and adults. Improvement in voice related quality of life has been demonstrated after vocal fold medialization in adults, but has not been investigated in children.[27] Delaying phonosurgical intervention until adulthood may be appropriate for some patients, but earlier intervention may benefit other children. Thyroplasty, injection laryngoplasty, and laryngeal reinnervation are three techniques of vocal fold medialization that can be performed in pediatric patients. Insight into etiology, workup, and prognosis of UVFI can help determine which patients will benefit from surgical intervention and which procedure is most suitable for each individual patient.

Methods of Vocal Fold Medialization

Injection Laryngoplasty

Injection laryngoplasty with Teflon was used first in children for aspiration. It was intended as a one-time permanent treatment.[1,28] Its use has fallen out of favor due to granuloma formation.[1] Nonpermanent materials are now used in children for both voice and aspiration.[3,4,12] With the advent of nonpermanent injectables, injection laryngoplasty is a more conservative option than other treatments. It is particularly advantageous in the early window when spontaneous recovery of vocal fold movement is possible. Children who want to test if medi-alization provides them with an improvement in aspiration or voice, may elect for injection laryngoplasty. The procedure can be repeated in a serial fashion if desired.

With the exception of a cooperative teenager, injection laryngoplasty is performed under general anesthesia in children. Injections with an undersized endotracheal tube in place, intermittent apneic ventilation, jet ventilation, laryngeal mask airway, or tubeless total intravenous anesthesia (TIVA) with topical lidocaine and spontaneous respiration are options (Figs 16–1 and 16–2). Major complications in endolaryngeal surgery are more common when jet ventilation is used.[29] The method chosen is dependent on the patient's medical status and the comfort level of surgeon and anesthesiologist.

There have been no major complications reported with injection laryngoplasty in children.[1,3,4,12,28] However, vocal fold hematoma, vocal fold inclusion cyst, laryngeal abscess, and tracheotomy have been reported in adults.[30,31] Airway compromise secondary to overinjection or complications due to poor intraoperative airway management are possible. Long-term effects of serial vocal fold injection, such as scarring, have not been studied.

There are myriad choices for materials in injection laryngoplasty (Table 16–3).[32] Micronized, acellular, cadaveric dermis (Cymetra) and bovine collagen (Zyplast) have produced results for 4 to 12 months.[33,34] Calcium hydroxylapatite (Radiesse) is purported to last 2 years, but we did not identify published work reporting follow-up longer than 6 months.[35,36] Recently, foreign body reaction has been reported after injection with calcium hydroxylapatite.[37] Autologous fat can work well, but has inconsistent results.[12,38] Porcine gelatin powder (Surgifoam) is reported to last a few weeks, but results up to several months have been described.[12,39]

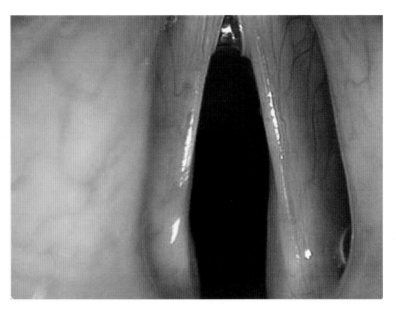

Fig 16–1. Image of suspension laryngoscopy with left vocal fold paralysis, note atrophy of left vocal fold.

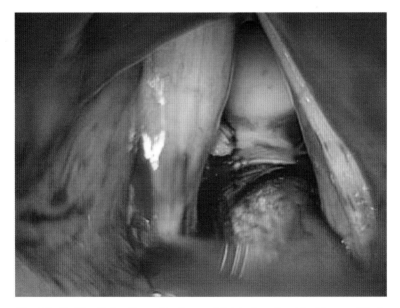

Fig 16–2. Postinjection of left vocal fold of patient in Figure 16–1, note improvement of medialization and bulk of cord. This patient underwent injection under suspension laryngoscopy with spontaneous breathing using total intravenous anesthesia (TIVA), but an endotracheal tube was temporarily placed to prevent an aspiration of injection material (calcium hydroxylapatite) into trachea.

Table 16–3. Table of Various Injectables

Material	Brand Name	Location of Injection	Over-injection	Duration	Cost ($/ml)
Fat	n/a	Lateral to vocal ligament	Yes	3–12 mos	n/a
Autologous Fascia	n/a	Lateral to vocal ligament	Yes	3 mos	n/a
Bovine Collagen	Zyplast	Lateral to vocal ligament	Yes	4–12 mos	300
Cadaveric Dermis	Cymetra	Lateral to vocal ligament	Yes	4–12 mos	271
Hyaluronic Acid	Restylane	In vibratory membrane	Slight	6–12 mos	212
Hydroxylapatite	Radiesse	Lateral to vocal ligament	Slight	12+ mos	295
Carboxymethylcellulose	Radiesse Voice Gel	In vibratory membrane	Yes	2–4 mos	245
Porcine Gelatin	Surgifoam	Lateral to vocal ligament	Yes	0.5–4 mos	100

Adapted from Grillone.[32]

Thyroplasty

There are 24 reported cases of pediatric thyroplasty, the youngest 2 years old.[1,3,12,40-42] Thyroplasty is ideally performed under local anesthesia where the patient can provide intraoperative feedback on implant placement. Thyroplasty improved voice, aspiration, and quality in three patients, but there are no large case series.[12] Adduction arytenoidopexy and cricothyroid joint subluxation may also be performed in a cooperative patient to further adjust vocal fold tension and posterior glottic position.[43] Several implant systems are available including prefabricated sized implants (Montgomery Implant System, Kapitex Healthcare, West Yorkshire, England), Gore-Tex ribbon (W.L. Gore and Associates, Newark, Del), and silicone blocks that can be customized by the surgeon (Netterville Thyroplasty Implant Set and PhonoForm Block, Medtronic, Miami, Fla). Choice of implant is largely a function of surgeon preference and training.

Most children cannot tolerate a thyroplasty while awake, especially prior to puberty or if developmental delay, neurologic disorder, or high vagal lesion is present. However, older adolescents can. Thyroplasty may also be combined with adduction arytenoidopexy (to provide better posterior glottic closure) and cricothyroid joint subluxation (to increase vocal fold tension on the affected side) in a method described by Zeitels (Video 16-1).[43]

Laryngeal mask airway with flexible fiberoptic laryngoscopy is an appropriate method of anesthesia for an uncooperative patient or a patient with impaired airway protection, but this method is inferior for obtaining optimum voice.[41] If thyroplasty is performed prior to puberty, revision surgery would likely be needed, but is technically difficult.[44] Long-term effects or results of thyroplasty placed in young children have not been reported. Aspiration pneumonia requiring intubation was reported in one pediatric patient after thyroplasty, accounting for the only major complication in the literature.[12] Implant displacement into the airway has not been reported in pediatric patients, but is of concern given the smaller airway.

Laryngeal Reinnervation Using Ansa Cervicalis to Recurrent Laryngeal Nerve Anastomosis (Ansa-RLN Anastomosis)

Recently, there has been some developing interest in ansa-RLN anastomosis to treat older children with UVFI. The goal of this procedure is not to produce a mobile vocal fold; rather it is to "reinnervate" the dennervated vocal fold, to restore its bulk, and to medialize to a position where the contralateral mobile vocal fold can make adequate contact and allow for appropriate glottal closure. The theoretic advantage of this procedure over traditional thyroplasty that makes it attractive for pediatric application stems from its being performed while the child is intubated under general anesthesia without the need for intraoperative patient compliance for vocal tuning. Performing the procedure under general anesthesia may also diminish the incidence of intraoperative aspiration and postoperative pneumonias.

The procedure is performed by identifying the ansa cervicalis nerve over the carotid sheath and then by identifying the recurrent laryngeal nerve. The ansa cervicalis can be readily identified at its origin off the hypoglossal nerve and traced throughout its course. We prefer to cut the ansa cervicalis at its posterior branch in an effort to preserve strap muscle innervation. The recurrent laryngeal nerve is located low in the neck, inferior to the thyroid. The neurorrhaphy is performed tension free under magnification using two 8-0 nylon sutures.

The results of ansa-RLN anastomosis may take 3 to 6 months to show evidence of effect. The time delay for reinnervation can be palliated by performing injection laryngoplasty at the same time as the reinnervation procedure.[12,45]

Reinnervation negates any chance of spontaneous recovery. Therefore it should be considered only after an observational period. In cases where neuropraxia is suspected, a period of 12 to 18 months is reasonable. If the nerve is known to be cut (neurontemesis), then earlier intervention is of consideration, although this hypothesis has not been tested. Laryngeal reinnervation does not restore normal motion to the vocal fold, rather the cord increases in tone and assumes a more median position.[46] It is unlikely to helpful in cases of vocal fold fixation. EMG may be of assistance in differentiating paralysis from fixation.[47]

Ansa cervicalis to recurrent laryngeal nerve reinnervation is an attractive method for treating unilateral vocal fold paralysis in children, particularly in the prepubertal child. The benefits of reinnervation may not be changed by child growth. This procedure is optimal under general anesthesia. The laryngeal skeleton is not altered; thus, additional phonosurgery is not compromised if needed later in life. Success with laryngeal reinnervation is reported in adults.[45,48,49] Recurrent laryngeal nerve and ANSA cervicalis neurorrhaphy has been used in two children with UVFI, both with improvement in quality of voice, range, and quality of life (Videos 16-2, 16-3, 16-4, and 16-5).[12]

CONCLUSIONS AND FUTURE DIRECTIONS

UVFI is an uncommon condition in pediatric patients; however, their management can be gratifying. Many children will recover or compensate without intervention. Injection laryngoplasty, thyroplasty, and ansa cervicalis recurrent laryngeal nerve reinnervation all have applications in the pediatric patient. Trials comparing applications with long-term follow-up are needed to better clarify the role of each method. Other methods of management, such as gene therapy, are being explored in animal models.[50,51]

VIDEOS ASSOCIATED WITH THIS CHAPTER

Video 16–1. Intraoperative placement of Gore-Tex for thyroplasty followed by further adjustment of vocal fold positioning with adduction arytenoidopexy and cricothyroid joint subluxation

Video 16–2. Preoperative recording of patient with unilateral vocal fold paralysis prior to reinnervation with ansa cervicalis to recurrent laryngeal nerve anastomosis.

Video 16–3. Preoperative stroboscopy (same patient as Video 16-2) with feeding tube in place.

Video 16–4. Three month postoperative recording of voice passage (same patient as Video 16-2).

Video 16–5. One-year postoperative stroboscopy (same patient as Video 16-2) after reinnervation.

REFERENCES

1. Daya H, Hosni A, Bejar-Solar I, Evans JNG, Baily CM. Pediatric vocal fold paralysis—long-term prospective study. *Arch Otolaryngol Head Neck Surg.* 2000;126:21-25.
2. de Gaudemar I, Roudaire M, Francois M, Narcy P. Outcome of laryngeal paralysis in neonates: a long-term retrospective study of 113 cases. *Int J Pediatr Otorhinolaryngol.* 2006;34:101-110.
3. Shah RK, Harvey-Woodnorth G, Glynn A, Nuss RC. Perceptual voice characteristics in pediatric unilateral vocal fold paralysis. *Otolaryngol Head Neck Surg.* 2006;134: 618-621.
4. Patel NJ, Kerschner JE, Merati AL. The use of injectable collagen in the management of pediatric vocal unilateral fold paralysis. *Int J Ped Otorhinolaryngol.* 2003;67:1355-1360.
5. Schindler A, Bottero A, Capaccio P, Ginocchio D, Adorni F, Ottaviani F. Vocal improvement after voice therapy in unilateral vocal fold paralysis. *J Voice.* 2006; Epub ahead of print.
6. Kelchner LN, Stemple JC, Gerdeman E, LeBorgne W, Adam S. Etiology, pathophysiology, treatment choices, and voice results for unilateral adductor vocal fold paralysis: a 3-year retrospective. *J Voice.* 1999;13: 592-601.
7. Gentile RD, Miller RH, Woodson GE. Vocal cord paralysis in children 1 year of age and younger. *Ann Otol Rhinol Laryngol.* 1986;95:622-625.
8. Altman JS, Benninger MS. The evaluation of unilateral vocal fold immobility: is chest x-ray enough? *J Voice.* 1997;11:364-367.
9. Chalian AA, Langlotz CP. Economic consequences of diagnostic imaging for vocal cord paralyis. *Acad Radiol.* 2001;8:137-148.

10. Scott A, Chong PST, Hartnick CJ. Simplifying larygneal EMG to assess pediatric vocal fold immobility: technical analysis and preliminary results. *Arch Otolaryngol Head Neck Surg.* In press.

11. Emery PJ, Fearon B. Vocal cord palsy in pediatric practice: a review of 71 cases. *Int J Pediatr Otorhinolaryngol.* 1984;8:147-154.

12. Sipp JA, Kershner JE, Braun N, Hartnick CJ. Phonosurgery for pediatric unilateral vocal fold paralysis: injection laryngoplasty, thyroplasty, or nerve reinnervation? *Arch Otolaryngol Head Neck Surg.* In press.

13. Pereira KD, Webb BD, Blakely ML, Cox CS, Lally KP. Sequelae of recurrent laryngeal nerve injury after patent ductus arteriosus ligation. *Int J Pediatr Otorhinolaryngol.* 2006;70:1609-1612.

14. Zbar RI, Chen AH, Behrendt DM, Bell EF, Smith RJ. Incidence of vocal fold paralysis in infants undergoing ligation of patent ductus arteriosus. *Ann Thorac Surg.* 1996;61: 814-816.

15. Clement WA, El-Hakim J, Phillipos EZ, Cote JJ. *Unilateral vocal cord paralysis following PDA ligation in extremely low birth rate infants: a benign complication?* Presented at American Society of Pediatric Otolaryngology (ASPO) San Diego, California, 2007.

16. Johns MM, Hoqikyan ND. Simultaneous vocal fold and tongue paresis secondary to Epstein-Barr virus infection. *Arch Otolaryngol Head Neck Surg.* 2000;126:1491-1494.

17. Driscol BP, Gracco C, Coelho C, et al. Laryngeal function in postpolio patients. *Laryngoscope.* 1995;105:35-41.

18. Schroeter V, Belz GG, Blenk H. Paralysis of recurrent laryngeal nerve in Lyme disease. *Lancet.* 1988;26:1245.

19. Steele NP, Myssiorek D. West Nile virus induced vocal fold paralysis. *Laryngoscope.* 2006;116:494-496.

20. Rafay MA. Turberculosis lymphadenopathy of superior mediastinum causing vocal cord paralysis. *Ann Thorac Surg.* 2000;70: 2142-2143.

21. Minhas SS, Watkinson JC, Franklyn J. Fourth branchial arch fistula and suppurative thyroiditis: a life-threatening infection. *J Laryngol Otol.* 2001;115:1029-1031.

22. Amin MR, Koufman JA. Vagal neuropathy after upper respiratory infection: a viral etiology? *Am J Otolaryngol.* 2001;22:251-256.

23. Burns BV, Shotton JC. Vocal palsy following vinca alkaloid treatment. *J Laryngol Otol.* 1998;112:485-487.

24. Khariwala SS, Lee WT Koltai PJ. Laryngeal consequences of pediatric cardiac surgery. *Arch Otolaryngol Head Neck Surg.* 2005; 131:336-339.

25. Tsunoda K, Kikkawa YS, Kumada M, Higo R, Tayama N. Hoarseness caused by unilateral vocal fold paralysis: how long should one delay for phonosurgery. *Acta Otolaryngol.* 2003;123:555-556.

26. Hudgins PA, Siegel J, Jacobs I, Abramowsky CR. The normal pediatric larynx. *AJNR Am J Neuroradiol.* 1997;18:239-245.

27. Gliklich RE, Glovsky RM, Montgomery WW. Validation of a voice outcome survey for unilateral vocal cord paralysis. *Otolaryngol Head Neck Surg.* 1999;120:153-158.

28. Levine BA, Jacobs IN, Wetmore RF, Handler SD. Vocal cord injection in children with unilateral vocal cord paralysis. *Arch Otolaryngol Head Neck Surg.* 1995;121:116-119.

29. Jaquet Y, Monnier P, Van Melle G, Ravussin P, Spahn DR, Chollet-Rivier M. Complications of different ventilation strategies in endoscopic laryngeal surgery: a 10-year review. *Anesthesiology.* 2006;104:52-59.

30. Laccourreye O, Papon JF, Kania R, Crevier-Buchman L, Brasnu D, Hans S. Intracordal injection of autologous fat in patients with unilateral laryngeal nerve paralysis: long-term results from the patient's perspective. *Laryngoscope.* 2003;113:541-545.

31. Zapanta PE, Bielamowicz SA. Laryngeal abscess after injection laryngoplasty with micronized Alloderm. *Laryngoscope.* 2004; 114:1522-1524.

32. O'Leary MA, Grillone GA. Injection laryngoplasty. *Otolaryngol Clin North Am.* 2006; 39:43-54.

33. Millstein CF, Akst LM, Hicks D, Abelson TI, Strome M. Long-term effects of micronized

alloderm injection for unilateral vocal fold paralysis. *Laryngoscope.* 2005;115:1691-1696.

34. Hertegard S, Hallen L, Laurent C, et al. Cross-linked hyaluron used as augmentation substance for treatment of glottal insufficiency: safety aspects and vocal fold function. *Laryngoscope.* 2002;112:2211-2219.

35. Hughes RGM, Morrison M. Vocal cord medialization by transcutaneous injection of calcium hydroxylapatite. *J Voice.* 2005;16:674-678.

36. Rosen CA, Thekdi AA. Vocal fold augmentation with injectable calcium hydroxylapatite: short-term results. *J Voice.* 2004;18:387-391.

37. Tanna N, Zalkind D, Glade RS, Bielamowicz SA. Foreign body reaction to calcium hydroxylapatite vocal fold augmentation. *Arch Otolaryngol Head Neck Surg.* 2006;132:1379-1382.

38. Kwon TK, Buckmire R. Injection laryngoplasty for management of unilateral vocal fold paralysis. *Curr Opin Otolaryngol Head Neck Surg.* 2004;12:538-542.

39. Shram VL, May M, Lavorato AS. Gelfoam paste injection for vocal cord paralysis: temporary rehabilitation of glottic incompetence. *Laryngoscope.* 1978;88:1268-1273.

40. Link DT, Rutter MJ, Liu JH, Willging JP, Myer CM, Cotton RT. Pediatric type I thyroplasty: an evolving procedure. *Ann Otol Rhinol Laryngol.* 1999;108:1105-1110.

41. Gardner GM, Altman JS, Balakrishnan G. Pediatric vocal fold medialization with Silastic implant: intraoperative airway management. *Int J Ped Otolaryngol.* 2000;52:37-42.

42. Tucker HM. Vocal cord paralysis in small children: principles in management. *Ann Otol Rhinol Laryngol.* 1986;95:618-621.

43. Zeitels SM, Mauri M, Daily SH. Adduction arytenopexy for vocal fold paralysis: indications and technique. *J Laryngol Otol.* 2004;118:508-516.

44. Maragos NE. Revision thyroplasty. *Ann Otol Rhinol Laryngol.* 2001;110:1087-1092.

45. Lee WT, Milstein C, Hicks D, Akst LM, Esclamado RM. Results of ansa to recurrent laryngeal nerve reinnervation. *Otolaryngol Head Neck Surg.* 2007;136:450-454.

46. Green DC, Berke GS, Graves MC. A functional evaluation of ansa cervicalis nerve transfer for unilateral vocal cord paralysis: future directions for laryngeal reinnervation. *Otolaryngol Head Neck Surg.* 1991;104:453-466.

47. Ysunza A, Landeros L, Pamplona MC, Prado H, Arrieta J, Fajardo G. The role of laryngeal electromyography in the diagnosis of vocal fold immobility in children. *Int J Pediatr Otorhinolaryngol.* 2007;71:949-958.

48. Su WF, Hsu YD, Chen HC, Sheng H. Laryngeal reinnervation by ansa cervicalis nerve implantation for unilateral vocal cord paralysis in humans. *J Am Coll Surg.* 2007;204:64-72.

49. Maronian N, Waugh P, Robinson L, Hillel A. Electromyographic findings in recurrent laryngeal nerve reinnervation. *Ann Otol Rhinol Laryngol.* 2003;112:314-323.

50. Araki K, Shiotani A, Watabe K, Saito K, Moro K, Ogawa. Adenoviral GDNF gene transfer enhances neurofunctional recovery after recurrent laryngeal nerve injury. *Gene Ther.* 2006;13:296-303.

51. Shiotani A, Saito K, Araki K, Moro K, Watabe K. Gene therapy for laryngeal paralysis. *Ann Otol Rhinol Laryngol.* 2007;116:115-122.

Pediatric Airway Reconstruction and the Voice

Karen B. Zur

INTRODUCTION

Pediatric airway reconstruction saw a surge in the early 1970s when Robin Cotton began applying surgical techniques that were developed in the adult population by Rethi and Feron, to manage children who suffered from laryngotracheal stenosis. His research and clinical work enabled technologically dependent children suffering from airway compromise due to acquired or congenital laryngotracheal pathology to lead a life without the need for a tracheostomy tube. Airway specialists throughout the United States and the world have adapted and expanded these techniques, allowing a significant rate of decannulation[1] and successful management of other airway disorders.

Now that the management of pediatric airway disorders has been mastered, attention is shifting toward the quality of life of these children. One of the main areas not previously addressed in a systematic fashion is the effect of airway disorders on a child's voice. Tracheostomy tube placement and airway reconstruction can lead to dysphonia, affecting a child's communication and quality of life. These voicing disturbances are due to multifactorial issues that are discussed at the end of this chapter.

Normally, the production of voice is related to the flow of air through the glottis, whose time-dependent shape is defined by the motion of the vocal folds and the translaryngeal pressure.[2] Airway lesions thus alter transglottic airflow patterns leading to either turbulent flow through the vocal folds or complete inability to cause vocal fold vibration due to a high-grade stenosis. Direct injury to the vocal folds may occur during intubation, use of the laser for management of myriad conditions affecting the airway, or open airway procedures (Fig 17–1).

The goal of this chapter is to introduce the reader to basic airway procedures and the voice-related issues following airway manipulation and reconstruction. A detailed description and definition of airway patholo-

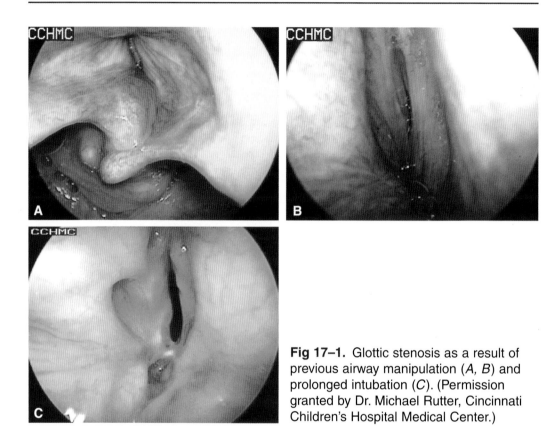

Fig 17–1. Glottic stenosis as a result of previous airway manipulation (*A, B*) and prolonged intubation (*C*). (Permission granted by Dr. Michael Rutter, Cincinnati Children's Hospital Medical Center.)

gies is beyond the scope of this chapter. The systematic, data-oriented paradigm of patient evaluation used by the author is discussed as well. This chapter focuses on the therapeutic interventions that are currently being used to rehabilitate these children.

OVERVIEW OF SURGICAL PROCEDURES TO IMPROVE AND/OR RECONSTRUCT THE AIRWAY

In cases of very mild subglottic or tracheal obstruction with no overt symptoms or complications, it is possible to closely observe the child. Interval endoscopies are performed to assess structural progression versus relative reduction of the obstruction. During the period of observation it is important to monitor underlying gastroesophageal reflux disease and eosinophilic esophagitis and to ensure optimal pulmonary status. In cases with more significant symptoms or obstruction, and following an adequate multidisciplinary evaluation, an appropriate intervention is chosen.

Tracheotomy

The indications for tracheotomy include: severe upper airway obstruction, long-term ventilation, and pulmonary toilet. When the tracheostomy is no longer medically necessary, the child will undergo a decannulation process to remove the tube. This will require another airway evaluation to ensure the airway caliber is adequate. Lesions that can be associated with chronic tracheostomies include suprastomal collapse and suprastomal granulation, and those should be managed prior to decannulation.

The greatest risk of an indwelling tracheostomy is death secondary to tube obstruction or an accidental dislodgement. Mortality related to the presence of a tracheostomy tube has been reported to approximate 0.5%.[3] It is therefore incumbent on the clinicians to educate the family and caretakers regarding proper care at home. Specific tracheotomy care protocols are often developed by many hospitals and medical centers.

Endoscopic Approaches to Repair of Glottic/Subglottic Stenosis

Certain conditions are amenable to endoscopic, "minimally invasive" approaches of repair. Discussion of the merits of various lasers (CO_2, KTP) versus "cold steel" is beyond the scope of this chapter. Base of tongue cysts/masses, glossoptosis (base of tongue collapse), recurrent respiratory papillomatosis (RRP), laryngomalacia, arytenoids prolapse, arytenoid subluxation leading to posterior glottic stenosis, small posterior glottic scar/web (Fig 17–2), bilateral vocal fold paralysis (Fig 17–3), small subglottic web, subglottic cysts and tracheal hemangiomas are but a few of airway lesions that may lead to stridor and airway compromise, and could potentially be managed transorally. All of these lesions can lead to dysphonia either due to the underlying

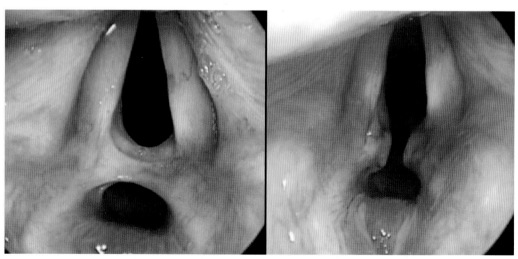

A   B

Fig 17–2. Endoscopic approach to manage a posterior glottic web. **A.** Preoperative view. **B.** Immediate postoperative view. This child had no sequelae from a voice or airway perspective.

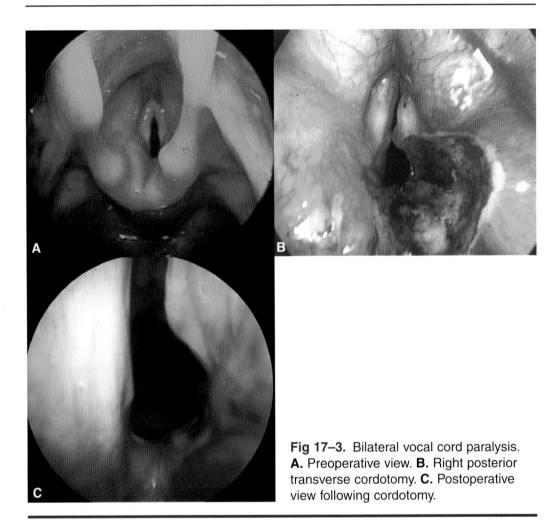

Fig 17–3. Bilateral vocal cord paralysis. **A.** Preoperative view. **B.** Right posterior transverse cordotomy. **C.** Postoperative view following cordotomy.

pathology or as a result of its management. For example, laryngotracheal recurrent respiratory papillomatosis, most commonly caused by HPV subtypes 6 and 11, often require numerous endoscopic debridements to maintain a safe airway (Fig 17–4). Several techniques have been utilized, including cold-dissection, laser techniques (CO_2, pulsed dye laser,[4] and KTP[5]) and the microdebrider.[6] The goal of management is to maintain a safe airway in the case of the obstructing papillomas, and to improve vocalization in milder situation by reducing the mass from the surface of the vocal fold. The goal of restoring mucosal wave without causing irreparable damage to the underlying vocal folds and mucosa is the basic tenet of management, as direct vocal fold and anterior commissure injury can lead to chronic vocal fold scarring, webbing of the larynx, and stenosis. To date, basic science research has been focused on the management and prevention of vocal fold scarring. Mitomycin C, an antifibroblast and antitumor agent, has been used, with variable success, to prevent scarring in the larynx. More innovative tissue engineering technologies utilize injectates to preserve the viscoelastic properties of

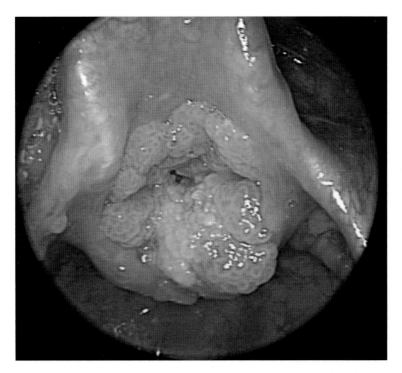

Fig 17–4. Laryngotracheal papillomatosis obstructing the airway.

the vocal folds. Prophylactic in vivo manipulation of the extracellular matrix with an injectable Carbylan-SX hydrogel appears to induce vocal fold tissue regeneration to yield optimal tissue composition and biomechanical properties favorable for phonation.[7] One hopes more clinical research and applications of these techniques will allow preservation of normal vocal fold morphology, while allowing proper management of the airway lesions, either endoscopically or via open surgical approaches.

Anterior Cricoid Split

Neonates who have been intubated for a prolonged period of time, who fail extubation due to minimal subglottic stenosis, and who meet strict eligibility criteria may benefit from performing a cricoid split to augment the airway.[8] This practice is falling out of favor in a population of neonates and infants who can avoid a tracheostomy tube placement. In this group, a thyroid ala graft is interposed between the cut ends of the cricoid cartilage (usually anteriorly) and the child remains intubated for a shorter duration than the cricoid split without the graft; this procedure is fondly referred to as the "mini-laryngotracheoplasty." Improved outcomes (88% success versus 83%) and shorter periods of intubation have made this procedure more favorable, whereas uncontrolled severe reflux, prematurity and low birth weight adversely affect the surgical results.[9]

Augmentation Procedures: Laryngotracheal Reconstruction (LTR)

Expansion procedures to aid in tracheostomy tube removal in the child with glottic/subglottic stenosis (Fig 17–5) include placement of anterior, posterior, or combined grafts to augment the cricoid and/or tracheal airway. Laryngotracheal reconstruction refers to an augmentation procedure with use of a graft(s). The aim of this surgical method is to re-establish airway continuity without the need for a tracheostomy tube and with preservation of laryngeal function for protection of the airway, swallowing, and voicing.[10] For this reason, the candidate for an LTR should have good pulmonary reserve, requiring no ventilatory support and be medically stable. The preoperative workup should include a comprehensive gastroenterological, pulmonary, and swallowing/aspiration evaluation.

Once the decision has been made to reconstruct, the surgical options include augmentation or resection. Resection is described in the next section. Another element that needs to be decided is whether or not the procedure should be single-staged or double-staged. A single-staged procedure means that at the conclusion of the surgery the tracheostomy tube will no longer be present, whereas a double-staged procedure implies that either a tracheostomy tube or a similar type of stent will be present at the end of the case (see next section).

The augmentation procedure involves placement of an autogenous cartilage graft between the split cricoid cartilage and/or split tracheal wall. Numerous graft materials have been reported in the literature over the years, but the most commonly used graft is the cartilaginous rib. Other sources of cartilage grafts, reported in both adult and pediatric literature, have included auricular cartilage, hyoid, thyroid ala, septal cartilage, and thyrotracheal autografts.[11-13] Regardless of the source of cartilage, studies have shown that autogenous cartilage used in the anterior and posterior pediatric larynx survives, grows and undergoes neovascularization.[14]

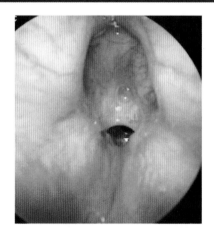

Fig 17–5. Laryngeal atresia. This patient underwent a tracheostomy tube placement at birth and is awaiting surgical reconstruction with a laryngotracheal reconstruction.

Resection Procedures: Partial Cricotracheal Resection

Patients with discrete levels of obstruction and those with high-grade stenoses (grade III-IV subglottic stenosis), often benefit from a graft-free resection procedure. Two resection procedures are used to manage either subglottic or tracheal stenosis; respectively, they are termed partial cricotracheal resection (CTR) or tracheal resection. This chapter focuses on the more complex CTR.

The CTR procedure involves: (1) resection of the anterior cricoid plate, remaining anterior to the cricothyroid joint; (2) resection of proximal tracheal stenosis, maintaining the first healthy tracheal ring intact; and (3) removing posterior cricoid scar in a submucosal plane, below the level of the cricoarytenoid joint. Once the scar is removed, the trachea is sutured to the posterior cricoid mucosa and to the anterior thyroid lamina (Fig 17–6). Chin to chest sutures are placed for 10 days to allow healing of the anastamosis without potential for head extension and tracheal separation in cases of patient agitation. The CTR, just like the LTR, can be performed in a single- or double-staged procedure, with similar indications for each as previously described.

AIRWAY RECONSTRUCTION AND THE VOICE

With the excellent decannulation rates discussed earlier in the chapter and the comfort of the pediatric airway surgeon in managing those cases, the focus of the multidisciplinary team caring for these children is now shifting toward improving their vocal quality of life. In his book *Odyssey of the Voice* Jean Abitbol states that " . . . feeling good about one's voice, just as feeling good about oneself, is essential for our communication with oneself and with others."[15] The ability

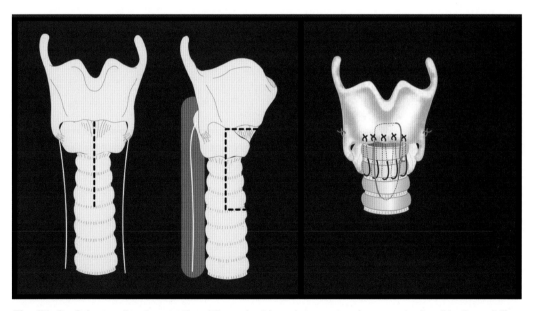

Fig 17–6. Cricotracheal resection. The cricoid and upper trachea are incised in the midline in a vertical fashion to allow exposure of the airway and to assess the stenotic lesion. At this point, the decision will be made whether an augmentation versus a resection procedure will be undertaken. For the partial CTR, the anterior cricoid plate and damaged tracheal rings are removed, anterior to the cricothyroid joint, with care to dissect in a subperichondrial plane, as to avoid the nearby recurrent laryngeal nerves. Once a circumferential dissection around the trachea is accomplished, sutures are placed between the trachea and inferior thyroid border, with two lateral detentioning sutures to secure the anastomosis. Hartley BE, Cotton RT. Pediatric Airway Stenosis: Laryngotracheal Reconstruction or Cricotracheal Resection? *Clin Otolaryngol Allied Sci.* 2000;25(5):342–349. Reprinted with permission.

to communicate effectively, effortlessly and with clarity is a secondary goal in the process of augmenting an airway. The focus of this section is on procedure-specific complications as they relate to the voice.

Chronic Tracheostomy

Dysphonia in children with tracheostomy tubes who can tolerate the placement of a Passy-Muir valve or cap, or in those children with a history of chronic subglottic stenosis who underwent surgical reconstruction, can be partly attributed to phonation patterns that involve the extensive use of supraglottic laryngeal structures.[16-19] When an individual has a tracheotomy tube in place, the direct airstream that can be utilized for vocal fold vibration is generated by inspiration through the tracheotomy tube. When the child is decannulated, he or she quite often continues the previously learned motor behavior for speech and breathing pattern. Reverse or inspiratory phonation is the compensatory speech characteristic used by children in this population.[21]

Glottic Insufficiency

Laryngofissure

A laryngofissure is created by incising the midline thyroid cartilage, splitting the vocal folds at the anterior commissure. Surgical procedures that require a laryngofissure such as those to manage laryngeal webs and high subglottic stenoses, can potentially lead to scarring and asymmetry at the level of the glottis. The laryngofissure is performed transcervically, often with the aid of an assistant surgeon who performs a simultaneous bronchoscopy to visualize the ante-

rior commissure. The author uses a No. 12 blade whose curvature and sharp tip allow direct placement of the knife at the commissure for lysis (Fig 17–7). During this maneuver, the vocal folds are at risk of direct injury and for asymmetric reapproximation of the vocal folds (Fig 17–8). This vertical asymmetry will lead to glottic insufficiency, wave irregularities, and potentially to breathy phonation. Furthermore, aggressive manipulation of the pre-epiglottic region could potentially lead to prolapse of the base (petiole) of the epiglottis (Fig 17–9).

The laryngofissure is often a component of the more extensive laryngotracheal surgery, providing an access to the posterior larynx when exposure of the posterior cricoid plate is limited in a young child, or when adjunct procedures are necessary at the level of the vocal process and arytenoids. In these circumstances, performing a revision laryngofissure, particularly in a

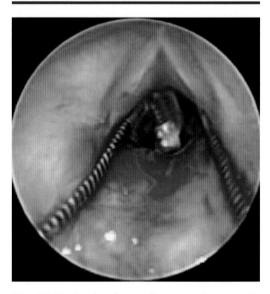

Fig 17–7. Lysis of anterior commissure utilizing simultaneous microlayngoscopy to assist in precise incision placement.

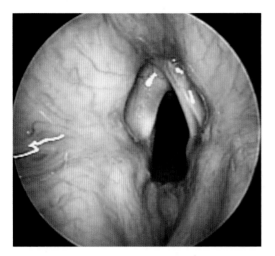

Fig 17–8. Asymmetric vocal fold height post-laryngotracheal reconstruction graft and a laryngofissure for management of a subglottic hemangioma.

young child, is unfavorable (Fig 17-10). Voice therapy techniques to minimize supraglottic compensation and to improve breath support and audibility should help in these cases. If voice therapy does not adequately augment the phonatory volume, augmentative or alternative communication devices should be considered. Another possible surgical option would be to plump a vocal fold with an injectate (such as Radiesse Gel, Cymetra, etc) to minimize the air escape through the glottis.

Glottic insufficiency can also result from prolonged intubation and a defect in the posterior glottis (Benjamin defect), preventing approximation of the arytenoids and vocal folds and leading to breathy dysphonia (Fig 17-11).

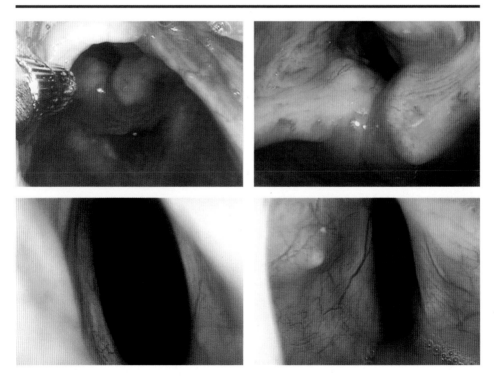

Fig 17–9. Intraoperative images of a patient long-term post-LTR with asymmetric vocal fold height, scarring, and petiole prolapse.

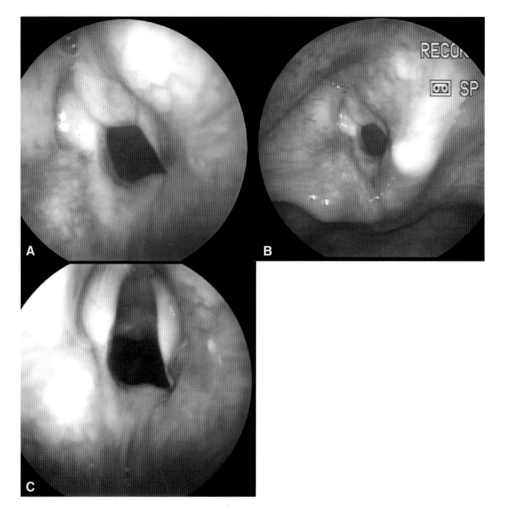

Fig 17–10. 14-year-old female, 30-week premature infant at birth with a history of prolonged intubation and resultant transglottic injury and grade 3 subglottic stenosis. She underwent a tracheostomy at 3 months of age and a subsequent LTR with anterior and posterior cartilaginous rib grafts at 2 years of age. Due to an anterior glottic stenosis at the commissure (*A,B*), she underwent a laryngofissure with a keel 2 years post-LTR. Five months later she was decannulated with a healthy airway (*C*) but a weak and breathy voice. Note the widened anterior commissure and mildly atrophic right vocal fold, slight asymmetric height approximation. On flexible transnasal stroboscopy she is noted to exhibit mild compression of ventricular folds and mild-moderate anterior-posterior compression with arytenoid prolapse. The vocal folds are mobile, but slightly atrophic.

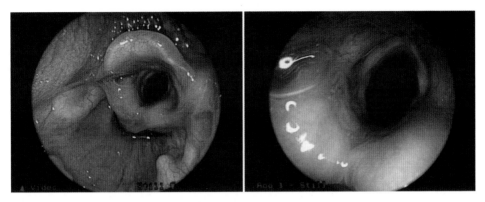

Fig 17–11. Intubation defect (Benjamin defect). One-week intubation history with associated breathy dyphonia due to a large posterior glottic chink.

Supraglottic Phonation

Posterior Cricoid Split

Surgical management of subglottic stenosis or posterior glottic stenosis may require a complete vertical division of the posterior plate to allow placement of a graft material or to allow fibrosis of a posterior cricoid split as described in the previous section. The posterior incision must be in the midline, to allow the proper placement of a posterior graft. This graft has to be of the proper vertical height to prevent postoperative posterior glottic/interarytenoid stenosis. Furthermore, the graft must not be too thick, in order to prevent postoperative dysphagia or extrusion (Fig 17-12).

A trend that has been noted by the author in over 200 dysphonic children evaluated following laryngotracheal reconstruction is anterior arytenoid prolapse with supraglottic compression. There are a couple of theories explaining the resultant prolapse. The first relates to destabilization of the arytenoid if the interarytenoid muscle is not cut during the posterior cricoid split.[20] Another issue related to placement of a posterior cricoid graft is the static distraction of the posterior glottis and the almost inevitable glottic insufficiency. To prevent air escape during phonation, a supraglottic sphincter is formed by the compensatory motion of the arytenoid cartilages onto the epiglottis. This is a child's natural way of adapting to the loss of volume generated at the level of the vocal folds, albeit creating a harsher tone with a deeper phonatory quality. In a recent study done ex vivo in excised larynges it was found that the false vocal folds and the epiglottis offer a positive contribution to the glottal resistance and sound intensity of the larynx. Also, vocal fold elongation and glottal medial compression caused an increase in glottal resistance. The pressure-flow relationships were approximately linear regardless of the structure.[21] It is the author's belief that early voice therapy techniques to minimize supraglottic compression can reduce these compensatory behaviors. It is imperative, however, to avoid placement of wider posterior grafts, to minimize overdistraction of this delicate region.

Supraglottic phonation in response to glottic insufficiency has also been shown

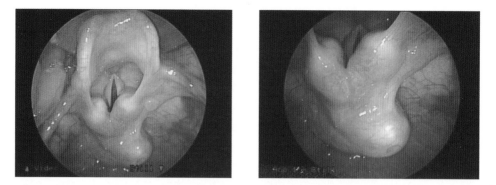

Fig 17–12. Images of a child who underwent a laryngotracheal reconstruction with a posterior cartilaginous rib graft. Both images depict a posterior cricoid bulge representing an extruded graft. It was subsequently removed and reimplanted with no long-term sequelae.

to promote formation of laryngoceles in a small group ($n = 5$) of children who previously underwent successful laryngotracheal reconstruction (Fig 17-13). Laryngocele formation represents the pathologic response of the larynx and supraglottis to increased intralaryngeal pressures. This is a well-recognized phenomenon in patients with laryngeal carcinoma, glass blowers, and those playing wind instruments.[22]

In a recent objective and subjective retrospective evaluation of postreconstruction dysphonia in a group of 12 patients it was shown that those children who used supraglottic structures for phonation were rated by experienced voice clinicians as demonstrating significantly more strain during voice production.[22] Hyperfunctional phonatory performance can adversely impact communication and social skills, as well as classroom performance. This was recently shown in a study utilizing the Pediatric Voice Handicap Index (pVHI), a proxy quality-of-life tool available for following dysphonia in children[23] (Appendix 17, pVHI). In this validation study, parents of 33 dysphonic children who underwent airway

reconstruction and had no voice therapy in the past, were asked to fill out a 23-item parental-proxy survey with a focus on the physical, emotional, and functional effects of their child's voice disorder. They were compared to a group of healthy controls without voicing issues. There was a statistically significant difference in the perception of a child's ability to integrate in school from an emotional and physical standpoint compared to a healthy child without a voice disorder.[23] The dysphonia group differed greatly from the control group on each subscale and on the total scores (Table 17-1).

Modulation and Pitch Range

Cricotracheal Resection (CTR)

The partial cricotracheal resection (CTR) involves the excision of the anterolateral cricoid plate and anastomosis of the distal tracheal ring to the proximal thyroid ala with suture lines placed in the posterior cricoid mucosa to attempt to reapproximate the trachealis to the more proximal cricoid

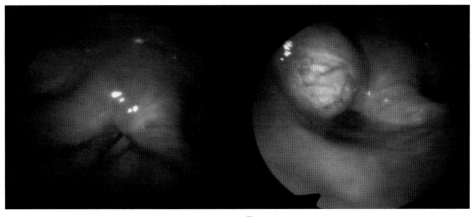

A   **B**

Fig 17–13. Glottic insufficiency with a chronic force of translaryngeal air and supraglottic compression may lead to laryngocele formation. **A.** View of the larynx at rest. **B.** With phonation, note the air-filled right aryepiglottic cyst and the muscle tension in the supraglottis. This is an 11-year-old female, 27-week premature infant at birth with a history of broncopulmonary dysplasia and prolonged intubation. She underwent a tracheostomy tube placement at the age of 4 months. She underwent a single staged laryngotracheal reconstruction with placement of anterior and posterior cartilaginous rib grafts following an unsuccessful tracheal resection and right laser arytenoidectomy the previous year. She has had an excellent airway, but experiences worsening dysphonia and loss of her soprano range.

Table 17–1. A Comparison of the Mean Scores Obtained for the Control Group and a Diverse Group of Dysphonic Airway Patients (*)

Scale	Control	Airway*
Functional	1.47	13.94
Physical	0.20	15.48
Emotional	0.18	12.15
TOTAL SCORE	1.84	41.58
Visual Analog Scale (VAS)		52.91

*The values reflect the pVHI subscales, total scores, and overall severity of the voice expressed by the child's parent (calculated from the visual analog scale, VAS). Reprinted from Zur KB, Cotton S, Kelchner L, Baker S, Weinrich B, Lee L. Pediatric Voice Handicap Index (pVHI): a new tool for evaluating pediatric dysphonia. *Int J Pediatr Otorhinolaryngol.* 2007;71(1): 77–82 with permission from Elsevier.

plate. This procedure is well suited for higher grade subglottic stenosis that has a healthy margin away from the vocal folds to allow for the proximal suture line.[24] Again, preservation of the vocal folds is imperative, and in the most complex of airway cases where there is an extension of the stenosis into the glottis, an extended CTR (eCTR) is often performed with judicious placement of a posterior cricoid graft.

It is intuitive that the CTR will lead to postoperative dysphonia due to obliteration of the cricothyroid membrane and removal of the cricothyroid muscle. Thus, patients are left with a deeper phonatory quality and loss of the higher pitch ranges. Furthermore, extensive scarring and manipulation of the prelaryngeal muscles during dissection, especially in revision laryngotracheal surgery, can render the patient dysphonic due to difficulties in modulating a sound.[25] Other potential complications may include arytenoid prolapse due to destabilization following manipulation of the lateral cricoarytenoid muscles, destabilization of the cricoarytenoid joint, and potential damage of the posterior cricoarytenoid ligament (if an extended CTR is performed with a posterior cricoid split).[26]

Additionally, vocal fold paralysis, albeit rare, may result if the dissection of the cricoid and trachea is not meticulous and the recurrent laryngeal nerve is injured. Other CTR-related complications that can lead to dysphonia include prolapse of the base (petiole) of the epiglottis leading to supraglottic phonation (Fig 17–14 and 17–15; Video 17–1), and restenosis of the airway and webbing on the undersurface of the vocal folds leading to turbulent airflow through the glottis (Fig 17–16).

Given the potential complications following reconstruction, it is incumbent on the surgeon to recognize the potential pitfalls of the reconstructions and to deliberately attempt to preserve laryngeal function when possible. In general, successful decannulation is reported to be as high as 95% for CTR;[25-26] however, data concerning voice outcomes are less well defined.

SYSTEMATIC APPROACH TO EVALUATION OF PEDIATRIC DYSPHONIA

There is a wide spectrum of voice disorders and laryngeal dysfunction presented by individuals requiring LTR, and a systematic documentation of communication ability, laryngeal condition, voicing, and potential for voicing pre- and postreconstruction surgery is essential. Complicating this issue is the fact that many of the children who undergo reconstruction, have spent the formative years of their life (birth to 3 years) with a tracheostomy tube. This is a critical period for language development and often these children exhibit delays.[27] Meticulous record keeping should provide valuable data to surgeons and speech-language pathologists regarding medical, surgical, and behavioral interventions' timing and planning. Careful adaptation of evaluation protocols and a team approach including patient, caregivers, otolaryngologist, and speech-language pathologist is essential to address all key assessment and subsequent management issues.[28]

The initial evaluation of a child with chronic laryngotracheal stenosis should include overall assessment of the child's communication, potential for voicing (ie, can the child phonate with the tracheotomy tube covered, ability of the child to tolerate and phonate with a Passy-Muir valve), and use of any form of alternative communication (ie, sign language). In the prelinguistic child a formal preoperative voice assessment may be difficult; however, the presence and the quality of stridor, a cry, breathing, or babbling may be documented. An awake-transnasal fiberoptic laryngoscopy may reveal information regarding vocal fold mobility during breathing and/or crying.

As already alluded to, the focus of the parents of a young child with laryngotracheal stenosis is to establish an adequate airway, successful decannulation, safe swallowing, and some type of functional voicing. However, once an adequate airway is well established and as the child ages, vocal quality becomes increasingly important to the family. In order to provide effective guidance and treatment, the effect of the child's current vocal quality on peer interactions and ability to function appropriately in school and extracurricular activities should be evaluated. Inquiry into the specific accommodations the classroom teacher has

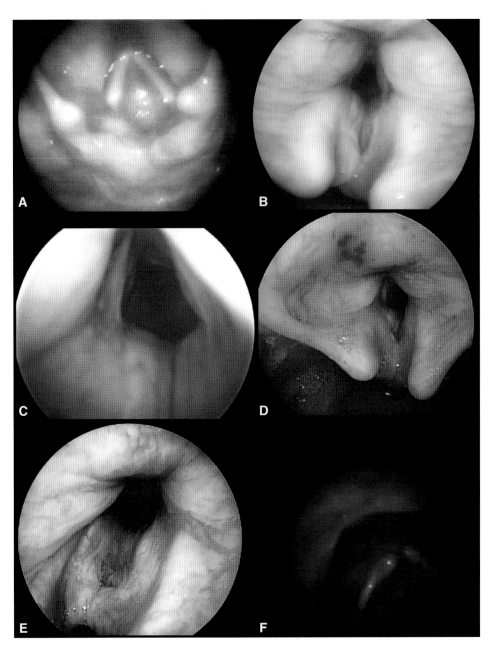

Fig 17–14. These images illustrate a potential pitfall from lack of voice therapy postcricotracheal resection. Note the progressive eversion of the false vocal folds with eventual loss of laryngeal architecture due to chronic supraglottic compensation. **A.** Preoperative view of a grade 4 subglottic stenosis **B.** Six months post-extended cricotracheal resection with laryngofissure and accidental injury to the right vocal fold **C.** Eighteen-months post-reconstruction **D.** Four-years post-reconstruction **E.** Ten-years postreconstruction. **F.** Ten-years postreconstruction, during flexible transnasal stroboscopy. See **Video 17–1.** This video of the patient described in Figure 17–15 illustrates the benefit of front focus phonation with a lip buzz. Please notice the irregular neocord vibration at the onset of the video. During the lip buzz maneuver, there is better regulation of the vibratory movement and a more crisp sound.

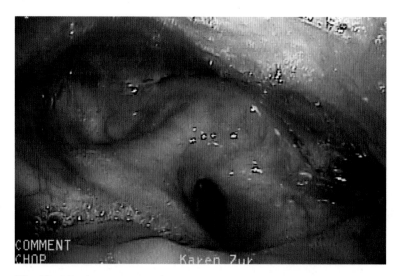

Fig 17–15. A teenager who presented with supraglottic stenosis and tracheostomy dependence. In the past, he underwent multiple laryngotracheal reconstructions with anterior and posterior cartilaginous grafts. This image is postsupraglottic reconstruction and petiole repositioning. He is decannulated and doing well. Transnasal stroboscopy reveals significant glottic insufficiency due to multiple prior reconstruction, supraglottic compression, and dysphonia.

made in order for the child to be heard and understood in class should also be made, as contact with the school's services can be made to help assist these children.[28]

Rating scales have recently been developed that can assist in determining these functional and social impact of voice impairment. Two such quality of life assessments include the pediatric Voice Handicap Index (pVHI)[23] and the Voice-Related Quality of Life Index (V-RQOL).[29] Whichever tool is used to monitor the quality of life of a child, it is important to include it as part of the evaluation and management of these triumphant children as visualization of the larynx is not necessarily reflective of a child's vocal performance (Fig 17-17; Video 17-2).

Although the potential exists for an increase of social, educational, and functional impairments for patients in the LTS population, as previously stated, it is not uncommon for caregivers and the child to view the vocal quality as a minor impairment when compared to previous airway concerns. Decannulation is the goal of airway reconstruction surgeries, and patients may or may not be prepared by the surgeon that the resulting vocal quality may not be normal. Further investigation of voice impairment scales in this population will assist in determining the impact of vocal quality, particularly throughout development into the adolescent years. Additionally, voice assessment teams will benefit from a better

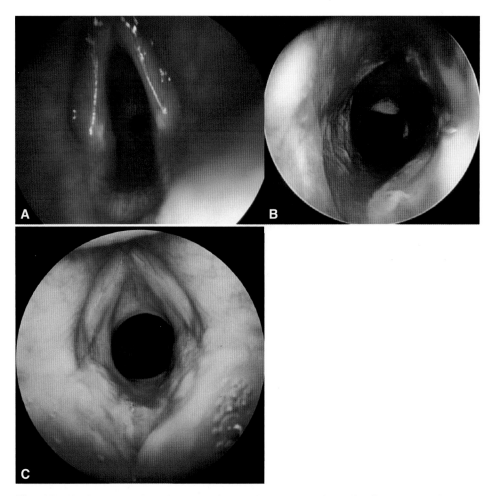

Fig 17–16. Laryngeal web postcricotracheal resection. **A.** Grade 3 subglottic stenosis and normal vocal fold appearance. **B.** Normal appearance of the airway postcricotracheal reconstruction. **C.** Small immediate subglottic web at the site of the thyrotracheal anastomosis. Minimal dysphonia noted in this child with an excellent airway. (Images courtesy of Dr. Mike Rutter, Cincinnati Children's Hospital Medical Center.)

understanding of the impact of the voice on daily function.[28]

Following quality of life survey and history, all patients undergo acoustic evaluations, utilizing a computer-based system (CSL, Visi-Pitch) and the visual analog scale-based expert consensus auditory perceptual evaluation of voice (CAPE-V). Voice recordings are obtained to document preoperative (when available) and postoperative voicing results, as well as progress with voice therapy. At the conclusion of the session, an endoscopic visualization of the larynx with or without stroboscopy is undertaken, again

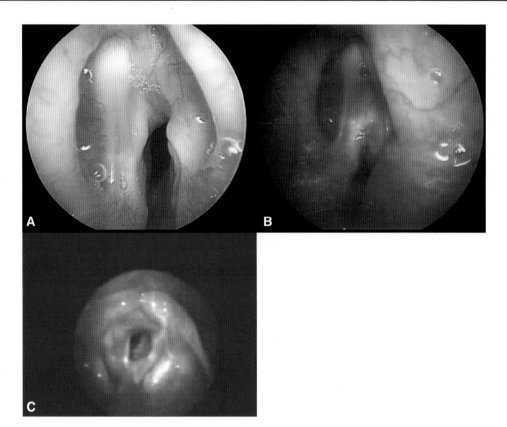

Fig 17–17 and **Video 17–2.** This is a 10–year-old female competitive athlete with a history of laryngeal atresia and subglottic stenosis (*A,B*). She underwent a tracheostomy tube placement at 10 days of age. She subsequently underwent a LTR with anterior and posterior rib grafts, and required a double-staged LTR with an anterior rib graft a year later in order to decannulate. She has no dyspnea on exertion, but her parents notice a quiet voice and difficulty being heard in classroom. (*C*) demonstrates laryngeal appearance during an office transnasal stroboscopy. Her left vocal fold exhibits normal mobility. The right arytenoid is mobile, but she has no true vocal fold. Instead, she is vibrating against a neocord and exhibits minimal lateral-medial compression with minimal dysphonia. The child is happy with her vocal performance and does not desire any voice therapy at this time. This case is illustrative of the importance of a perceptual evaluation in this population, as appearance does not always correspond to function.

photodocumenting altered voicing patterns. The goal of these evaluations is to capture the essence of their risk of dysphonia postoperatively, and to begin voice therapy intervention prior to development of supraglottic compression (Fig 17-18).

THE FUTURE

Prospective, comprehensive and close long-term follow-up of "airway children" with dysphonia will provide more powerful data

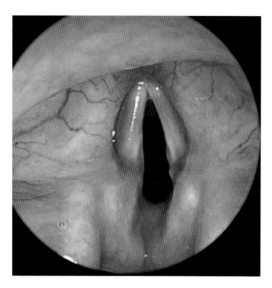

Fig 17–18. This is a 6-year-old female post-lye injection and interarytenoid scarring. She presented with inspiratory stridor and breathy phonation due to posterior glottic stenosis. She underwent a single-staged laryngotracheal reconstruction with a posterior cartilaginous rib graft. Voice therapy instituted several weeks postoperatively. She presents with a normal airway, no stridor on phonation, and no evidence of supraglottic compression 1 year postreconstruction.

on the effects of various surgical procedures on voicing. Currently, the available studies are limited and lack a combination of objective and subjective data to evaluate surgery-specific effects, utility of early voice therapy, benefits of various therapeutic maneuvers, and effectiveness of ancillary surgical interventions such as vocal fold injections to reduce glottic insufficiency.

The bottom line is providing a forum for management of dysphonic children following and during the perioperative reconstructive period to allow them to quickly integrate or reintegrate into their social setting and allow for as flawless a transition as

possible and to restore a normalized childhood. Future research will allow the surgeon to pinpoint and avoid surgical maneuvers that increase the risk of voice disturbances postoperatively as well as incorporate tissue engineering to rehabilitee or prevent vocal fold scarring which is at times encountered during these procedures.

CONCLUSION

In conclusion, a comprehensive and multidisciplinary evaluation and management should provide valuable information to surgeons and voice therapists regarding medical, surgical, and behavioral intervention timing and planning. The evaluation should be precise and stringent, to allow consistent data collection among and within patients.

The field of medicine involves constant progress and innovation. With the maturation of laryngology as a subspecialty and with the advent of technologic innovation and interventions in the younger populations, it is incumbent on the pediatric specialist to nourish the field of pediatric laryngology to help carry these children to a healthy and integrated life.

REFERENCES

1. Hartnick CJ, Hartley BE, Lacy PD, et al. Surgery for pediatric subglottic stenosis: disease-specific outcomes. *Ann Otol Rhinol Laryngol.* 2001;110(12):1109–1113.
2. Kucinschi BR, Scherer RC, Dewitt KJ, Ng TT. An experimental analysis of the pressures and flows within a driven mechanical model of phonation. *J Acoust Soc Am.* 2006; 119(5 pt 1):3011–3021.
3. Wetmore RF, Marsh RR, Thompson ME, et al. Pediatric tracheostomy: a changing

procedure? *Ann Otol Rhinol Laryngol.* 1999;108:695-699.

4. Valdez TA, McMillan K, Shapshay SM. A new laser treatment for vocal cord papilloma—585-nm pulsed dye. *Otolaryngol Head Neck Surg.* 2001;124(4):421-425.

5. Tasca RA, McCormick M, Clarke RW. British Association of Paediatric Otorhinolaryngology members experience with recurrent respiratory papillomatosis. *Int J Pediatr Otorhinolaryngol.* 2006;70(7):1183-1187.

6. Schraff S, Derkay CS, Burke B, Lawson L. American Society of Pediatric Otolaryngology members' experience with recurrent respiratory papillomatosis and the use of adjuvant therapy. *Arch Otolaryngol Head Neck Surg.* 2004;130(9):1039-1042.

7. Hansen JK, Thibeault SL, Walsh JF, Shu XZ, Prestwich GD. In vivo engineering of the vocal fold extracellular matrix with injectable hyaluronic acid hydrogels: early effects on tissue repair and biomechanics in a rabbit model. *Ann Otol Rhinol Laryngol.* 2005;114(9):662-670.

8. Cotton R. Management of subglottic stenosis. *Otolaryngol Clin North Am.* 2000;33:111-130.

9. Forte V, Chang MB, Papsin BC. Thyroid ala cartilage reconstruction in neonatal subglottic stenosis as a replacement for the anterior cricoid split. *Int J Pediatr Otorhinolaryngol.* 2001;59(3):181-186.

10. Smith ME, March JH, Cotton RT, et al. Voice problems after pediatric laryngotracheal reconstruction: videolaryngostroboscopic, acoustic, and perceptual assessment. *Int J Pediatr Otorhinolaryngol.* 1993;25:173-181.

11. Cotton R. The problem of pediatric laryngotracheal stenosis: a clinical and experimental study on the efficacy of autogenous cartilaginous grafts placed between the vertically divided halves of the posterior lamina of the cricoid cartilage. *Laryngoscope* 1991;101:1-34.

12. Caputo V, Consiglio V. The use of patient's own auricular cartilage to repair deficiency of the tracheal wall. *J Thorac Cardiovasc Sur.* 1961;41:594-596.

13. Zur KB, Urken ML. Vascularized hemitracheal autograft for laryngotracheal reconstruction: a new surgical technique based on the thyroid gland as a vascular carrier. *Laryngoscope.* 2003;113:1494-1498.

14. Pashley N, Jaskunas J, Waldstein G. Laryngotracheoplasty with costochondral grafts—a clinical correlate of graft survival. *Laryngoscope.* 1984;94:1493-1496.

15. Abitbol J. *Odyssey of the Voice.* 1st ed. San Diego, Calif: Plural Publishing, 2006.

16. Weinrich B, Baker S, Kelchner L, et al. Examination of aerodynamic measures and strain by vibratory source. *Otolaryngol HNS.* 2007;136:455-458.

17. Clary RA, Pengilly A, Bailey M, et al. Analysis of voice outcomes in pediatric patients following surgical procedures for laryngotracheal stenosis. *Arch Otolaryngol Head Neck Surg.* 1996; 122:1189-1194.

18. MacArthur CJ, Kearns GH, Healy GB. Voice quality after laryngolotracheal reconstruction. *Arch Otolaryngol Head Neck Surg.* 1994;120:641-647.

19. Zalzal GH, Loomis SR, Fischer M. Laryngeal reconstruction in children: assessment of voice quality. *Arch Otolaryngol Head Neck Surg.* 1993;119:504-507.

20. Rutter MJ, Yellon RF, Cotton RT. Management and prevention of subglottis stenosis in infants and children. In: Bluestone CD, Stool SE, eds. *Pediatric Otolaryngology.* Vol. 2. 4th ed. Philadelphia, Pa: Saunders; 2003.

21. Alipour F, Jaiswal S, Finnegan E. Aerodynamic and acoustic effects of false vocal folds and epiglottis in excised larynx models. *Ann Otol Rhinol Laryngol.* 2007; 116(2):135-144.

22. Zur KB, Cotton RT, Willging JP, Rutter MJ. *Laryngocele Formation Following Pediatric Laryngotracheal Reconstruction.* Abstract and oral presentation, European Society of Pediatric Otolaryngology, June 2006.

23. Zur KB, Cotton S, Kelchner L, Baker S, Weinrich B, Lee L. Pediatric Voice Handicap Index (pVHI): a new tool for evaluating pediatric dysphonia. *Int J Pediatr Otorhinolaryngol.* 2007;71(1):77-82.

24. Rutter MJ, Hartley BE, Cotton RT. Cricotracheal resection in children. *Archives Otol Head Neck Surg.* 2001;127(3); 289-292.

25. Monnier P, Lang F, Savary M. Partial crico-tracheal resection for pediatric subglottic stenosis: a single institution's experience in 60 cases. *Eur Arch Otorhinolaryngol.* 2003;260:295-297.

26. Rutter MJ, Link DT, Hartley BE, et al. Arytenoid prolapse as a consequence of crico-tracheal resection in children. *Ann Otol Rhinol Laryngol.* 2001;110:210-214.

27. Simon BM, Fowler SM, Handler SD. Communication development in young children with long-term tracheostomies: preliminary report. *Int J Pediatr Otorhinolaryngol.* 1983; 6(1): 37-50.

28. Baker S, Kelchner L, Weinrich B, et al. Pediatric laryngotracheal stenosis and airway reconstruction: a review of voice outcomes, assessment, and treatment issues. *J Voice.* 2006;20(4):631-641.

29. Hartnick CJ. Validation of a pediatric voice quality-of-life instrument. *Arch Otolaryngol HNS.* 2002;128:919-922.

APPENDIX 17

Pediatric Voice Handicap Index

Subject Number: _____   Date: _____

I would rate my/my child's talkativeness as the following (circle response)	To be filled out by Staff:

I would rate my/my child's talkativeness as the following (circle response)

1	2	3	4	5	6	7
Quiet Listener			Average Talker			Extremely Talkative

To be filled out by Staff:

F= _____
P= _____
E= _____
Total= _____

Talkativeness: _____

Instructions: These are statements that many people have used to describe their voices and the effects of their voices on their lives. Circle the response that indicates how frequently you have the same experience.

0=Never   1=Almost Never   2=Sometimes   3=Almost always   4=Always

Part I - F

1) My child's voice makes it difficult for people to hear him/her   0 1 2 3 4

2) People have difficulty understanding my child in a noisy room   0 1 2 3 4

3) At home, we have difficulty hearing my child when he/she calls through the house.   0 1 2 3 4

4) My child tends to avoid communicating because of his/her voice.   0 1 2 3 4

5) My child speaks with friends, neighbors, or relatives less often because of his/her voice.   0 1 2 3 4

6) People ask my child to repeat him/herself when speaking face-to-face.   0 1 2 3 4

7) My child's voice difficulties restrict personal, educational and social activities.   0 1 2 3 4

Part II – P

1) My child runs out of air when talking   0 1 2 3 4

2) The sound of my child's voice changes throughout the day   0 1 2 3 4

3) People ask, 'What's wrong with your child's voice?"   0 1 2 3 4

4) My child's voice sounds dry, raspy, and/or hoarse   0 1 2 3 4

5) The quality of my child's voice is unpredictable   0 1 2 3 4

6) My child uses a great deal of effort to speak (eg, straining)   0 1 2 3 4

7) My child's voice is worse in the evening   0 1 2 3 4

0=Never   1=Almost Never   2=Sometimes   3=Almost always   4=Always

8) My child's voice "gives out" when speaking   0 1 2 3 4

9) My child has to yell in order for others to hear him/her.   0 1 2 3 4

Part III – E

1) My child appears tense when talking to others because of his
    or her voice.   0 1 2 3 4

2) People seem irritated with my child's voice   0 1 2 3 4

3) I find other people don't understand my child's voice problem   0 1 2 3 4

4) My child is frustrated with his/her voice problem   0 1 2 3 4

5) My child is less outgoing because of his/her voice problem   0 1 2 3 4

6) My child is annoyed when people ask him/her to repeat   0 1 2 3 4

7) My child is embarrassed when people ask him/her to repeat   0 1 2 3 4

Overall Severity Rating of Voice
(Please place "X" mark anywhere along this line to indicate the severity of your child's voice; the verbal descriptions serve as a guide)

_____

Normal   Severe

Reprinted from Zur KB, Cotton S, Kelchner L, Baker S, Weinrich B, Lee L. Pediatric Voice Handicap Index (pVHI): a new tool for evaluating pediatric dysphonia. *Int J Pediatr Otorhinolaryngol.* 2007;71(1):77–82 with permission from Elsevier.

Functional and Spasmodic Dysphonias in Children

Marshall E. Smith
Nelson Roy
Cara Sauder

INTRODUCTION

The voice is an indicator of health, emotion, gender, and age. It forms part of one's individual identity and personality and is a primary means of communication and expression. In children this organ is developing in physical structure in concert with the rest of the speech mechanism. At this same time also proceeds the neurocognitive, behavioral growth and maturation of the child. As the larynx has highly developed neural connections it is not surprising that the voice is sensitive to neural input and control. This includes input derived from emotional centers in the brain. The larynx has been labeled "the valve of emotion."[1] It is highly responsive to emotional state and stress at all ages.

Studies of voice disorders in children have suggested that the majority of dysphonias are due to vocal abuse and misuse. The common manifestation of these is vocal nodules.[2,3] This disorder can be thought of as "functional" due to underlying dysfunction as the cause of tissue trauma that creates the nodules. That being said, there occasionally arises in children dysphonias for which no structural or physical pathologic change to the vocal folds can be identified. In this chapter, a functional voice disorder is defined as a voice disturbance which occurs in the absence of structural or neurologic laryngeal pathology. In adult voice clinics these disorders may account for up to 40% of cases.[4] In pediatric series, functional voice disorders occur less frequently. A series of 427 children referred to a tertiary pediatric voice disorders clinic reported that 7% of cases had a functional etiology.[2] In another recent series, only 4% of 136 children with voice disorder were labeled as functional or neurogenic.[3] In this review, the major manifestations of functional voice disorders in children are discussed. These include muscle tension dysphonia (MTD) and aphonia, and puberphonia or mutational falsetto.

Neurogenic dysphonias in children are due to a variety of causes, the most common of which is vocal fold paralysis. This chapter discusses other neurogenic movement disorders that affect the larynx. The major one is known as laryngeal dystonia or spasmodic dysphonia (SD). Other types of central neurologically based laryngeal disorders include essential vocal tremor and spastic dysarthrias, such as that associated with cerebral palsy. Laryngeal spasticity may affect the voice and airway in these patients.

FUNCTIONAL VOICE DISORDERS

MTD has gained common usage as a diagnostic label for functional dysphonias thought to be due to dysregulated or imbalanced laryngeal and paralaryngeal activity.[4] A variety of glottic and supraglottic patterns of laryngeal closure have been described.[5,6] Their diagnostic utility, however, has come into question because these closure patterns are not unique to MTD, and do not reliably distinguish them from normal speakers, or other voice disorders.[7]

The predominant auditory perceptual feature of MTD is a strained voice quality, disordered pitch (usually pitch elevation), and reduced loudness. These features may lead to diagnostic confusion with SD.[8] Periods of aphonia may also be present. These may be intermittent or persistent. Another feature that may be present in MTD is that periods of normal voice may occur in between the dysphonic intervals. On physical examination, exquisite tenderness to palpation in the thyrohyoid space, and narrowing of the thyrohyoid space are frequently encountered.

There have been a variety of explanations offered for MTD, including technical misuse due to excessive vocal demands, altered adaptation following upper respiratory infection, increased laryngeal tone due to local irritative conditions such as gastroesophageal reflux, compensation for underlying glottic insufficiency, and psychologic or personality traits that express excess laryngeal tension.[4]

The psychological traits of MTD patients have been studied in some depth. In the most extensive studies by Roy et al, personality profiles were obtained in large groups of patients with MTD, SD, vocal fold paralysis, vocal nodules, and normal controls.[9-11] MTD subjects scored high on dimensions of introversion, anxiety, depression, and emotionality. Vocal nodule patients scored similarly on anxiety and emotionality scales; however, instead of introversion (quiet, unsociable, passive, careful), they demonstrated extroversion (dominant, sociable, active). Patients with SD, vocal fold paralysis, and normal speakers demonstrated no distinguishing personality traits. MTD is described as muscularly inhibited voice production in the context of individuals with personality traits of introversion and neuroticism. In response to certain environmental cues or triggers elevated laryngeal tension creates incomplete or disordered vocal production in a structurally and neurologically intact larynx.[4]

Despite the above issues that involve the cause of MTD, successful treatment of MTD through behavioral management has been demonstrated in a number of reports.[5,12,13] This focuses on the proximate causes of the dysphonia and rebalancing the laryngeal mechanism to produce normal voice. The most effective technique in our experience is manual circumlaryngeal massage and laryngeal reposturing to lower the larynx.[5,12,14] This can yield remarkable improvement, with two-thirds of patients achieving normal voice return from a single treatment session. Successful treatment with behavioral therapy in nearly all patients is expected. Recalcitrant or resistant cases may respond after several sessions of therapy. In a case series of pediatric patients treated for "muscle tension dysphonia" recently published, seven of the eight children had vocal nodules with supraglottic hyperfunction seen on laryngoscopy.[15] One patient had aphonia without lesions. All patients improved with voice therapy. As an adjunct treatment for severe MTD, Dworkin et al reported the use of topical lidocaine spray to the larynx followed by voice therapy.[16] We have found this to be effective in pediatric patients (see case report below). We also used lidocaine block of the recurrent laryngeal nerve to facilitate phonation in a case of recalcitrant functional aphonia in an adolescent.[17] Sensory or motor perturbation of the laryngeal mechanism may relax excessive laryngeal muscle tension and help the patient gain confidence that they have the capacity to produce normal voice.

Case Report 1

A 14-year-old female had a 7-year history of voice loss, including both dysphonia and aphonia. She had been to several ENT physicians and speech pathologists but had not been able to regain her voice. On physical exam, the patient was mouthing words with articulation, but had no marked phonation and even had some difficulty whispering. She did not have a normal cough. A fiberoptic laryngoscopy revealed during phonation the vocal folds in a bowed posture and some abduction of the vocal fold observed during attempts at phonation, but normal vocal fold adduction during breath holding and Valsalva maneuver. The neck exam was remarkable for severe thyrohyoid region tenderness. As she was traveling

from a long distance, she worked with the speech pathologist for an extended therapy session on initiating glottal stops and vegetative glottal sounds. She returned 2 months later and underwent a laryngeal lidocaine wash given transcervically via the cricothyroid space. This was immediately followed by an extended therapy session, during which time she made considerable improvement. On follow-up examination 2 months later she demonstrated normal voice quality (Video 18-1).

Case Report 2

A 9-year-old female was brought by her mother for a second opinion regarding complete voice loss of sudden onset when the child awoke 1 month earlier. She also complained of a sore throat and constant throat pain. She saw her primary care doctor and was treated with Augmentin® for 2 weeks. She saw a pediatric otolaryngologist who did a fiberoptic laryngoscopy and showed "no problems" and referred her to a speech pathologist. She also saw a school psychologist who reported that she had no psychological impairments. She had normal activity level and was active in tumbling and had no history of trauma to the neck. Her only notable health condition is that she was small for her age, below the fifth percentile for height and weight. On examination, the patient was noted to have aphonia with soft voice and slight whispering. Occasional phonatory sounds can be elicited with cough, throat clearing, and inhalatory phonation. Transnasal fiberoptic laryngoscopy showed the vocal folds positioned in a hyperadducted whispering posture with an open posterior chink, and mild true vocal fold edema was observed. The patient was treated with a course of prednisone without improvement. She underwent three weekly sessions of behavioral voice therapy using inhalation phonation, throat clear with phonation, glottal fry, throat focused /r/ phonation, and manual reposturing. These were also without progress. A transnasal fiberoptic laryngoscopy and lidocaine wash were then performed, with 4% lidocaine spray of the larynx and hypopharynx utilizing the curved spray atomizer (MAD 600, Wolfe-Tory, Inc, Salt Lake City, Utah). This provided excellent topical anesthesia of the vocal folds which were able to be palpated with the fiberscope and the subglottic larynx and trachea inspected through the vocal folds without any gagging or coughing. The speech pathologist then immediately worked with the patient on voice therapy techniques of inhalatory/exhalatory phonation and nasal voiced consonants with aggressive and persistent practice. After 30 minutes she was able to phonate and left the clinic speaking with a normal voice (Video 18–2).

The voice of adolescence is characterized by pitch instability. This is true for both males and females but more so in males. In a study of children ages 10 to 17 without and with vocal complaints, acoustic measures of pitch stability on sustained vowel phonation were not found to statistically distinguish the normal from several disordered voice groups.[18] However, the group diagnosed with puberphonia had the most variability of frequency and amplitude. Puberphonia is a voice disorder of adolescent males. It has also been labeled mutational falsetto, adolescent male transitional dysphonia, incomplete mutation, and persistent falsetto. It can be seen in early adolescence, or can persist into late adolescence or adulthood. The voice does not successfully accomplish pitch change during puberty, between 12 and 14 years of age. The voice has been described as weak, thin, breathy, and hoarse in quality.[6,12] A recent study in a large patient group with puberphonia measured the average speaking F_0 at 241 Hz.[19] It is frequently accompanied by downward pitch breaks into chest register. Coughing sound is also in chest register.[6] The voice of puberphonia may be described as a habituated use of falsetto register accompanied by pitch breaks rather than maintenance of the preadolescent voice. This pattern is commonly seen in MTD, so in our view, puberphonia is considered a variation of MTD seen in adolescent males. The larynx is generally positioned high in the neck, and excessive thyrohyoid tenderness and a narrow thyrohyoid space are found on palpation. Laryngeal lowering maneuvers, including head dorsiflexion, depression of the mandible, hyoid pushback and laryngeal pull-down, are combined with vocalization.[12] This may create a surprised patient and his mother when his normal deep chest register voice is produced for the first time.

The first-line treatment of puberphonia is behavioral voice therapy.[6,12] The same techniques of laryngeal lowering and reposturing combined with vocal cues that are used for MTD apply to the treatment of puberphonia. Ideally, this is conducted by a speech pathologist experienced in this approach. These techniques facilitate lowering of the larynx to engage the chest register and thyroarytenoid muscle activity. This lowers the pitch of the voice to the patient's normal male range. A recent study of 45 patients with puberphonia included 16 patients ages 11 to 15 years and 29 patients ages 16 to 40 years. All patients were treated successfully with behavioral therapy techniques with maintenance of improvement documented at 6 months.[19] For recalcitrant cases of puberphonia, novel approaches have been tried. These include a case report of the use of botulinum toxin to relax cricothyroid muscle function.[20]

Pitch lowering phonosurgical procedures including type III thyroplasty[21] and hyoid detachment/laryngeal lowering laryngoplasty[22] have also been described.

Case Report 3

An 18-year-old male complained of a 4-year history of voice problems. These coincided with onset of puberty. He was treated with speech therapy in schools for 1 year without improvement. He also was treated for allergies with fexofenadine, which did not affect his voice. On examination the voice demonstrated roughness, pitch breaks, and decreased loudness. An improvement in voice with engagement of the chest register was elicited with laryngeal reposturing maneuvers. Laryngostroboscopy demonstrated a normal laryngeal mechanism.

The patient was seen for a single session of voice therapy. Initially, laryngeal reposturing maneuvers were used to cue the patient to create chest register phonation during vegetative vocalizations and sustained vowels. Then the vocalizations were shaped into use with connected speech. The "new" voice was reinforced by having the patient read out loud, and by negative practice (temporarily reverting to the "old" voice and then back again). By the end of the therapy session he was able to consistently produced normal chest register phonation at normal male vocal pitch. He required no further therapy sessions (Video 18–3).

The negative impact of these voice problems in children can be substantial. It may affect their ability to form and maintain social relationships with peers and adults, to communicate in school and home environments, and to enter the world of work. Although they are labeled "functional" because no underlying disease process involving the organs of voice and speech is found, the significance of the problem should not be minimized. The organs of voice and speech are neurally controlled, and this neural control is profoundly influenced by central nervous system controls involving emotional state, personality, and stress response as described above. The impact of voice disorders in children on their social, emotional, and physical function is just beginning to be investigated (see Chapter 9 on pediatric voice quality of life measures). Providers caring for these children need to aggressively advocate for needed services, such as voice and speech therapy provided by experienced clinicians. Documentation by video and audio recordings, patient-based quality of life measures, and references from peer-reviewed publications may all be needed in making appeals to insurance providers to cover speech therapy services for these patients.

LARYNGEAL DYSTONIA

Dystonia is a neurologic disorder in which sustained muscle contractions cause twisting and repetitive movements or abnormal postures.[23] It occurs in several forms depending on how localized in the body are the symptoms. Focal dystonia affects an isolated part of the body. Examples include blepharospasm, writer's cramp, and laryngeal dystonia, also known as spasmodic dysphonia (SD). As more areas of the body are affected the manifestations are segmental (affecting adjoining parts of the body), multifocal, or generalized to the whole body. SD usually occurs as a focal dystonia. In the largest published series of over 900 patients, SD occurred as a focal condition in 64% of cases.[24] Others occurred with segmental or generalized symptoms, which is the usual presentation in children. Dystonia can occur as a primary disorder without underlying cause, or may be secondary to other causes such as neurologic disease, or exposure to drugs known to cause acquired dystonia (eg, phenothiazines). In Blitzer et al's series, 82.5% of their patients had primary dystonia, 17.5% had secondary dystonia. They also reported that 12% of their patients presenting with primary dystonia that included involvement of the larynx had symptom onset before age 20 years; 4% had symptom onset at or under 10 years of age. However, the initial symptoms did not usually involve the larynx.[23] In another prospective study of 168 patients, the youngest age of laryngeal symptom onset was 13 years.[25] Laryngeal dystonia has a high female preponderance, from 63 to 79%. Its onset has been associated with following an upper respiratory infection, and a history of childhood mumps or measles.[25] Females have a predominance of autoimmune diseases; however, an association of dystonia with specific autoimmune disease has not been made.

Although most dystonia patients are focal and primary, children usually present with more generalized symptoms.[23] Limb and axial symptoms are more commonly seen in children than cranial and cervical-based manifestations. They often have underlying neurologic conditions, including, but not limited to, Wilson's disease, Huntington's chorea, spinocerebellar ataxia, primary torsion dystonia, dopa-responsive dystonia (Segawa disease), and PANDAS. Primary torsion dystonia may present in adolescence in familial and nonfamilial forms. DYT gene mutation testing is recommended for these patients.[26] Dystonia presenting in childhood usually does not involve SD as a presenting feature.[27] However, cervical symptoms may occur and can include SD.[28,29] When there is no other identifiable etiology for the dystonia a trial of levo-dopa is recommended.

Some cases can be responsive to levo-dopa even in the absence of a positive genetic testing for dopa-responsive dystonias, for example, GTP-cyclohydrolase deficiency.[29]

Another movement disorder that may present in adolescence is essential tremor (ET). The age of onset has bimodal peaks in late adolescence/young adulthood and in older adulthood.[23] ET is the most common movement disorder. It is familial in at least 50 to 70% of cases. Transmission is autosomal dominant, with incomplete penetrance. In its classical form, a bilateral, largely symmetric postural or kinetic tremor involving hands and forearms is visible and persistent, with possible additional or isolated tremor in head but absence of abnormal posturing. Isolated tremor of the voice occurs in about 15% of cases. The effect on the voice can cause voice breaks similar to that of SD. Medications that are prescribed for ET, for example, propranolol and primidone, may not be helpful for voice tremor. For severe cases that create voice breaks and increased vocal effort, laryngeal botulinum toxin A injection can be effective.

SD manifests in several subtypes, including the adductor (vocal folds closing) or ADSD and abductor (vocal folds opening) or ABSD varieties. An irregular tremor, called dystonic tremor is present in about 25% of cases.[23] Rarely, it occurs during respiration, with symptoms of dyspnea. In the most common ADSD type, the speaker experiences intermittent overclosure of the vocal folds during speech. This creates debilitating voice breaks and an effortful, strain-strangled voice quality. A signature feature of dystonia is task specificity. This means that the symptoms are provoked by certain movements, postures, or tasks. Examples in SD include the observations that singing and whispering are less effortful and sound better than speaking. The same is often true for sustained vowel phonation versus connected speech. Task specificity in laryngeal dystonia implies that the frequency and severity of laryngeal spasms may vary with the specific voice or speech context.[30] Performance differences on speech tasks have been identified in ADSD patients comparing connected speech with sustained vowel phonation,[8] and sentences loaded with voiced versus voiceless consonants.[31,32] Patients with MTD generally do not display this task-dependent differential performance, for example, the voice sounds as poorly on sustained vowel phonation as on connected speech. When proposed in 1976, unilateral lidocaine block of the recurrent laryngeal nerve was described as a diagnostic test to identify candidacy for recurrent laryngeal nerve section for ADSD.[33] This positive effect was confirmed in a prospective study of ADSD patients using a combination of blinded listener, patient-based, and acoustic measures.[34] Unfortunately, in a subsequent prospective study the lidocaine block test was found not to distinguish MTD from ADSD patients with these measures.[35] Both groups responded positively to the lidocaine block, so it cannot be recommended as a method to separate the two disorders. At this time, the diagnosis of SD remains a clinical one, based on perceptual features as described above and examination for other manifestations of dystonia.

Treatment for SD may involve behavioral therapy, medications, injections, or surgery.[23] Behavioral therapy does not have a major role, but can help patients with mild symptoms compensate for the disorder or prolong the effect of botulinum toxin injections.[36] The current gold standard treatment of SD is laryngeal botulinum toxin injection.[37] For the ADSD form injections are placed into the laryngeal adductor muscles. ABSD is treated with injections in the posterior cricoarytenoid muscles.[38]

These are technically more difficult, and the response to injections is overall not as dramatic as the ADSD form. Patients with vocal tremor improve, but not to the degree that those without tremor do. Medications used to treat dystonia, for example, anticholinergics, clonazepam, may also ameliorate SD symptoms.[23] In surgical treatment of SD, unilateral RLN section is not generally performed now due to a high late relapse rate. A variation on this concept, the selective laryngeal adductor denervation-ansa reinnervation, (introduced in 1999), shows promising results.[39,40]

Case Report

A 22-year-old female complained of voice problems for the last 2 years. She described her voice as choppy and reports that the onset was gradual. She also noticed a shaking feeling in her body since age 14 and has noted a tremor in her head for at least the last 2 years. She complained of a chronically tense neck that sometimes causes the head to turn to the right, mildly shaking handwriting, and the occasional feeling of cramps in legs and feet. She had no family history of movement disorders. For her voice problem she saw an otolaryngologist who diagnosed her with reflux laryngitis and gave her some antireflux medicine. This did not help her voice at all and she discontinued the medication. On examination she had a notable strained-strangle quality to her voice with intermittent hypernasality and a fast irregular tremor audible both in running speech and sustained vowel phonation. She demonstrated a notable turning of the head to the right with side-to-side head tremor. Voice symptoms were more prominent when the head tremor was worse. Oral reading of task specific sentences revealed much more difficulty on voiced consonants and vowels than with those containing voiceless consonants. The voice was fluent and spasm-free in falsetto and whisper. On physical exam, marked tightness in the right sternocleidomastoid region was noted. A transnasal fiberoptic laryngoscopy was performed and this demonstrated notable tremor of the pharynx, larynx and palate during phonation attempts with interruption of vibration due to adductor spasms. Her Voice Handicap Index score was 108 (normal 0–5), and she rated her voice problem as severe. A diagnosis of adductor spasmodic dysphonia was made. The patient had a dystonic laryngeal tremor and segmental dystonia with torticollis. The SD was treated with laryngeal injections of botulinum toxin A with marked improvement in her voice. She was referred to a neurologist for treatment of torticollis with cervical muscle injections of botulinum toxin A.

OTHER NEUROLOGIC CONDITIONS AFFECTING THE LARYNX

Myriad neurologic disorders exist which can affect the voice and speech mechanism. This is expected, due to the extensive neural connections to the structures of the larynx and the rest of the speech articulatory system. Neurologic disorders of voice and speech are traditionally classified by site of lesion based on location. From peripheral to central, these include muscle, neuromuscular junction, lower motor neuron, upper motor neuron, extrapyramidal sytem, cortex, subcortex, and cerebellum.[41] A neurologic disorder that affects the neuromuscular junction is myasthenia gravis. In children, juvenile onset myasthenia gravis usually does not present with isolated voice weakness, but with other symptoms of fatigue, eyelid drooping, and difficulty swallowing or chewing. Dystonia is an example of a neurologic disorder localized to the extrapyramidal system. Other neurologic conditions that may affect the voice and speech of children, especially those with cerebral palsy, involve the upper motor neuron, cerebellar, and cortical and subcortical systems. Upper motor neuron lesions create spasticity which causes a strained, harsh, and hypernasal voice quality. The effects of speech and voice from cerebellar lesions are felt to be a breakdown in integration and alterations in motor programming (ataxia).[42] Causes of cerebellar lesions include cerebellar degeneration, infarcts, hemorrhage, or neoplasm. The characteristics of speech and voice in ataxic dysarthria included harsh voice, monopitch, monoloudness, and poor pitch or loudness control (bursts of loudness).[43] Lesions of the cortex and subcortical regions, such as those caused by stroke, head injury, or tumor, can produce apraxia of phonation, in conjunction with apraxia of respiration and articulation.[44] Apraxia is a loss of ability to program the coordinated movements of speech in the absence of other peripheral motor or sensory impairment. Phonatory characteristics can vary from mutism to trial-and-error nonspeech to whispered speech, with or without airflow.[45] Verbal and nonverbal vocalizations may be encountered in Gilles de la Tourette syndrome (TS). TS is a rare, chronic disorder of involuntary motor tics that begins in childhood and persists in adulthood.[46] It is seen predominantly in men, often runs in families, and may have an autosomal dominant mode of inheritance. The involuntary vocalizations in TS range from unintelligible nonverbal noises to verbal tics including coprolalia (repetition of obscene words), echolalia (repetition of the last syllable, word, or sentence spoken by others), or palilalia (repeating by the patient of the last word or sentence in a phrase). Laryngeal botulinum toxin injection has been used to reduce vocal volume and the social embarrassment of vocal tics.[47,48]

Some neurologic conditions may impair the abductory function of the vocal folds and obstruct the airway. The most common examples are bilateral vocal fold paralysis and cerebral palsy. The pediatric airway can also be treated with botulinum toxin A to the vocal folds. Children with cerebral palsy can develop laryngospasm. Bilateral vocal fold paralysis patients may develop laryngeal synkinesis, whereby the laryngeal adductor muscles activate during inspiration. These conditions may benefit from vocal fold botulinum toxin injection to improve the airway through relaxation of the thyroarytenoid muscles.[49,50]

VIDEOS ASSOCIATED WITH THIS CHAPTER

Video 18–1. A 14-year-old female with severe muscle tension dysphonia had a 7-year history of voice loss, including both dysphonia and aphonia. The voice at the initial evaluation and therapy session after lidocaine wash demonstrating voice recovery is seen. The maintenance of voice 2 months after therapy session is also demonstrated.

Video 18–2. A 9-year-old female with severe functional aphonia was brought by her mother for a second opinion regarding complete voice loss of sudden onset when the child awoke 1 month earlier. The evaluation, lidocaine wash technique, and therapy session is demonstrated, showing recovery of voice.

Video 18–3. An 18-year-old male with a 4-year history of voice problems who has puberphonia, a form of muscle tension dysphonia in adolescent males. The evaluation and a single therapy session are demonstrated, including laryngostroboscopy before and after the voice is restored.

REFERENCES

1. Roy N, McGrory JJ, Tasko SM, Bless DM, Heisey D, Ford CN. Psychological correlates of functional dysphonia: an investigation using the Minnesota Multiphasic Personality Inventory. *J Voice.* 1997;11:443–451.
2. Campbell TF, Dollaghan CA, Yaruss JS. Disorders of language, phonology, fluency, and voice in children: indicators for referral. In: Bluestone CD, Stool SE, et al, eds. *Pediatric Otolaryngology.* 4th ed. Philadelphia, Pa: Saunders; 2003:1773–1787.
3. Wuyts FL, Heylen L, Mertens F, et al. Effects of age, sex, and disorder on voice range profile characteristics of 230 children. *Ann Otol Rhinol Laryngol.* 2003;112:540–548.
4. Roy N. Functional dysphonia. *Curr Opin Otolaryngol Head Neck Surg.* 2003;11: 144–148.
5. Roy N, Ford CN, Bless DM. Muscle tension dysphonia and spasmodic dysphonia: the role of manual laryngeal tension reduction in diagnosis and treatment. *Ann Otol Rhinol Laryngol.* 1996;105:851–856.
6. Morrison MD, Rammage LA. *The Management of Voice Disorders.* San Diego, Calif: Singular Publishing Group; 1994.
7. Sama A, Carding PN, Price S, et al. The clinical features of functional dysphonia. *Laryngoscope.* 2001;111:458–463.
8. Roy N, Gouse M, Mauszycki SC, Merrill RM, Smith ME. Task specificity in adductor spasmodic dysphonia versus muscle tension dysphonia. *Laryngoscope.* 2005;115:311–316.

9. Roy N, Bless DM. Toward a theory of the dispositional bases of functional dysphonia and vocal nodules: exploring the role of personality and emotional adjustment. In: Kent RD, Bass MJ, eds. *Voice Quality Measurement.* San Diego, Calif: Singular Publishing Group; 2000:461–480.

10. Roy Bless DM, Heisey D. Personality and voice disorders: a superfactor trait analysis. *J Speech Lang Hear Res.* 2000;43:749–768.

11. Roy N, Bless DM, Heisey D. Personality and voice disorders: a multitrait-multidisorder analysis. *J Voice.* 2000;14:521–548.

12. Aronson AE. *Clinical Voice Disorders: An Interdisciplinary Approach* 3rd ed. New York, NY: Thieme-Stratton; 1990.

13. Ramig LO, Verdolini K. Treatment efficacy: voice disorders. *J Speech Lang Hear Res.* 1998;41:S101–S116.

14. Roy N, Leeper HA. Effects of the manual laryngeal musculoskeletal tension reduction technique as a treatment for functional voice disorders: perceptual and acoustic measures. *J Voice.* 1993;7:242–249.

15. Lee EK, Son YI. Muscle tension dysphonia in children: voice characteristics and outcome of voice therapy. *Int J Pediatr Otorhinolaryngol.* 2005;69:911–917.

16. Dworkin JP, Meleca RJ, Simpson ML, et al. Use of topical lidocaine in the treatment of muscle tension dysphonia. *J Voice.* 2000; 14:567–574.

17. Smith ME, Darby KP, Kirchner K, Blager FB. Simultaneous functional laryngeal stridor and functional aphonia in an adolescent. *Am J Otolaryngol.* 1993;5:366–369.

18. Boltezar IH, Burger ZR, Zargi M. Instability of voice in adolescence: patholgic condition or normal developmental variation? *J Pediatr.* 1997;130:185–190.

19. Kagli M, Sati I, Acar A, et al. Mutational falsetto: intervention outcomes in 45 patients. *J Laryngol Otol* . In press.

20. Woodson GE, Murry T. Botulinum toxin in the treatment of recalcitrant mutational dysphonia. *J Voice.* 1994;8:347–351.

21. Li GD, Mu L, Yang S. Acoustic evaluation of Isshiki type III thyroplasty for treatment of mutational voice disorders. *J Laryngol Otol.* 1999;113:31–34.

22. Pau H, Murty GE. First case of surgically corrected puberphonia. *J Laryngol Otol.* 2001; 115:60–61.

23. Brin MF, Fahn S, Blitzer A, Ramig LO, Stewart C. Movement disorders of the larynx. In: Blitzer A, Brin MF, Sasaki CT, Fahn S, Harris KS, eds. *Neurologic Disorders of the Larynx.* New York, NY: Thieme; 1992: 248–278.

24. Blitzer A, Brin MF, Stewart CF. Botulinum toxin management of spasmodic dysphonia (laryngeal dystonia): a 12-year experience in more than 900 patients. *Laryngoscope.* 1998;108(10):1435–1441.

25. Schweinfurth JM, Billante M, Courey MS. Risk factors and demographics in patients with spasmodic dysphonia. *Laryngoscope.* 2002;112:220–223.

26. Fasano A, Nardocci N, Elia AE, Zorzi G, Bentivoglio AR, Albanese A. Non-DYT1 early-onset primary torsion dystonia: comparison with DYT1 phenotype and review of the literature. *Mov Disord.* 2006;21(9):1411–1418.

27. O'Riordan S, Raymond D, Lynch T, Saunders-Pullman R, Bressman SB, Daly L, Hutchinson M. Age at onset as a factor in determining the phenotype of primary torsion dystonia. *Neurology.* 2004;63(8):1423–1426.

28. Boseley ME, Gherson S, Hartnick CJ. Spasmodic dysphonia in an adolescent patient with an autoimmune neurologic disorder. *Am J Otolaryngol.* 2007;28:140–142.

29. Schneider SA, Mohire MD, Trender-Gerhard I, et al. Familial dopa-responsive cervical dystonia. *Neurology.* 2006;66:599–601.

30. Bloch CS, Hirano M, Gould WJ. Symptom improvement of spastic dysphonia in response to phonatory tasks. *Ann Otol Rhinol Laryngol.* 1985;94:51–54.

31. Erickson M. Effects of voicing and syntactic complexity on sign expression in adductor spasmodic dysphonia. *Amer J Speech Lang Pathol.* 2003;12:416–424.

32. Roy N, Mauszycki SC, Merrill RM, Gouse M, Smith M. Toward improved differential diagnosis of adductor spasmodic dysphonia and

muscle tension dysphonia. *Folia Phoniatr Logop.* 2007;59:83-90.

33. Dedo HH. Recurrent laryngeal nerve section for spastic dysphonia. *Ann Otol Rhinol Laryngol.* 1976;85:451-459.

34. Smith ME, Roy N, Wilson C. Lidocaine block of the recurrent laryngeal nerve in adductor spasmodic dysphonia: a multi-dimensional assessment. *Laryngoscope.* 2006;116:591-595.

35. Roy N, Smith ME, Allen B, Merrill RM. Adductor spasmodic dysphonia versus muscle tension dysphonia: examining the diagnostic value of recurrent laryngeal nerve lidocaine block. *Ann Otol Rhinol Laryngol.* 2007;116:161-168.

36. Murry T, Woodson GE. Combined-modality treatment of adductor spasmodic dysphonia with botulinum toxin and voice therapy. *J Voice.* 1995;9:460-465.

37. Sulica L. Contemporary management of spasmodic dysphonia. *Curr Opin Otolaryngol Head Neck Surg.* 2004;12:543-548.

38. Woodson G, Hochstetler H, Murry T. Botulinum toxin therapy for abductor spasmodic dysphonia. *J Voice.* 2006;20:137-143.

39. Berke GS, Blackwell KE, Gerratt BR, Verneil A, Jackson KS, Sercarz JA. Selective laryngeal adductor denervation-reinnervation: a new surgical treatment for adductor spasmodic dysphonia. *Ann Otol Rhinol Laryngol.* 1999;108:227-231.

40. Chhetri DK, Mendelsohn AH, Blumin JH, Berke GS. Long-term follow-up results of selective laryngeal adductor denervation-reinnervation surgery for adductor spasmodic dysphonia. *Laryngoscope.* 2006;116:635-642.

41. Smith ME, Ramig LO. Neurological disorders and the voice. In: Rubin JS, Sataloff R, Korovin G, eds. *Diagnosis and Treatment of Voice Disorders.* 2nd ed. New York, NY: Thomson/Delmar Learning; 2002:409-433.

42. Kent RD, Netsell R, Abbs JH: Acoustic characteristics of dysarthria associated with cerebellar disease. *J Speech Hear Res.* 1979; 22:627-648.

43. Zwirner P, Murry T, Woodson GE: Phonatory function in neurologically impaired patients. *J Commun Disord.* 1991;24:287-300.

44. Aronson AE. *Clinical Voice Disorders.* 3rd ed, New York, NY: Thieme; 1990.

45. Duffy J. Apraxia of speech. In: Duffy J. *Motor Speech Disorders: Substrates, Differential Diagnosis, and Management.* St. Louis, Mo: Mosby; 1995:259-281.

46. Tolosa E, Peña J: Involuntary vocalizations in movement disorders. *Adv Neurol.* 1988;49: 343-363.

47. Salloway S, Stewart CF, Israeli L, et al. Botulinum toxin for refractory vocal tics. *Mov Disord.* 1996;11:746-748.

48. Porta M, Maggioni G, Ottaviani F, Schindler A. Treatment of phonic tics in patients with Tourette's syndrome using botulinum toxin type A. *Neurol Sci.* 2004;24:420-423.

49. Worley G, Witsell DL, Hulka GF. Laryngeal dystonia causing inspiratory stridor in children with cerebral palsy. *Laryngoscope.* 2003;113:2192-2195.

50. Smith ME, Park AH, Muntz HR, Gray SD. Airway augmentation and maintenance through laryngeal chemodenervation in children with impaired vocal fold mobility. *Arch Otolaryngol Head Neck Surg.* 2007;133:610-612.

Paradoxical Vocal Fold Motion

Venu Divi
Mary J. Hawkshaw
Robert T. Sataloff

INTRODUCTION

Diagnosis and treatment of paradoxical vocal fold motion (PVFM) are challenging for the otolaryngologist and especially for the pediatric otolaryngologist. Commonly referred to as vocal cord dysfunction (VCD), PFVM is now the preferred term for the affliction. PVFM involves episodic, inappropriate adduction of the vocal folds during the inspiratory phase of the respiratory cycle resulting in intermittent (usually partial) glottic obstruction. It is important to distinguish between those patients with a true laryngeal disorder and those with other conditions that may appear to cause similar symptoms. In order to determine the etiology of this complex disorder, comprehensive neurolaryngologic evaluation, usually including dynamic laryngeal assessment, strobovideolaryngoscopy, and laryngeal electromyography (LEMG), is essential. Consultation with a neurologist, pulmonologist, and gastroenterologist are required often. Psychological and voice therapy evaluations have proven useful, as well.

OVERVIEW

PVFM is a diagnosis that has been used widely, but the patients receiving this diagnosis may actually be suffering from one or more of a variety of disorders that may appear to impair upper respiratory tract function. Moreover, many patients who have paradoxical vocal fold adduction have been diagnosed incorrectly as having asthma. Originally described by Patterson et al[1] in 1974 as Munchausen's stridor, the etiology was first thought to be psychogenic. Other causes and exacerbating factors have been identified since that time, as well as other disorders that may present with similar symptoms. Maschka et al[2] described a classification scheme for paradoxical vocal fold motion based on seven categories (Table 19–1), providing useful descriptions of the presenting symptoms associated with each of these diagnoses.

In addition to psychogenic causes and those listed in Table 19–1, other common diagnoses in patients referred to laryngologists for suspected PVFM include respiratory

Table 19–1. Maschka et al Classification Scheme for Paradoxical Vocal Fold Motion

Feature	History	Associated Signs and Symptoms
Brainstem compression	Often otherwise unremarkable	Vagal dysfunction (velopharyngeal insufficiency, GERD)
Severe cortical injury	Static encephalopathy or cerebrovascular accident	Sialorrhea, upper airway obstruction, poor neuromuscular control
Nuclear or lower motor neuron injury	Medullary infarction, amyotrophic lateral sclerosis, myasthenia gravis	Other neurologic signs related to underlying etiology
Movement disorders	Exacerbated by stress or exertion	Other focal dystonias, tremors, rigidity, bradykinesia, decreased reflexes
Gastroesophageal reflux*	Otherwise unremarkable	May occur during calm, crying, or feeding
Factitious symptoms or malingering	Conscious effort to deceive	Underlying secondary gain
Somatiziation/conversion disorder	Unconscious manifestation of stress	Well-motivated, high achievers

*= Reflux is associated more commonly with laryngospasm than with true paradoxical adduction, in our experience (VD, MJH, RTS), and usually is accompanied by symptoms and signs of laryngopharyngeal reflux (LPR).

dystonia, laryngospasm, increased laryngeal irritability (usually due to reflux), and supraglottic collapse. All of these conditions are seen fairly commonly in children and adults; but in our experience, treatable organic etiologies are much more prevalent than psychogenic or serious neurologic causes.

Neurologic

Respiratory dystonia is a particularly important cause of PVFM. The condition is related to spasmodic dysphonia, but it affects respiration rather than voice. Dystonias that affect the respiratory function of the larynx may be accompanied primarily by other dystonic movements such as blepharo-spasm, mandibular dystonia, torticollis, spasmodic dysphonia, or upper-extremity tremors. This type of PVFM typically is better with sleep and worsens with stress and exertion. However, usually dystonic PVFM occurs alone and is called respiratory dystonia.[3,4] Patients with rhythmic adduction and abduction of the vocal folds may be found to have an associated palatal myoclonus. Kelman and Leopold[5] reported a patient with a brainstem lesion abnormality causing PVFM and suggested that the proximity of adductor and abductor neurons to each other in the nucleus ambiguus may permit inappropriate stimulation from the respiratory centers. The series reported by Maschka et al[4] also documented two patients with known central neurologic etiologies for their laryngeal movement disorders that were characterized by stridor and paradoxical vocal fold adduction during inspiration; but the patients had normal phonation.

Respiratory dystonia should be differentiated from psychogenic stridor and reflux-induced laryngeal spasm. Patients with true respiratory dystonia tend to demonstrate fairly consistent patterns of paradoxical vocal fold movement (adduction during inspiration) during respiratory and speech tasks, although the severity may vary. Many patients have worsening of their symptoms during stress and exertion. They differ from patients with reflux-induced laryngospasm who usually have acute episodes of sudden airway obstruction due to forceful vocal fold adduction, rather than chronic adduction associated with inspiration. They also differ often from patients with psychogenic causes in their consistency even when they are not being observed.

In children and adults, intracranial etiologies also must be investigated. Several intracranial abnormalities have been reported to give rise to PVFM, including Arnold-Chiari malformation, cerebral aqueductal stenosis, and compression of the nucleus ambiguus.[4] We have seen it associated with multiple sclerosis as well. Static encephalopathy also may be associated with PVFM and may be accompanied by global developmental delay, hypertonia, spastic diplegia, and sialorrhea. These patients typically present as older children or adolescents, whereas those suffering from brainstem compression present typically during infancy or early childhood. The diagnosis in patients with cerebral compromise may be complicated by a narrowed airway at the level of the nasopharynx or oropharynx which causes increased inspiratory pressures and, therefore, may mimic PFVM or actually cause paradoxical adduction through the Bernoulli effect. Correction of the upper airway obstruction may result in improvement at the level of the glottis in some cases.

Psychiatric

Patients may suffer episodes of airway obstruction in response to emotional stress or anxiety; and any past psychiatric history should be noted. "Munchausen's stridor," Patterson et al's[1] original description of unclassified stridor, has been supported by multiple other reports.[4,6-7] It is likely that some of those reports inadvertently included patients with organic disorders such as respiratory dystonia that have been recognized much more recently. Vocal fold dysfunction of psychiatric origin has been called by many other names in the past including psychogenic stridor, functional stridor, and functional upper airway obstruction. It is imperative that the clinician rule out organic causes of airway obstruction and vocal fold dysfunction before attributing the respiratory symptoms to a nonorganic cause. Psychogenic PVFM is most common in young women and in members of the health care profession.[7] Over half of patients meet the diagnostic criteria for a psychological disorder, and up to 18% have a history of prior factitious disorder.[6,7] Other disorders such as anxiety, depression, personality disorders, stress disorders, or a history of sexual abuse may be present. Many of these patients have a characteristic worsening of symptoms on observation and abatement of symptoms when they believe that they are not being observed. The main difference between a factitious/malingering disorder and a conversion disorder is that factitious/malingering disorders are expressed for secondary gain. According to the DSM-IV-TR,[8] a factitious disorder requires the presence of (1) intentional production or feigning of physical or psychological signs or symptoms, (2) motivation for the behavior is to assume the sick role, and (3) absence of external incentives for the behavior (eg, economic gain, avoiding legal responsibility, improving physical well-being, as in malingering). Malingering is not considered a medical condition and is described as the intentional production of false or exaggerated symptoms motivated by external incentives, such as obtaining compensation or drugs. Patients with conversion disorder typically have a preceding psychological or emotional incident that may have triggered an episode, although expert psychotherapy may be needed to identify the incident. Unlike malingering patients, those suffering from a conversion disorder are not aware that any underlying psychological insult is associated with their complaints. They are typically well motivated and compliant with therapy. Extensive testing in patients with conversion disorder typically yields no organic origin. Altman et al[9] documented a psychiatric illness in 70% of their patients presenting with PVFM, and other case reports have supported this observation.[6,7] This lends support to the original supposition that psychogenic or "conversion" disorder is present in some patients. However, it is not clear immediately in many cases whether there is a causal relationship between psychiatric abnormalities and PVFM, and thorough evaluation for psychiatric and organic causes is required in all cases.

Increased Laryngeal Irritability

Recent upper respiratory tract infection (URI) may have preceded the onset of symptoms and been associated with increased airway irritability that may lead to PVFM, especially if laryngopharyngeal reflux (LPR) is also present. Laryngeal hyperreactivity may be induced by LPR even without an URI, and the clinician should inquire about symptoms of laryngopharyngeal reflux including cough, throat clearing, hoarseness, globus sensation, "postnasal drip," and excess mucus production. LPR is a known cause of laryngeal irritability and has been reported in some studies to be present in up to 80% of patients with PVFM.[7,10]

The increased laryngeal irritability caused by LPR contributes to the laryngeal hypersensitivity seen in some patients with PVFM or laryngospasm mistaken for PVFM. Treatment of LPR must be accompanied by treatment of any other concomitant disorders. Several inhaled antigens have been shown to increase laryngeal irritability and may trigger PVFM. Previously described triggers include air pollutants (dust, smoke), perfumed products (perfume, soap, detergents, and deodorants), chemical agents (paint), animal fur, and pollen.[10] Any relation between symptoms, environment, and potential exposure should be investigated. An associated history of irritant exposure may be present as may a history of food or environmental allergies. A full allergy workup is warranted in patients in whom inhaled irritants are a suspected trigger. Caution must be exercised in associating PVFM with multiple chemical sensitivity disorder because of the controversies and complexities surrounding this diagnosis.

Supraglottic Collapse and Vocal Fold Hypomobility

Cystic fibrosis, partial airway obstruction, and other conditions that require high inspiratory pressures may draw the vocal folds or the supraglottic tissues toward the midline into the airway, through the Bernoulli effect.[11] Careful observation should be made to see if supraglottic collapse is resulting in obstruction of airflow. This may be caused by conditions in which the laryngeal skeleton or tracheobronchial tree is weakened, such as tracheomalacia or laryngomalacia. However, supraglottic (aryepiglottic fold and false vocal fold) collapse also may occur in children with tissue redundancy or laxity in the absence of any other abnormality. In addition, bilateral vocal fold paralysis commonly results in vocal fold adduction on inspiration. The narrow glottis causes high airflow, which in turn draws the vocal folds to the midline during inspiration (Bernoulli effect). Conditions such as cricoarytenoid joint dysfunction causing vocal fold hypomobility may present with stridor that can be confused with PFVM as well. However, the symptoms usually are less dramatic in these patients because they have innervated vocal folds with muscle tone that helps resist the Bernoulli effect. So, passive paradoxical adduction of the vocal folds usually is not seen in patients with normally innervated vocal folds.

EVALUATION

History and Physical Examination

Specific areas of questioning are necessary when working up a patient with suspected PVFM. Patients are seen commonly for otolaryngologic evaluation after they have been treated for refractory asthma unresponsive to bronchodilator or steroid therapy, or after an episode of acute respiratory distress. The patients have a history of emergency room visits for dyspnea treated with intubation and occasionally even tracheotomy. In children, the episodes of respiratory distress often are associated with strenuous exercise, prompting an evaluation for asthma. However, unless asthma is present concurrently, methacholine challenge test may have been negative, but occasionally may be falsely positive for asthma (as discussed below). PVFM presents commonly in children during high levels of exertion, particularly in high-performance athletes. This may have very severe ramifications. For example, patients may be striving to achieve an athletic scholarship and require evaluation for safety of continued participation in sports. Failure to achieve an accurate diagnosis and effective treatment may be life altering. Initially, symptoms typically are present during exertion or stress. However, as the condition progresses, symptoms may be present even at rest. PVFM episodes may be associated with stridor interpreted as wheezing, suprasternal retractions, dysphonia, or aphonia. The dysphonia or aphonia may precede the acute episode and linger after its resolution. Exercise-induced reflux may cause intermittent laryngospasm that can be mistaken for PVFM during the eliciting athletic activity as well. If this condition is suspected, athletic activity should be performed with a multichannel pH-impedance monitor in place to confirm the diagnosis. Due to the demand of their schedules, many school athletes are prone to eating habits which may promote LPR, including eating late at night or immediately prior to an athletic event.[12,13]

A full allergic history should be taken including any respiratory inhalant allergens that have an association with the patient's dyspnea. The physician should inquire about recent respiratory infections as they may cause increased laryngeal irritability. A focused psychiatric history should be obtained with any positive answers pursued with a potential referral to a psychiatrist. Specific questions should be asked regarding stress levels and any correlation of social stress or other psychological factors with onset of respiratory symptoms. A history of throat clearing, globus sensation, excessive mucus, and hoarseness may indicate LPR as a potential etiology. Additional historical aspects of each topic are discussed with various specific etiologies.

Physical examination is the gold standard for diagnosing PVFM. A full head and neck examination should be performed including testing of the functions of all cranial nerves. Dynamic endoscopic laryngeal examination should note signs of reflux including posterior pachydermia, arytenoid erythema and edema, subglottic fullness, and vocal fold edema. Vocal fold motion should be documented and signs of upper aerodigestive tract collapse noted. Strobovideolaryngoscopy should be included even in patients who are not hoarse because the traumatic vocal fold contact that occurs during PVFM, laryngospasm, and other respiratory obstructive events results in vocal fold injury in many patients.

The presence of PVFM is confirmed through observation of vocal fold adduction during the inspiratory phase of respiration. Typically the anterior two-thirds of the vocal folds medialize leaving a diamond-shaped posterior glottic chink, although near-complete glottic closure occurs in some patients. Observation of supraglottic or other structural collapse associated with symptoms also establishes a diagnosis. Although observation of active vocal fold adduction on inspiration confirms the diagnosis (Video 19–1), the office examination may be normal if the patient is not placed in a situation that elicits the respiratory distress. Therefore, for patients who complain of airway distress during exercise, facilities should be present to allow the patient to perform physical

activity with intensity equal to the eliciting activity. Cardiac and respiratory monitoring may be beneficial, although not necessary in all patients. This will allow for evaluation of any concomitant cardiac arrhythmias that may be present. There are case reports of patients who develop ventricular tachycardia during exertion which presents as airway obstruction (personal communication, Michael Johns, MD, 2007). In this situation, inspiration against glottic adduction allows a decrease in intrathoracic pressure which increases venous return in order to maintain cardiac output. Other maneuvers, such as repetitive rapid deep inspirations, alternating phonating the /i/ vowel and sniffing, and other speaking tasks may elicit the abnormal laryngeal movement in some patients.[5]

LEMG provides information regarding neuromuscular function which can be used to determine whether adductor muscles are active during the inspiratory phase of the respiratory cycle. EMG gives information regarding the amount of muscle contraction and synchrony of paired firing. In patients with a spasmodic dysphonia, a condition related to respiratory dystonia, EMG demonstrates an increase in discharge from the vocalis muscle at rest and during phonation as well. Warnes and Allen[14] utilized EMG to determine the effectiveness of biofeedback and voice therapy. They showed that during a course of treatment, electrical discharge from the laryngeal musculature at rest decreased until a normative level was reached. This was achieved with surface electrodes which significantly increases feasibility over needle electrodes when treating children. To the best of our knowledge, similar therapy has not been tried for respiratory dystonia, but the concept seems worthy of investigation.

Airway fluoroscopy also may be used in diagnostic evaluation to determine the presence of diaphragmatic dys-synergism with the vocal folds. This results in an uncoordinated depression of the diaphragm while the vocal folds are still in the midline.

Flow-volume spirometry is very useful in supporting the diagnosis of PVFM, too. During an acute episode, "flattening" of the inspiratory limb is seen, demonstrating an extrathoracic upper airway obstruction (Fig 19-1). When the patients are asymptomatic, the flow-volume loop will return to normal. The expiratory/inspiratory flow ratio is typically greater than 2.[15] Unlike asthma and other forms of intrathoracic small airway obstruction in which FEV_1 is reduced, the FEV_1 is preserved in PVFM. Pulmonary function testing also may be used in association with methacholine challenge or bronchodilator medication to rule out concomitant asthma. Guss and Mirza[15]

published a report of seven patients sent to an otolaryngology clinic for choking and dyspnea. Only three patients in the study were found to have a 20% reduction in their FEV_1 consistent with the presence of asthma. Three of the other patients developed documented PVFM with methacholine challenge typically utilized for diagnosis of asthma. This is most likely due to excessive laryngeal hypersensitivity, although the mechanism has not been proven. These patients may be misdiagnosed with asthma and found to be nonresponsive to treatment. Although these patients were not the same ones diagnosed with PVFM, Newman et al[7] found that 53 of 95 patients with confirmed PVFM suffered from asthma as well. Table 19-2 compares the various features of PVFM versus asthma.[12]

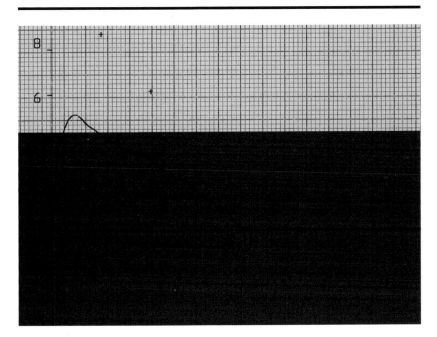

Fig 19–1. The flow-volume loop above demonstrates flattening of the inspiratory limb, demonstrating an extrathoracic airway obstruction as seen in PVFM.

Table 19–2. Distinguishing Diagnostic Features of PVFM and Asthma[12]

Diagnostic Feature	PVFM	Asthma
Chest tightness	Yes/No	Yes
Throat tightness	Yes	No
Stridor with inhalation	Yes	No
Wheezing with expiration	No	Yes
Types of triggers	Exercise, extreme temperature (hot or cold), airway irritants (GERD), emotional stressors	Exercise, extreme temperature (hot or cold), airway irritants, allergens, emotional stressors
Number of triggers	Usually one	Usually multiple
Usual onset of symptoms after beginning exercise	<5 min; however, can be variable	>5–10 min
Recovery period	5–10 min	15–60 min
Response to bronchodilators and/or systemic corticosteroids	No response	Good response
Nocturnal awakening with symptoms	Rarely	Almost always
Female preponderance	Yes	No

TREATMENT

Patients who present to the emergency room with an acute episode of respiratory distress typically are treated as a patient suffering from an asthma attack or an acute airway obstruction. Many patients receive beta-2 agonists and corticosteroids. If the symptoms do not abate, intubation, and at times emergency tracheotomy, is used to control the airway. Heliox, a combination of helium and oxygen, which has a lower molecular weight and is less dense than oxygen, can ease the dyspnea of patients with respiratory distress.[16] The lighter molecular weight gas results in less turbulence across the narrowed glottis. Christo-pher et al[17] found that the wheezing and dyspnea resolved in all patients suffering from laryngospasm when a 20% helium/oxygen mixture was administered. However, these emergency treatments usually are used in patients in whom the diagnosis of PVFM has not been made or even suspected.

There are many different treatment approaches for the treatment of PVFM, and the most appropriate modalities depend upon the cause. Biofeedback is an effective method for retraining some patients to manage an acute episode. Laryngeal image biofeedback, initially described by Bastian and Nagorsky[18], has been shown to be an effective learning tool for patients to mimic target tasks. This study demonstrated that patients can reliably alter laryngeal movements and postures using laryngeal image feedback in the absence of auditory-perceptual cues. Visual laryngoscopic biofeedback in association with speech therapy has been effective as definitive treatment in some patients, although it is only partially effective in most. A variety of other noninvasive therapeutic approaches have been used with varying success including respiratory retraining, psychological educational approaches, and other techniques to restore sensory and motor function and control. Behavioral management may be partially effective in some cases. For example, many patients have less prominent paradoxical adduction during nasal breathing than during oral breathing, especially patients who do not have respiratory dystonia. Focusing on nasal breathing is very helpful for such patients in managing a crisis situation. Martin et al[19] described a speech therapy program which divided treatment of the acute episode into seven steps. These steps were designed around the concepts of pitch change, diaphragmatic breathing, and extrinsic muscle tension reduction. A summary of the seven steps is included in Table 19–3.

When patients have a psychiatric component to their respiratory distress, it is

Table 19–3. Seven-Step Behavioral Treatment for PVFM[19]

1. Providing the patients slow direction and acknowledging the patients' fear and helplessness and that the stridor is real
2. Utilizing a behavioral approach to exercises, so that with self-awareness and good breathing patterns, the patients will be prepared to voluntarily control an attack when it occurs.
3. Advising use of diaphragmatic breathing, such as is used by professional singers, directs attention away from the larynx. This gives the patients a place to focus body awareness, so respiratory effort can be utilized without producing laryngeal, clavicular, or thoracic tension. The patient concentrates on pushing the lower abdomen out with inspiratory descent of the diaphragm. On expiration, the patient concentrates on utilizing support from the lower abdominal muscles.
4. Advising use of "wide-open throat" breath, concentrating on having the lips closed, the tongue lying flat on the floor of the mouth behind the lower front teeth, with the buccal areas of the mouth relaxed, releasing the jaw gently, and using diaphragmatic inhalation and exhalation techniques.
5. Advising the patient to focus on exhalation interrupts the patients' tendency to feel that they are unable to get any more breath and to hold onto their breath. They are taught to exhale, release their breath, and then allow inhalation to follow effortlessly. They are allowed to develop an exhalation count, so they know they can maintain exhalation up to that number of counts, and avoid gasping for air.
6. Increasing self-awareness of the breathing sequence of inhalation and exhalation decreases the feeling of helplessness via increased self-awareness of the correct sequence of the breathing process.
7. Interrupting effortful breathing is fostered by developing the attitude that their breathing does not have to be actively performed but is part of a natural body process that can be gradually trusted and practiced.

often helpful not to imply initially that they have a psychiatric illness which is causing their problem. First, the psychological symptoms may be secondary. Second, even if they are not, many patients and families are more willing to accept psychological consultation if it develops as an outgrowth of good rapport with a laryngologist and voice pathologist. If patients are told abruptly that their illness is psychiatric in origin, they may be resistant to voice therapy and psychotherapy. In addition, the diagnosis may prove to be wrong. Although both speech-language pathologists and psychologists have a role in behavioral treatment of PVFM, a speech-language pathologist is more appropriately suited for initial treatment. In addition to addressing the emotional issues associated with this illness, speech-language pathologists are instrumental in teaching the patient how to avoid and/or deal with an acute episode of dyspnea. Initial referral to a psychologist may imply to the patient and family members that the physician believes the problem to be "in the patient's head." The anxiety associated with PVFM and related disorders is a significant component of the disorder. The need for psychologic evaluation and treatment for both the patient and the family is a concept that should be introduced gradually to ensure that the patient is openly receptive to the treatment.

Botulinum toxin has been used with success to treat respiratory dystonia. This concept was introduced in 1992 by Brin et al.[3] In their series of 7 patients with PVFM, 4 were offered vocalis muscle Botox injections with outstanding relief of laryngeal symptoms. Five of the 10 patients reported by Altman et al[9] responded at least partially to botulinum toxin injected into the thyroarytenoid muscle, and two of them had other dystonias. In our experience, EMG-confirmed adductor muscle activity during respiration, in combination with other findings that suggest respiratory dystonia, indicates that Botox has a higher likelihood of being an effective treatment. Interestingly, respiratory dystonia which is not accompanied by dysphonia responds extremely well to low doses of botulinum toxin injected into the thyroarytenoid muscle, although associated respiratory dysrhythmia may persist.

More aggressive airway management strategies have been described. Lloyd and Jones[20] have described a patient in whom an arytenoidectomy and partial cordectomy were performed. PVFM persisted 2 weeks after the procedure, and the patient then underwent a stitch lateralization of the vocal fold. The percutaneous stitch was removed after 6 weeks and the patient was symptom free for 1 year. Eventually, she did require tracheotomy and completion arytenoidectomy. This treatment, although seemingly aggressive, may be necessary to decannulate patients who have refractory PVFM, but such intervention should be needed in exceedingly rare cases (none, in our experience).

Soft-tissue surgery has proven very helpful in patients with supraglottic collapse. Excision of redundant supraglottic tissue (usually using a CO_2 laser) eliminates the collapsing tissue and alters aerodynamics resulting in cure of the symptoms in most cases.

CONCLUSION

PVFM is uncommon but not rare. Dystonic and psychogenic causes are encountered frequently and can be treated effectively. Supraglottic tissue collapse, reflux, other causes of laryngeal hyperirritability, and other conditions that may produce PVFM must be differentiated from true paradoxic adduction. Organic etiologies should be sought in all patients. Botulinum toxin provides effective control for patients with respiratory dystonia, and voice therapy and psychological intervention are valuable in many cases. Surgery is necessary only rarely for PVFM, but is curative in most patients with isolated supraglottic collapse. Otolaryngologists should be able to diagnose and treat effectively virtually all patients who present with symptoms consistent with PVFM in collaboration with an expert team of therapists and consulting physicians in other specialties.

VIDEOS ASSOCIATED WITH THIS CHAPTER

Video 19–1. Video of example of PVFM seen on videolaryngoscopy and demonstration of relief with biofeedback exercises.

REFERENCES

1. Patterson R, Schatz M, Horton M. Munchausen's stridor: non-organic laryngeal obstruction. *Clin Allergy.* 1974;4:307–310.
2. Maschka D, Bauman N, McGray P, Hoffman H, Karnell M, Smith R. A classification scheme for paradoxical vocal cord motion. *Laryngoscope.* 1997;107:1429–1435.
3. Brin MF, Blitzer A, Stewart C, Fahn S. Treatment of spasmodic dysphonia (laryngeal dystonia) with local injections of botulinum toxin: review and technical aspects. In: Blitzer A, et al, eds. *Neurologic Disorders of the Larynx.* New York, NY: Thieme; 1993: 225.
4. Morrison M, Rammage L, Emami AJ. The irritable larynx syndrome. *J Voice.* 1999;13: 447–455.
5. Kellman RM, Leopold DA. Paradoxical vocal cord motion: an important cause of stridor. *Laryngoscope.* 1982;92:58–60.
6. O'Connell M, Sklarew P, Goodman D. Spectrum of presentation of paradoxical vocal cord motion in ambulatory patients. *An Allergy Asthma Immunol.* 1995;14:341–344.
7. Newman KB, Mason UG, Schmaling KB. Clinical features of vocal cord dysfunction. *Am J Resp Crit Care Med.* 1995;152: 1382–1386.
8. American Psychiatric Association. *Diagnostic and Statistical Manual of Mental Disorders*, 4th ed. Washington DC: Author; 1994:683.
9. Altman K, Mirza N, Ruiz C, Sataloff R. Paradoxical vocal fold motion: presentation and treatment options. *J Voice.* 2000;14:99–103.
10. Andrianopoulos M, Gallivan G, Gallivan H. PVCM, PVCD, EPL, and irritable larynx syndrome: what are we talking about and how do we treat it? *J Voice.* 2000;14:607–618.
11. Sataloff RT, Deems D. In: *Professional Voice: The Science and Art of Clinical care.* 3rd ed. San Diego, Calif: Plural Publishing; 2005: 887–902.
12. Sandage MJ, Zelany SK. Paradoxical vocal fold motion in children and adolescents. *Language, Speech, and Hearing Services in Schools.* 2004;35,4:353–362.
13. McFadden ER, Zawadski DK. Vocal cord dysfunction masquerading as exercise-induced asthma. *Am J Res Crit Care Med.* 1996;153: 942–947.
14. Warnes E, Allen K. Biofeedback treatment of paradoxical vocal fold motion and respiratory distress in an adolescent girl. *J Appl Behav Anal.* 2005;38:529–532.
15. Guss J, Mirza N. Methacholine challenge testing in the diagnosis of paradoxical vocal fold motion. *Laryngoscope.* 2006;116:1558–1561.
16. Gallivan G, Hoffman L, Gallivan H. Episodic parxysmal laryngospasm: voice and pulmonary function assessment and management. *J Voice.* 1996;10:93–105.
17. Christopher KL, Wood RP, Eckert RC, Blager FB, Raney RA, Soudhrada JF. Vocal cord dysfunction presenting as asthma. *N Eng J Med.* 1983;308:1566–1570.

18. Bastian R, Nagorsky M. Laryngeal image bio-feedback. *Laryngoscope.* 1987;97:1346–1349.

19. Martin RJ, Blager FB, Gay ML, Wood RP II. Paradoxic vocal cord motion in presumed asthmatics. *Sem Resp Med.* 1987;8:332–337.

20. Lloyd RV, Jones NS. Paradoxical vocal fold movement: a case report. *J Laryngol Otol.* 1995;109:1105–1106.

20

Psychiatric and Psychological Interventions for Pediatric Voice Disorders

Abigail L. Donovan
Bruce J. Masek

INTRODUCTION

In medicine, there is great temptation to classify disease as "organic" or "psychiatric."[1] However, there are many illnesses that straddle these boundaries and require a dual approach, that is, an approach informed by both medical and psychological factors. These illnesses, including pediatric voice disorders such as habit cough and paradoxical vocal fold movement (PVFM), reside somewhere in between the mind and the body. In some cases, organic disease may trigger the voice symptom, which is then maintained by psychological factors; in other cases, psychological stresses or primary psychiatric illnesses may be predominantly manifested in voice symptoms. Thus, these pediatric voice disorders are diseases in which psychological factors may play a significant role in the onset, exacerbation, or maintenance of the illness. Moreover,

these disorders have been found to be responsive to psychological and psychiatric interventions when medical interventions have been unsuccessful.

BACKGROUND

Habit cough is also sometimes referred to as psychogenic cough, as the disorder frequently co-occurs with the advent of an emotional stressor in the patient's life. Habit cough typically develops after a respiratory infection, although the cough persists after the resolution of the infection for weeks, months, and, in some cases, years.[2] One hypothesis is that the physical illness triggers an irritation in the throat that leads to cough; the ongoing cough then leads to further throat irritation, which in turn produces more cough, creating a positive feedback loop. Habit cough is characterized by a repetitive, nonproductive cough which is "seal-like" or "honking." The cough can occur up to several hundred times an hour while the patient is awake, it frequently improves when the patient is distracted, and it is usually absent when the patient is asleep.[3] Adolescents account for 90% of reported cases.[4] Approximately 3 to 10% of children with a cough of unknown origin for greater than 1 month will receive a diagnosis of habit cough.[5] Chest radiographs and pulmonary function testing are usually normal and the cough is unresponsive to bronchodilators, anti-inflammatory medications, and cough suppressants. The intensity and frequency of the cough can vary greatly from patient to patient. Some patients are able to continue functioning normally, whereas others may be unable to attend school or participate in social activities.

Paradoxical vocal fold movement (PVFM), also known as vocal fold dysfunction (VFD), is characterized by the paradoxical adduction of the anterior two-thirds of the vocal cords during the inspiratory phase of the respiration cycle. PVFM presents clinically as episodic inspirational stridor and the episodes may start and resolve abruptly.[6] The episodes occur more frequently during the daytime and improve while the patient is asleep or distracted.[6] PVFM is commonly initially misdiagnosed as asthma, although it should be noted that the two disorders are not mutually exclusive. In one study of patients hospitalized for PVFM, greater than 50% also had asthma.[7] However, the symptoms of PVFM do not improve with inhaled bronchodilators or anti-inflammatory medications. The clinical presentation can be quite dramatic and may also mimic the stridor characteristic of a foreign body aspiration. The diagnosis of PVFM can be made definitively by utilizing laryngoscopy to visualize the adducted folds in the inspiration phase, during an acute episode. The adduction is not visible when the patient is asymptomatic; thus, a normal laryngoscopy does not exclude PVFM.

In pediatrics, PVFM is most commonly seen in adolescents and it is thought to occur more frequently in females.[7,8] It has also been reported to occur in elite athletes with acute onset during sporting events.[9] One study estimates a 5% prevalence of PVFM in elite athletes.[10] PVFM may be associated with anxiety, as pediatric patients with PVFM have been found to have higher levels of anxiety and a higher number of anxiety related diagnoses by structured interview.[11]

CASE STUDIES

The most complex cases of voice disordered pediatric patients are treated at tertiary academic medical centers. The availability of pediatric otolaryngologists, pulmonologists, psychologists, and child psychiatrists allows for the multidisciplinary approach to treatment, as is illustrated in the following two cases.

Case 1: Philip

Philip is a 12-year-old Korean boy, adopted by white parents as an infant, who developed an incessant, nonproductive cough which caused him to miss 2 months of school. The medical evaluation, including larygnoscopy and endoscopy, revealed no abnormalities. Immediately prior to the onset of his cough, Philip had been asking his adoptive parents specific questions about his adoption and birth parents. Philip was diagnosed with habit cough and underwent laryngeal botulinum toxin injection, which led to a complete resolution of his cough for 10 weeks. Although he had been referred for psychiatric evaluation, he was not evaluated until his cough returned. This reoccurrence transpired shortly after his mother received information regarding abnormal lab values related to her kidney transplant, although she had been healthy for the previous 12 years.

At the time of reoccurrence, Philip was evaluated by a psychologist specializing in behavioral medicine who agreed with the diagnosis of habit cough. Philip then underwent 6 sessions of biofeedback training, with complete resolution of his symptoms. He was also referred for psychotherapy to address psychological issues related to his adoption. He remains free of symptoms 12 months after treatment.

Case 2: Mary

Mary is a 13-year-old girl with a learning disorder who was medically healthy until she developed stridor suddenly while on a school field trip. During the field trip, Mary complained of inhaling some dust. She developed inspiratory stridor that occurred with every inhalation and was absent only during sleep. Thorough medical evaluation, including neck and chest X-ray, revealed no abnormality. Laryngoscopy revealed paradoxical vocal fold movement. Mary subsequently underwent botulinum toxin injection to the thyroarytenoid muscle on two separate occasions, without relief from her symptoms. After the first injection, she was referred for biofeedback training, although treatment was discontinued after 3 sessions as her symptoms were slightly worse.

Mary then underwent four sessions of hypnosis and practiced self-hypnosis in between sessions. Each session produced a measurable decrease in both the frequency

and the intensity of her stridor that lasted progressively longer (hours to days) between sessions. Concurrently, she participated both in individual psychotherapy and in family therapy. Her individual therapy was partially focused on increasing her coping skills for anxiety and stress, particularly school-based symptoms. In addition, Mary was prescribed risperidone and citalopram, to address issues of anxiety and depression. After the fourth session of hypnosis, with psychotherapy and medication, Mary's symptoms resolved completely, and have not returned at 6-month follow-up.

ASSESSMENT

Prior to referral to a mental health specialist, a thorough medical evaluation must be completed, in order to accurately make the diagnosis of habit cough or PFVM, as well as to rule out any medical illnesses. Medical evaluation should assess for asthma, infection, foreign body aspiration, chronic sinusitis, laryngopharyngeal reflux, subglottic stenosis, tracheomalacia, and adenotonsilitis. Both habit cough and PVFM may be triggered or exacerbated by medical conditions, which should be appropriately treated prior to psychological treatment. Specifically, PVFM may be triggered or exacerbated by postnasal drip, GERD, and asthma,[12,13] whereas habit cough may be triggered by a variety of infections.

Once a definitive diagnosis is made, not every patient with habit cough or PVFM will require evaluation and treatment by a mental health professional. Speech therapy can teach the patient relaxed throat breathing and diaphragmatic breathing and has been shown to be effective treatment for PVFM.[14] Reassurance by medical professionals that the symptom does not represent serious physical illness may also be therapeutic.

For patients that do require treatment by a mental health professional, appropriate referral is critical and delay can be potentially detrimental. The pediatric voice specialist should consider referral to a mental health professional under the following circumstances: when no organic etiology is found after thorough medical evaluation, when the symptoms have not responded to conventional treatment, when speech therapy has failed to produce adequate results, when the symptoms are clearly triggered by stress, when the patient appears to derive secondary gain from the symptoms, such as when school refusal is present, or when the symptoms are disproportionate to the physical signs of illness. Although there may be new and innovative procedures for the treatment of these disorders, for the patient who has failed standard treatment, it is wise to consider psychological evaluation, if available in a timely manner, prior to initiation of experimental procedures.

Research has indicated that some patients with PVFM have high levels of anxiety[11]; however, the prevalence of other psychiatric disorders in this population is not currently known. As a result, it is difficult to determine specific criteria for referral to a mental health provider in this population. Thus, the pediatric voice specialist must determine the need for psychological assessment on a case by case basis. The specialist should observe for obvious signs of anxiety or depression, as well as for the presence of clear social stressors or family discord, all of which should prompt referral to a mental health professional. However, in the absence of obvious psychopathology or psychological distress, it is wise to proceed with medical treatment and speech therapy, until these modalities of treatment have been proven unsuccessful. In addi-

tion, mental health services for children are scarce, especially outside of large medical centers. For the otolaryngologist who practices within a large medical center, it is reasonable to secure the services of a mental health practitioner for more rapid psychological assessment and ancillary treatment.

A psychological assessment of the voice disordered patient will contain standard elements. The first is a detailed Functional Behavioral Assessment (FBA) of the symptom in the context of the patient's environment. This type of assessment examines the role that the symptom plays in the patient's life and the impact that it has on the patient's environment. For example, an adolescent with habit cough may be excused from music lessons, gym class, or the entire day of school due to the cough. If the adolescent is motivated to miss these activities, then the "medical excuse" of habit cough represents a powerful negative reinforcer, as it allows escape from an undesirable aspect of the patient's environment. Or, the young child whose habit cough occurs in a specific situation in response to the attention it draws from her parents.[15] In this case, it was determined through behavioral observation and reinforcement that the frequency of the cough could be manipulated by parents using social attention or tangible rewards. By shifting their attention to cough-free intervals, they quickly extinguished the symptom permanently. Understanding the role that the symptom plays in the world of the patient may in turn lead to possible therapeutic interventions. The function of the symptom is frequently not consciously known by the patient and an explanation of the clinician's hypothesis, in nonjudgmental language, is often helpful. Then, alternative means for meeting the patient's needs must be explored. For the patient with school refusal, the reason for the school refusal needs to be examined.

This issue is often complex and a detailed assessment will need to examine the possibility of an undiagnosed learning disorder, as was the case with Mary, or social stress at school, such as bullying. This type of patient may then benefit from increased academic or social support at school. For the patient who consciously or unconsciously needs more time with a parent, setting up a schedule of daily, dedicated one-on-one time may be a successful intervention.

The second element of the psychological assessment will be a thorough evaluation of stressors in the environment that coincide with the onset of symptoms. Careful analysis is important, as adolescents may have become so desensitized to the circumstances that sometimes they do not even recognize them as stressful. In addition, thoughts and feelings about potentially stressful events may be suppressed by adolescents and denied as a cause of distress. Nonjudgmental and open-ended questions are important tools for eliciting information without putting the adolescent in a defensive position. Pertinent examples of environmental stressors from clinical practice include divorce or separation of the parents, significant medical or psychiatric illness in a parent or sibling, as was the case with Philip, moving or changing schools, and the loss of a relative or friend. Some children and adolescents are unable to express their distress in words and, therefore, unconsciously express distress through physical symptoms, such as habit cough or other voice disorders. This process is entirely unconscious and should not be confused with malingering or a factitious disorder. These patients may benefit from time-limited therapy to have an opportunity to express their distress in words, thus obviating the need for the symptom.

The third element of the psychological assessment will be a thorough evaluation for the presence of psychopathology. It should be noted that not all patients with voice disorders will have major psychopathology, but rather this group is a distinct minority. Psychiatric disorders that have been associated with voice disorders include major depressive disorder, generalized anxiety disorder, and conversion disorder. In fact, patients with PVFM may be more likely to have generalized anxiety disorder and anxiety-related diagnoses, such as Separation anxiety, when compared to asthmatic controls.[11] In addition, the symptoms of Tourette's disorder, transient tic disorder, and chronic tic disorder may mimic the symptoms of both PVFM and habit cough and should be thoughtfully evaluated by the mental health clinician.

MANAGEMENT

The psychological management of pediatric voice disorders can be divided into several categories: biofeedback, self-hypnosis, psychotherapy, and medication. Currently, there have been no clinical studies assessing the efficacies of the various treatment modalities compared to each other. However, they have individually been found to be successful with a wide variety of cases. Thus, the choice of which modality to use for a given patient is at the discretion of the clinician. Moreover, if one modality fails to produce remission of the symptoms, a second or third modality can be tried.

In addition to primary psychological management of the symptoms, patients will also benefit from regular follow-up visits with the voice specialist. These follow-up visits allow for ongoing objective assessments of symptom severity and serve to reassure the patient that no major medical illness is present. Reassuring the patient and the family on an ongoing basis is critical to the success of any psychological symptom management.

Some patients and families may be reluctant to accept the absence of organic causes or "physical" findings, or may be reluctant to accept referral to a mental health clinician for a "medical" condition. For these patients and families, it may be helpful to frame the role of psychological treatment as important for coping with illness, or with the stress that ongoing symptoms cause.

Biofeedback

A scattering of case reports document the usefulness of biofeedback alone, and in combination with psychological therapies, to treat VFD,[16,17] PVFM,[18] and habit cough.[4,19] In only two studies did biofeedback training target specific muscles thought to be involved in the production of symptoms.[16,17]

The most common application of biofeedback training is to facilitate learning relaxation techniques to modulate arousal and control muscle hypertonicity. In this paradigm, measurement of physiologic activity is achieved using noninvasive sensor technology to record muscle activity, heart rate, skin temperature, and respiration. Signals are processed by a computer and "fed back" to the patient as a readily interpretable analogue representation on a computer monitor. With this information, patients learn to lower sympathetic arousal and refine control of skeletal muscle activity as they are taught and practice relaxation techniques. How biofeedback works is a matter of conjecture, but presumably learning to control physiologic responses is educational and reinforcing.

Biofeedback has been used in the treatment of a wide range of medical and psychiatric disorders in children and adolescents. Patients as young as 7 years of age can learn to control maladaptive physiologic responses with the aid of biofeedback. With few exceptions, sensors attach to skin that is readily accessible using adhesive disks, Velcro, or paper tape. Patients are seated in a reclining chair facing a computer monitor in a room controlled for ambient light and sound. Initially, it is important for a parent to be present to observe the procedural aspects of biofeedback and to help the child process the learning experience outside of the session.

In Philip's case, biofeedback sessions started with attaching three self-adhesive EMG electrodes to his throat over the laryngeal muscle area, which had been wiped with an alcohol prep; a photoplethysmograph was fastened with Velcro to the volar surface of his right middle finger; and a thermistor was taped to the volar surface of his right index finger. Total preparation time of approximately 3 minutes allowed for 30 minutes of biofeedback training per session.

In all but the mildest of cases, habit cough is an intrusive and distressing symptom for the individual and those in proximity. As a result, child and adolescent patients often find themselves segregated with a 1:1 tutor outside of their normal classroom and soon thereafter with home tutoring. Philip was still attending school in his regular classroom because the symptom occurred at a low rate (1 to 2 times per minute). His ability to concentrate and retain information was deemed reasonably intact, which was an important consideration before starting treatment. In addition, his resting baseline EMG activity was well above the upper normal limit, such that it was feasible to use biofeedback training as a focused learning tool to decrease EMG activity to normal limits.

In contrast, Mary's inspirational stridor occurred 20 to 30 times per minute and was quite audible above normal room conversation. The symptom proved to be too big a distraction during biofeedback training, which made her more anxious because she had high expectations for the treatment to be successful.

Self-Hypnosis

The portrayal of hypnosis in popular culture bears little resemblance to the self-hypnosis utilized in a therapeutic setting. Hypnosis does not involve mind control, or the hypnotist causing people to perform actions against their will. In a therapeutic setting, hypnosis is more accurately described as self-hypnosis, as the patient is the active agent and actually hypnotizes him- or herself. Hypnosis is best understood as a natural mental state characterized by deep relaxation. Children may be exceptionally good candidates for the therapeutic use of hypnosis given their ability to engage in imaginary play.

Self-hypnosis has been shown to be an effective treatment for habit cough. In one recent study, 78% of patients with habit cough had complete resolution of their symptoms after a single session and an additional 12% within the next month.[2] The mechanism of action of self-hypnosis, although not fully understood, likely relates to the promotion of increased relaxation and an alteration in the perception of the cough trigger.[2] Self-hypnosis also promotes patient autonomy and self-reliance and restores the locus of control to the patient.

Self-hypnosis has also been shown to be an effective treatment for vocal fold dysfunction. At a pediatric pulmonary center, 38% percent of pediatric patients with vocal fold dysfunction had a complete resolution of their symptoms, and an additional 31% had significant improvement in their symptoms, after a single hypnosis session.[20]

In the case of Mary, self-hypnosis was successful in reducing and, with the aid of psychotherapy and medication, eventually completely resolving her symptoms after 4 sessions. Mary found self-hypnosis to be a successful coping skill and she developed a sense of mastery and self-confidence based on her ability to effectively cope with the stress in her environment.

Psychotherapy

Psychotherapy may be useful for the pediatric voice disorder patient. Psychotherapy can be used to explore the stressors in a patient's life and suggest means for modifying them. For example, the talented and highly competitive teenage athlete with PVFM may be unable to initially identify the stress that athletic performance plays in his or her life. The issue may further be complicated by the confidence that athletic achievement can bring, subtle or unspoken parental pressure to perform, or even the necessity of college scholarships. As another example, the child with habit cough may be unable to cope with the stress of a divorce and the parent's new romantic relationship. This social stress may be further complicated by feelings of jealousy, and a wish to see the parents reunite. Psychotherapy can be instrumental in untangling these compelling forces and discovering alternative solutions.

Psychotherapy may also be useful in offering the patient alternative means to cope with stress. Some patients may benefit from learning concrete methods for coping with stress, such as visualization, deep breathing, progressive muscle relaxation, and distraction. Other patients may find that the act of participating in psychotherapy, having a place to discuss the difficulty in their lives, may be a successful coping skill itself. In addition, the psychotherapist may function as a useful mediator between parents and child, and can advocate on behalf of the child for reducing or eliminating environmental stress in the form of advanced classes, highly competitive sports teams, or overly high expectations.

Medication

There has been only extremely limited research on the role of psychiatric medications in the treatment of pediatric voice disorders. There is no FDA-approved medication for the treatment of habit cough or PVFM. However, this does not mean that some patients with PVFM or habit cough will not benefit from the judicious use of psychiatric medication.

It has been reported in the literature that patients with PVFM are more likely to have anxiety disorders.[11] However, research indicates that anxiolytic medication is no more effective than placebo when treating the general population of patients with PVFM.[8] Therefore, the use of anxiolytic medication should be reserved for a smaller subset of voice disorder patients who display symptoms of anxiety independent of their voice disorder. For patients who meet full diagnostic criteria for an anxiety disorder, pharmacologic management is also indicated.

There are several pharmacologic options for the treatment of anxiety in this population, including benzodiazepines and selective serotonin reuptake inhibitors (SSRIs). Short-term use of benzodiazepines, such as lorazepam (Ativan) and clonazepam (Klonopin), may provide immediate relief, given their quick onset of action; however, the physiologic dependence associated with these medications makes them less ideal for long-term therapy. SSRIs, including fluoxetine (Prozac), paroxetine (Paxil), sertraline (Zoloft), citalopram (Celexa), or escitalopram (Lexapro), have a more favorable side-effect profile for long-term therapy for anxiety disorders, although they can take up to 6 to 8 weeks to show efficacy. Low doses of atypical antipsychotic medications, such as risperidone (Risperdal), quetiapine (Seroquel), or olanzapine (Zyprexa), although not FDA approved for the treatment of anxiety, may also be helpful. When prescribing these medications, laboratory values such as fasting glucose, cholesterol, and prolactin may need to be monitored regularly. There is a case report of pimozide (Orap), a typical antipsychotic, being curative for habit cough,[21] although the side-effect profile, including the risk for tardive dyskinesia, makes this medication an unattractive option for most pediatric patients.

Some patients with voice disorders may endorse symptoms of anxiety that fall below the threshold of diagnosis. There has been no research examining the use of anxiolytic medication in this subpopulation, although one might hypothesize that medication could be beneficial in relieving their anxiety symptoms and decreasing their level of distress.

A subset of patients may also experience symptoms of depression either preceding their voice disorder or as a result of the voice disorder. These patients may benefit from antidepressant therapy, after thorough psychiatric evaluation. In this case, first-line therapy for uncomplicated depression would be an SSRI. Given that these medications have potentially serious side effects, they should only be prescribed by a physician well trained in their use.

CONCLUSION

Pediatric voice disorders originate in both the mind and the body. Furthermore, successful treatment may include medical interventions, psychological interventions, or both. One major quandary is when to refer pediatric voice disordered patients to behavioral medicine. The otolaryngologist should consider referral to a behavioral medicine specialist if no organic etiology is determined, if traditional medical interventions and treatments have failed to produce adequate symptom relief, or if symptoms are disproportionate to the degree of physical illness. In addition, the otolaryngologist should strongly consider referral to a behavioral medicine specialist, despite the severity or course of symptoms, if the patient has clear symptoms of anxiety or depression or severe psychosocial stress. It may be beneficial for the otolaryngologist to cultivate a strong relationship with a local mental health provider for ease of referral, to ensure ongoing communication and to promote consistent, quality care for the pediatric voice disorder patient.

REFERENCES

1. Moran MG. Vocal cord dysfunction. A syndrome that mimics asthma. *J Cardiopulm Rehabil.* 1996;16:91-92.
2. Anbar RD, Hall HR. Childhood habit cough treated with self-hypnosis. *J Pediatr.* 2004; 144:213-217.
3. Weinberg EG. "Honking": psychogenic cough tic in children. *SAMJ, S Afr Med J.* 1980: 198-200.
4. Riegel B, Warmoth JE, Middaugh SJ, et al. Psychogenic cough treated with biofeedback and psychotherapy. A review and case report. *Am J Phys Med Rehabil.* 1995;74: 155-158.
5. Holinger LD, Sanders AD. Chronic cough in infants and children: an update. *Laryngoscope.* 1991;101:596-605.
6. Julia JC, Martorell A, Armengot MA, et al. Vocal cord dysfunction in a child. *Allergy.* 1999;54:748-751.
7. Newman KB, Mason UG, Schmaling KB. Clinical features of vocal cord dysfunction. *Am J Respir Crit Care Med.* 1995;152: 1382-1386.
8. Kuppersmith R, Rosen DS, Wiatrak BJ. Functional stridor in adolescents. *J Adolesc Health.* 1993;14:166-171.
9. McFadden ER, Zawadski DK. Vocal cord dysfunction masquerading as exercise-induced asthma. a physiologic cause for "choking" during athletic activities. *Am J Respir Crit Care Med.* 1996;153:942-947.
10. Rundell KW, Spiering BA. Inspiratory stridor in elite athletes. *Chest.* 2003;123:468-474.
11. Gavin LA, Wamboldt M, Brugman S, Roesler TA, Wamboldt F. Psychological and family characteristics of adolescents with vocal cord dysfunction. *J Asthma.* 1998;35: 409-417.
12. Balkissoon R. Vocal cord dysfunction, gastroesophageal reflux disease, and nonallergic rhinitis. *Clin Allergy Immunol.* 2007; 19:411-426.
13. Wood RP 2nd, Milgrom H. Vocal cord dysfunction. *J Allergy Clin Immunol.* 1996;98: 481-485.
14. Anbar RD, Hehir DA. Hypnosis as a diagnostic modality for vocal cord dysfunction. *Pediatrics.* 2000;106:E81.
15. Watson TS, Sterling HE. Brief functional analysis and treatment of a vocal tic. *J App Behav Anal.* 1998;31: 471-474.
16. Altman KW, Mirza N, Ruiz C, et al. Paradoxical vocal fold motion: presentation and treatment options. *J Voice.* 2000;14:99-103.
17. Earles J, Kerr B, Kellar M. Psychophysiologic treatment of vocal cord dysfunction. *Ann Allergy Asthma Immunol.* 2003;90: 669-671.

18. Warnes TS, Allen KD. Biofeedback treatment of paradoxical vocal fold motion and respiratory distress in an adolescent girl. *J App Behav Anal*. 2005;38:529–532.

19. Labbe EE. Biofeedback and cognitive coping in the treatment of pediatric habit cough. *Appl Psychophysiol Biofeed*. 2006;31:167–172.

20. Anbar RD. Hypnosis in pediatrics: applications at a pediatric pulmonary center. *BMC Pediatrics*. 2002;2:11.

21. Ojoo JC, Kastelik JA, Morice AH. A boy with a disabling cough. *Lancet*. 2003;361:674.

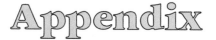

Appendix

Pediatric Laryngeal Electromyography Supplement

Andrew R. Scott
Christopher J. Hartnick

CASE

DM was a 2-month-old ex 27-week prema-ture infant who was intubated for respira-tory distress shortly after birth and mechan-ically ventilated for 6 weeks in the neonatal intensive care unit. At 7 weeks of age she had persistent stridor and otolaryngology was consulted. Flexible laryngoscopy dem-onstrated bilateral vocal fold immobility. She underwent direct laryngoscopy, bron-choscopy, and suspension laryngoscopy with intraoperative laryngeal electromyog-raphy (LEMG) with the NIM 2 system. Find-ings were notable for vocal folds which were mobile to palpation. LEMG during spontaneous respiration demonstrated motor unit action potentials (MUAP) in the left thyroarytenoid (TA) muscle, but no activity in the right TA muscle (Fig A–1A). The par-ents refused tracheotomy, and the child remained in the hospital under close obser-vation for management of complications related to bronchopulmonary dysplasia.

Four weeks later the patient was again taken to the operating room. Direct laryn-goscopy and bronchoscopy findings were unchanged, however intraoperative LEMG was now notable for the presence of MUAP in both TA muscles (Fig A–1B). Repeat flex-ible laryngoscopy while the patient was awake demonstrated persistent right vocal fold paralysis; however, the left vocal fold was now mobile.

Over the next 4 weeks the child contin-ued to improve clinically. Flexible laryngos-copy performed in the office at a one-month follow-up appointment confirmed return of function of both vocal folds with full and symmetric movement.

BACKGROUND

Chapter 8 clearly describes the limitations of electromyographic evaluation of children with laryngeal dysfunction. The utility of per-forming LEMG in patients under anesthesia

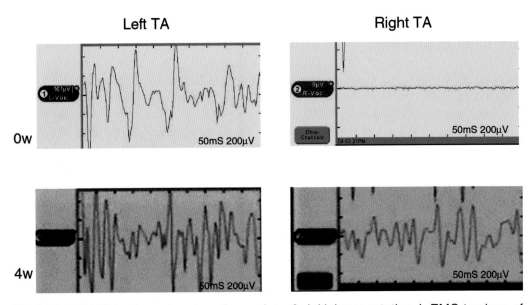

Fig A–1. L-EMG tracings at various time points. **A.** Initial presentation. L-EMG tracings of the right and left TA muscles using monopolar paired electrodes and NIM 2 Response system; gain set to 200 μV with a sweep speed of 5 ms/division. Normal MUAP in the left TA muscle and electrical silence in the right TA muscle. **B.** 4-week follow-up. L-EMG tracings of the right and left TA muscles using monopolar paired electrodes and the NIM 2 Response system set at a gain of 200 μV with a sweep speed of 5 ms/division. Normal MUAP in both TA muscles.

remains controversial. The significance of MUAPs produced during respiratory variation as this activity pertains to voluntary laryngeal function is still unknown. Often, however, children will not comply with office based, awake, volitional, task-focused laryngeal EMG and the question remains whether operative laryngeal EMG has any clinical role to play. Our institution and others continue to perform intraoperative LEMG in select cases, such as children with bilateral vocal fold immobility where any hint of recovery of function would have clinical utility or children with stable bilateral vocal fold immobility when a surgeon is deciding which side to perform a cordotomy. These procedures require the use of electromyography equipment in the operating room, which often must be further modified for use in the pediatric larynx.[1-5] Chapter 8 presents a brief review of a simplified technique for intraoperative LEMG in children using nerve monitoring equipment, which has made electromyography more accessible at our institution. This Appendix introduces this simplified technique to the interested practitioner so as to spur more thought and research into developing modalities by which LEMG can best be performed in children.

TECHNIQUE

Anesthesia and Exposure

An IV is placed after mask-induction, and adequate general anesthesia is obtained using a remifentanil and propofol infusion. A single intraoperative dose of dexamethasone (0.5 mg/kg) is given. The glottis is exposed using a Lindholm laryngoscope (Fig A–2A) and the child is placed in suspension. Anesthesia is lightened until the patient is breathing regularly and spontaneously.

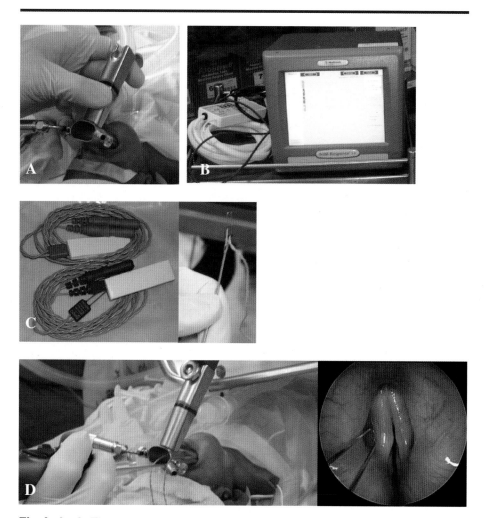

Fig A–2. A. The pediatric Lindholm laryngoscope is used to expose the larynx. **B.** The NIM Response 2.0 monitor and attached "patient interface" cord. **C.** Paired subdermal electrodes, which are inserted using laryngeal alligator forceps. **D.** Endoscopic placement of electrodes into the TA muscle.

Technique of Laryngeal Electromyography

The NIM Response system (Medtronic ENT USA, Inc., Jacksonville, Fla) is used to perform laryngeal EMG (Fig A–2B). A monopolar grounding electrode (Medtronic ENT USA, Inc., Jacksonville, Fla) is placed subcutaneously into the right shoulder. Paired, monopolar, subdermal monitoring needle electrodes (Fig A–2C) from the NIM 2 Response kit (Medtronic ENT USA, Inc. Jacksonville, FL) are placed endoscopically into each thryoarytenoid (TA) muscle using laryngeal alligator forceps (Fig A–2D/Video A1). Intraoperative LEMG is recorded from both TA muscles during spontaneous respiration. Recordings are taken using the NIM 2 Response monitor (Factory settings: EMG display: 80 Hz–2 kHz (–6 +3 dB @ 500 Hz), EMG Audio: 120 Hz –1.7 kHz (–6 +3 dB @ 500 Hz), sweep speed 50 ms (5 ms per division), and gain values of 50 μV and 200 μV) (Video A2).

In order to capture data for later analysis by a consulting neurologist, video and audio recordings are made using a digital video recorder (Med X Change DRS2, Med X Change, Inc, Bradenton, Fla), which is connected to the NIM 2 Response monitor via audio and video outputs using a video converter (TView MicroXGA, Focus Enhancements, Inc, Campbell, Calif). The acoustic signal and video data are stored and later reviewed by a neurologist with electromyography training. Once recordings have been made, the child is taken out of suspension and allowed to recover from anesthesia.

Although pediatric intraoperative L-EMG is not routinely performed at referral centers, the small body of literature on the subject and our own experience suggest that the technique is safe and can be performed as an outpatient procedure.[3,5]

CRITIQUES

Currently, pediatric LEMG remains primarily a research tool and no standard application has been widely accepted. Possible reasons for this relate to technical challenges in performing intraoperative LEMG as well as a lack of data in regard to the utility of electromyography in accurately predicting vocal fold recovery. Additionally, there is no accepted, standardized technique for performing intraoperative LEMG and no established normal values or outcome measures exist for pediatric patients. Issues relating to children that further complicate electromyographic evaluation of vocal fold paralysis (VFP) include understanding the pathophysiology behind congenital and idiopathic VFP and how the standard adult model, which was developed primarily for iatrogenic injury, may or may not be applicable to this disease process.

Our simplified method for intraoperative LEMG addresses many of the problems described above; however, some disadvantages remain. Improvements over previously-described protocols include the use of standardized equipment that does not require intraoperative modification. For example, placement of paired electrodes from the NIM Response 2 kit using laryngeal forceps is far less difficult than endoscopic placement of needle electrodes or hooked-wire electrodes described in prior studies. The paired, subdermal electrodes were chosen because the 2.5-mm spacing between the two monopolar electrodes allows thorough sampling across the length of the TA muscle. Additionally, the paired electrodes allow for two-point fixation within the muscle, resulting in less waveform variability with body motion than is observed with standard, single-needle electrodes. The electrodes are ready-made, requiring no further modification for use in the pediatric larynx.

Utilizing nerve monitoring equipment that is already present in most operating rooms obviates the need for obtaining commercial EMG equipment. The use of a digital video recorder allows for the storage of both audiovisual data for future viewing by a consulting neurologist, thereby negating the need for intraoperative interpretation of acoustic signals and electromyographic data.

The limitations of our technique should be noted as well. As with any intraoperative LEMG technique, the procedure requires general anesthesia and measures EMG activity that is nonvolitional, correlating with respiratory variation rather than phonatory effort. Additionally, the NIM 2 Response system uses a sweep speed of 50 ms, or 5 ms per division, which is different from the standard display setting for most laryngeal EMG protocols. This intraoperative L-EMG protocol also only samples the TA muscles, as the paired electrodes are not optimally shaped for sampling the posterior cricoarytenoid (PCA) muscles. Finally, there are no established criteria for differentiating background noise from a true motor unit action potential using the NIM system. The waveform generated with the NIM system is lower in amplitude and has a "blunted" quality in comparison to waveforms recorded with concentric, monopolar electrodes (Fig A–3).

FUTURE DIRECTIONS

One way around the conundrum of assessing voluntary RLN function under anesthesia is through the use of evoked laryngeal electromyography (ELEMG), in which a nerve stimulator is used to deliver a preset current to the RLN and laryngeal muscles.

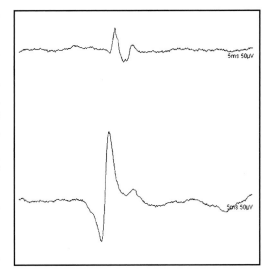

Fig A–3. A side-by-side comparison of MUAP wave morphology using paired subdermal electrodes (*top*) and a standard concentric, monopolar electrode (*bottom*). Measurements were made simultaneously from the left deltoid muscle; both electrodes are sampling the same, single motor unit. Recording with the TECA system: sweep speed of 5 ms per division; gain set to 50 µV.

A technique for the use of ELEMG on awake adults was first described by Satoh in 1978 and had the added benefit of potentially localizing lesions along the course of the recurrent laryngeal nerve.[6] The method of delivering a standardized stimulus to the RLN rather than relying on volitional movement or respiratory variation allows for the possibility of quantifying the level of innervation of laryngeal muscles. ELEMG has many parallels to evoked EMG of facial muscles, or electroneurography (ENoG). In the same way that ENoG plays a role in predicting return of facial nerve function, ELEMG may hold promise for prognosticating RLN recovery. Investigation is already underway in the development of a practical and reproducible

ELEMG technique. Zealear et al performed an investigative study in 24 canines and determined that a relatively noninvasive technique was possible.[7] Both Zealear's technique and the original method described by Satoh require the use of a percutaneous needle stimulator, which may provoke anxiety in patients and cause some discomfort with repeated nerve stimulation. This technique may actually be better suited for children, who must be anesthetized for any form of LEMG. Furthermore, the simplified technique of intraoperative LEMG described herein involves modifying the use of a machine that is, in fact, designed primarily for recording evoked waveforms.

REFERENCES

1. Jacobs IN, Finkel RS. Laryngeal electromyography in the management of vocal cord mobility problems in children. *Laryngoscope.* 2002;112:1243-1248.

2. Koch BM, Milmoe G, Grundfast KM. Vocal cord paralysis in children studied by monopolar electromyography. *Pediatr Neurol.* 1987;3:288-293.

3. Gartlan MG, Peterson KL, Hoffman HT, Luschei ES, Smith RJH. Bipolar hooked-wire elctromyographic technique in the evaluation of pediatric vocal cord paralysis. *Ann Otol Rhinol Laryngol.* 1993;102:695-700.

4. Berkowitz RG. Laryngeal electromyographic findings in idiopathic congenital vocal cord paralysis. *Ann Otol Rhinol Laryngol.* 1996; 105:207-212.

5. Wohl DL, Kilpatrick JK, Leschner RT, Shaia WT. Intraoperative pediatric laryngeal electromyography: experience and caveats with monopolar electrodes. *Ann Otol Rhinol Laryngol.* 2001; 110:524-531.

6. Satoh I. Evoked electromyographic trest applied for recurrent laryngeal nerve paralysis. *Laryngoscope.* 1978;88:2022-2031.

7. Zealear DL, Swelstad MR, Fortune S, et al. Evoked electromyographic technique for quantitative assessment of the innervation status of laryngeal muscles. *Ann Otol Rhinol Laryngol.* 2005;114(7):563-572.

Index